D0890072

Retrospective Assessment of Mental States in Litigation

Predicting the Past

Retrospective Assessment of Mental States in Litigation

Predicting the Past

Edited by

Robert I. Simon, M.D.

Daniel W. Shuman, J.D.

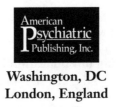

Washington, DC
London, England

Note: The authors have worked to ensure that all information in this book concerning drug dosages, schedules, and routes of administration is accurate as of the time of publication and consistent with standards set by the U.S. Food and Drug Administration and the general medical community. As medical research and practice advance, however, therapeutic standards may change. For this reason and because human and mechanical errors sometimes occur, we recommend that readers follow the advice of a physician who is directly involved in their care or the care of a member of their family. A product's current package insert should be consulted for full prescribing and safety information.

Books published by American Psychiatric Publishing, Inc., represent the views and opinions of the individual authors and do not necessarily represent the policies and opinions of APPI or the American Psychiatric Association.

Manufactured in the United States of America on acid-free paper
06   05   04   03   02   5   4   3   2   1
First Edition

American Psychiatric Publishing, Inc.
1400 K Street, N.W.
Washington, DC 20005
www.appi.org

Library of Congress Cataloging-in-Publication Data
Retrospective assessment of mental states in litigation : predicting the past / edited by Robert I. Simon, Daniel W. Shuman. — 1st ed.
    p. ; cm.
    Includes bibliographical references and index.
    ISBN 1-58562-001-7 (alk. paper)
    1. Forensic psychiatry.   I. Simon, Robert I.   II. Shuman, Daniel W.
    [DNLM: 1. Forensic Psychiatry. 2. Mental Competency. 3. Retrospective Studies. 4. Risk Assessment. W 740 R438 2002]
    RA1151 .R445 2001
    614'.1—dc21
                     2001045873

British Library Cataloguing in Publication Data
A CIP record is available from the British Library.

*To our parents, who taught us the importance
of the past to our future.*

—R.I.S. and D.W.S.

Doubt is not a very pleasant condition,
but certainty is absurd.

—*Voltaire*

Contents

Contributors

Daniel Brown, Ph.D.
Assistant Clinical Professor of Psychology, Harvard Medical School, Boston, Massachusetts

Jamie Caploe, Ed.M., J.D.
Private practice, San Francisco, California

Edward J. Frischholz, Ph.D.
Affiliate Staff Psychologist, Rush North Shore Medical Center, Department of Psychiatry, Skokie, Illinois

Liza H. Gold, M.D.
Clinical Assistant Professor, Program in Psychiatry and Law, Georgetown University School of Medicine, McLean, Virginia

Thomas G. Gutheil, M.D.
Professor of Psychiatry, Harvard Medical School; Co-Director, Program in Psychiatry and the Law, Massachusetts Mental Health Center, Boston, Massachusetts; Past President of the American Academy of Psychiatry and the Law

Michael R. Harris, M.D.
Assistant Professor, Division of Forensic Psychiatry, Case Western Reserve University School of Medicine, Cleveland, Ohio

Sarah E. Henderson, B.Sc. (Hons)
Doctoral student, Department of Psychology, University of Aberdeen, Aberdeen, United Kingdom

Roy B. Lacoursiere, M.D.
Private practice; Visiting Professor, Washburn University School of Law, Topeka, Kansas

Amina Memon, Ph.D.
Professor, Department of Psychology, University of Aberdeen, Aberdeen, United Kingdom

Phillip J. Resnick, M.D.
Professor of Psychiatry and Director of Forensic Psychiatry, Case Western Reserve University School of Medicine, Cleveland, Ohio

Richard Rogers, Ph.D., A.B.P.P.
Professor of Psychology, University of North Texas, Denton, Texas

John Z. Sadler, M.D.
Department of Psychiatry, University of Texas Southwestern Medical Center, Dallas, Texas

Alan W. Scheflin, J.D., LL.M., M.A.
Professor of Law, Santa Clara University School of Law, Santa Clara, California

Daniel W. Shuman, J.D.
Professor of Law, Dedman School of Law, Southern Methodist University, Dallas, Texas

Robert I. Simon, M.D.
Clinical Professor of Psychiatry; and Director, Program in Psychiatry and the Law, Georgetown University School of Medicine, Washington, D.C.

Ralph Slovenko, J.D., Ph.D.
Professor of Law and Psychiatry, Wayne State University Law School, Detroit, Michigan

A. J. Stephani, J.D.
Director, Glenn M. Weaver Institute of Law and Psychiatry; and Adjunct Professor, University of Cincinnati College of Law, Cincinnati, Ohio

Kenneth Tardiff, M.D., M.P.H.
Professor of Psychiatry and Public Health, Department of Psychiatry, Weill Medical College of Cornell University, New York, New York

Nancy E. Walker, Ph.D., M.L.S.
Associate Director, Institute for Children, Youth, and Families, Michigan State University, East Lansing, Michigan

Glen Weissenberger, J.D.
Joseph P. Kinneary Professor of Law and Trustee, Glenn M. Weaver Foundation, University of Cincinnati College of Law, Cincinnati, Ohio

Acknowledgments

Dr. Simon thanks Ms. Polly Brody for her invaluable assistance. Professor Shuman gratefully acknowledges Dean John Attanasio at the SMU School of Law and the M.D. Anderson Research Fund, which generously supported this work. Michale Heinlin provided excellent research assistance in the preparation of Professor Shuman's chapters. Dr. Simon and Professor Shuman both are indebted to all the contributing authors, who brought their excellent scholarship to bear on a topic of great importance to the mental health professions and the law.

Introduction

Ralph Slovenko, J.D., Ph.D.

The various authors in this book, edited by Dr. Robert I. Simon and law professor Daniel W. Shuman, explore the role of the psychiatrist or psychologist as an expert witness when called on in the legal arena to render a retrospective judgment of the mental state of an individual. The law requires evidence of mental state at the time of the commission of a crime, of suicide intent in civil litigation, of mental capacity in contract litigation, and of testamentary capacity. All of these situations call for a retrospective reconstruction. Dr. Simon calls it a "daunting task." At one time, to explain a misdeed, the answer was simple—it was always "the devil made him do it." The mentally ill were regarded as possessed by demons; hence the expression "to beat the devil out of a person." The Talmud said, "No man commits a crime except when a spirit of madness has entered into him." Freud introduced the death instinct, although he acknowledged the lack of confirming evidence in favor of his hypothesis.

In the clinical arena involving the treatment of a patient, a therapist is not bound by the historical truth that is called for in the legal arena. Freud's celebrated analysis of the "Wolf Man" (Sergei Petrov Pankejeff, a Russian aristocrat ruined by the revolution) involved an interpretation that in early childhood he had observed his parents having sexual intercourse. The explanation was designed to explain the cause of his bowel malfunction and his sexual compulsion. Freud eventually arrived at the view that he would never know the historical truth about any particular patient's experience. To the question of whether the Wolf Man actually saw his parents in a primal scene, Freud concluded that in therapy the important concern is the construct in the patient's mind.

Psychoanalyst Theodor Reik argued that psychoanalysis has no contribution to make in ascertaining what is real (i.e., veridical) because it is concerned with mental (inner) reality rather than material (outer) reality. The psychoanalyst—ordinarily concerned with the patient's view of reality rather than with the actual reality—does not cross-examine the patient. Indeed, some psychoanalysts say that outside information about the patient actually interferes with their clinical work, and they prefer to close their eyes to it. By and large they learn the "truth" only through the eyes of the patient. Conversely, the forensic expert must be a detective, but how can he or she assess the past mental state of an individual? Can the forensic expert, as a result of interviews that take place long after the event, and often with an individual who has benefited from treatment (not to mention legal advice), discern what went through the individual's mind at the time in question?

A much-publicized evaluation of psychiatric postdiction involved the mental status of exiled Pyotr Grigorenko, the Red Army major general who took up the cause of the Crimean Tartars, when he was confined to a mental institution in his country in 1963. Was the confinement warranted? Several prominent American psychiatrists, on the basis of interviews with Grigorenko when he was in the United States in 1979, claimed that he was not mentally ill when he was confined in 1963, some 16 years earlier. On the basis of the interviews, the American team reported that they found no evidence in Grigorenko's history consistent with mental illness in the past. Without available contemporaneous evidence, oral or written, as was the case, what was the probative value of that psychiatric postdiction?

A question is raised: What is the validity of a diagnosis of past mental illness based on a person's current mental status? Is it just a guess? In countries around the world, some forensic psychiatrists want to depend on or are asked to depend on only their examination, without any outside information. An opinion about mental state at some previous time, however, cannot be determined solely on the basis of an examination several months or years after the event. Mental illness, like physical disease, is classified as active or acute, latent, or chronic. People have their ups and downs from day to day and year to year. Was the illness, if ever actually present, in remission, as psychiatrists say, at the time in question? Was it a brief reactive psychosis? Was it transient? Did an alleged dissociation occur before or after the offense? DSM-IV-TR states that "In determining whether an individual meets a specified legal standard (e.g., for competence, criminal responsibility, or disability), additional information is usually required beyond that contained in the DSM-IV diagnosis" (American Psychiatric Association 2000, p. xxxiii).

In medicine it is said, "The diagnosis has been made; let the treatment begin." Diagnosis informs treatment interventions but not necessarily legal decisions. When defense lawyers claim that an accused person is mentally ill, the prosecution lawyers or the court asks for a diagnosis, but even if a retrospective judgment of mental illness is made, it is not dispositive of a legal issue. An individual may be given a diagnosis of schizophrenia or mania but still be civilly or criminally responsible for a wrongdoing. To claim exemption from responsibility for a criminal act, an accused person must assert two conditions: 1) that at the time he or she had a mental disease or defect and 2) that it impaired his or her cognition or control. In the making of a will, there may be a "lucid interval," as the law puts it.

To make a retrospective judgment, lay evidence at the time of the act, police reports, and mental disability history must be evaluated. Under the law of evidence, an expert can consider "facts or data" of the type "reasonably relied upon by experts in the particular field in forming opinions or inferences upon the subject" (Federal Rules of Evidence, Rule 703). Lay witnesses may give testimony on observed symptoms of mental disease, but these witnesses may testify only on the basis of facts known to them; they may not make a retrospective judgment.

In a tort (personal injury) case the etiology (as well as prognosis) of a plaintiff's mental disorder is questioned. After examining the plaintiff, the forensic psychiatrist will provide a diagnosis, one that appears in DSM-IV-TR. However, unlike a medical diagnosis, a psychiatric diagnosis does not inform about the etiology and pathogenesis of an illness—with the notable exception of posttraumatic stress disorder, which is attributed to a traumatic event that involved a threat of "death or serious injury, or a threat to the physical integrity of self or others" (American Psychiatric Association 2000, p. 467). DSM-IV-TR states that whatever the cause of a mental disorder, "it must currently be considered a manifestation of a behavioral, psychological, or biological dysfunction in the individual" (American Psychiatric Association 2000, p. xxxi). It does not identify the biological or environmental contribution to a disorder. It does not state whether a biological factor, if any, is a genetic defect, a predisposition, an abnormal chemistry, or a statistically unusual but normal variant. The silence reflects lack of knowledge as to etiology and pathogenesis of the various disorders. DSM-III (American Psychiatric Association 1980) and its later incarnation in DSM-III-R (American Psychiatric Association 1987) and DSM-IV (American Psychiatric Association 1994) place great diagnostic emphasis on signs and symptoms of low inference, which is designed to ensure high interrater reliability but does not ensure validity. DSM diagnosis is based on phenomenology and therefore does not meet the medical standard for a diagnosis.

There is controversy over the admissibility of "syndrome evidence"— a concurrence of several symptoms—in criminal or tort cases to establish that a particular traumatic event or stressor actually occurred. In a child abuse case, for example, a psychiatrist or psychologist testifies that the child has the characteristics of a sexually abused child and that, by implication, the child was sexually abused. In medical diagnosis, of course, the individual's symptoms are compared with a pattern, and a conclusion is drawn about etiology. As diagnosis moves from more objective criteria of identifiable and measurable pathology to symptom presentation only, it changes from disease to syndrome. A syndrome is more likely to include arbitrary or subjective criteria.

Certain assumptions about psychological evidence to ascertain a stressor are particularly questionable. One assumption is that a certain posttraumatic stress syndrome is the pathway of a particular kind of stressor. In actuality a wide variety of stressors may result in the trauma. A second assumption is that victims of a particular stressor react in the same manner. In actuality the effect of a stressor depends on the interaction between predisposition and environmental influence. In short, not all victims react with the same characteristics, and many persons with these characteristics have not been abused but instead may be experiencing something else or may be malingering or acting "hysterically." Thousands of people have claimed that parental abuse in childhood produced major psychological trauma, the repressed memory of which was recovered, thanks to the ministrations of their therapists. The "revival of memory" therapists, as well as some forensic experts, link the symptoms of eating disorders and dissociation to childhood sexual abuse.

Whether an alleged victim's observed emotional trauma supports the allegation about the stressor is highly questionable. In the usual tort or criminal case, an act is not in dispute (e.g., an automobile accident); rather, causation and damages are in dispute. In a turnaround, in cases involving syndrome evidence, symptoms are offered as evidence that a certain act occurred. During a therapy session, the poet Anne Sexton asked, "Do I make up a trauma to go with my symptoms?"

The editors of this book begin the final chapter with the apt observation, "Of all the tasks that the legal system asks psychiatrists and psychologists to perform, retrospective assessment of mental states is likely the most problematic and, ironically, the least critically examined." Compounding the problem, the legal system, in some instances, asks for information about a person's mental state without the expert ever having had the opportunity to examine the person (as in the case of testamentary capacity when the testator is deceased). The American Medical Association's Principles of Medical Ethics, annotated by the American Psychiatric Association to apply to psychiatry, state that it is unethical for psychiatrists to offer a professional opinion unless they have conducted an examination and have been granted proper authorization for such a statement. Nevertheless, a retrospective assessment often is essential to the resolution of a controversy, so regardless of its shortcomings, there is no way to do without it. Ethically, examiners are obliged to clarify the effect of their limited information on the reliability and validity of their reports and testimony, and they should appropriately limit the nature and extent of their conclusions or recommendations.

For the development of guidelines for more reliable evaluations of past mental states, the editors have brought together leading commentators in law and psychiatry. The authors provide a wake-up call to the problems involved in retrospective assessment of mental states.

References

American Psychiatric Association: Diagnostic and Statistical Manual of Mental Disorders, 3rd Edition. Washington, DC, American Psychiatric Association, 1980

American Psychiatric Association: Diagnostic and Statistical Manual of Mental Disorders, 3rd Edition, Revised. Washington, DC, American Psychiatric Association, 1987

American Psychiatric Association: Diagnostic and Statistical Manual of Mental Disorders, 4th Edition. Washington, DC, American Psychiatric Association, 1994

American Psychiatric Association: Diagnostic and Statistical Manual of Mental Disorders, 4th Edition, Text Revision. Washington, DC, American Psychiatric Association, 2000

Note on Terminology

In the text, in page citations of direct quotations from legal material, the term *at* preceding page number(s) indicates the exact page(s) on which the quotation is located. In reference lists, in page citations of legal material, the term *at* indicates the page where the reference begins.

1

Retrospective Assessment of Mental States in Criminal and Civil Litigation

A Clinical Review

Robert I. Simon, M.D.

Introduction

St. Paul spoke of our uncertain knowledge in this life when he wrote: "For now we see in a mirror dimly; but then we will see face to face. Now I know only in part; then I will know fully, even as I have been known" (1 Cor. 13:12 NRSV). Descartes, Locke, Berley, Hume, and other philosophers also struggled with the correspondence of perception and reality (Magee 1997). Beyond the difficulty of sorting out the accuracy of our own perceptions of events is the problem of sorting out our perceptions of the behavior of others. Specifically, we cannot have direct access into the mental states of others. Nonetheless, in legal matters, psychiatrists and psychologists are asked to determine future mental capacity (e.g., employability, dangerousness), current competency (e.g., guardianship, competence to stand trial), and retrospective capacity (e.g., testamentary capacity, mental state at time of offense). The determination of mental state at the time of a crime, suicide intent in civil litigation, mental capacity in contract litigation, and testamentary capacity require retrospective reconstruction. Confounding the fundamental problem of learning about another's thoughts or feelings, such assessments—often done without benefit of direct examination—are daunting tasks, due to the passage of time, the uncertain credibility of witnesses, the paucity of collateral sources of information, and often the death of the person in question.

The Forensic Examination

For all the advancements in the study of human behavior, knowledge about the human mind is still limited and imperfect. Scientifically validated explanations for legally relevant behavior rarely exist. Research advances in the biochemistry of mental disorders, for example, do not purport to explain a defendant's behavior on a specific occasion. Instead, forensic examiners must rely on circumstantial evidence confounded by the inherent limitations on all our perceptions.

The forensic examiner's task is mercifully much less ambitious than the psychoanalyst's goal to unearth the unconscious. The limited task of reconstruction is difficult enough without the additional burden of an expansive inquiry into the litigant's mind. Reconstructing an individual's mental state is a limited, task-specific procedure in regard to a defined legal issue. It bears a certain analogy to a biopsy, which is specifically intended to determine the diagnosis but is not itself major surgery.

What, then, can psychiatrists and psychologists legitimately do regarding the retrospective assessment of mental states? The answer may turn, in part, on the use of diagnostic categories. Psychiatrists and psychologists are trained in making psychiatric diagnoses using DSM-IV (American Psychiatric Association 1994). This diagnostic manual, whose latest version is a text revision (DSM-IV-TR; American Psychiatric Association 2000), is a work in progress involving the participation of hundreds of mental health professionals and the referencing of thousands of peer-reviewed articles related to psychiatric diagnoses. The reliability among psychiatrists for the diagnosis of Axis I major mental disorders is high, although the validity is undetermined, as noted in DSM-III-R (American Psychiatric Association 1987, pp. 470–471). The diagnosis of Axis II personality disorders, however, is less reliable because the diagnostic criteria are not as well defined. For many diagnoses listed in DSM-IV-TR, the cause is unknown and the long-term course uncertain. Psychiatric diagnoses are undergoing constant study and revision based on evolving research.

DSM-IV-TR warns about the risks of misunderstanding and the misuse of psychiatric diagnoses for forensic purposes. The dangers arise from the imperfect fit between the law, psychiatry, and psychology. DSM-IV-TR states that, "In most situations, the clinical diagnosis of a DSM-IV mental disorder is not sufficient to establish the existence for legal purposes of a 'mental disorder,' 'mental disability,' 'mental disease,' or 'mental defect.' In determining whether an individual meets a specified legal standard (e.g., for competence, criminal responsibility, or disability), additional information is usually required beyond that contained in the DSM-IV diagnosis" (American Psychiatric Association 2000, p. xxxiii).

First, it is important that a diagnosis, by itself, not be allowed to cast a dominating spell on the court. Diagnosis used appropriately informs treatment interventions but not necessarily legal decisions. Legal criteria do not make the existence of a psychiatric diagnosis alone dispositive. For example, an individual may be schizophrenic but still be civilly or criminally responsible for his or her actions.

Diagnosis is nevertheless important in the retrospective reconstruction of mental states. Mental disorders are threshold requirements in mental state reconstructions because there is some degree of association between psychiatric diagnosis and impaired mental capacity. Moreover, an extensive psychiatric literature is opened up to the fact-finder whenever a diagnosis is made. However, a diagnosis by itself does not establish that an individual lacks mental capacity in regard to a specific legal standard. Functional mental capacity or impairment must be assessed separately. Even without a psychiatric diagnosis, an individual may meet an insanity defense test (e.g., automaton defenses). The diagnosis of a psychiatric disorder is a necessary but insufficient reason for exculpation under various legal tests and standards.

Diagnosis in the retrospective assessment of mental states presents levels of complexity. Although the reliability of a current psychiatric diagnosis is reasonably high, the reliability of a retrospectively reconstructed diagnosis is much more problematic. It is also possible that a diagnosis may obfuscate or confuse the issue when a significant disparity exists between a mental disorder and the functional impairment it allegedly caused. Nevertheless, diagnosis may act as a restraint on wild speculations about an individual's mental state in the past. The *credible* expert can see but darkly through the retrospective glass, providing opinions based only on observable data. The *expansive* expert uses the same glass as a kaleidoscope, reporting bright and florid detail based on ungrounded speculation.

Even after careful assessment, it may not be possible to determine the presence or absence of a psychiatric diagnosis retrospectively. The forensic examiner must exercise extreme caution in determining an individual's past ley by reason of insanity for attempting to assassinate President Ronald Reagan, the United States Congress passed the Comprehensive Crime Control Act (CCCA; 18 USC, § 20). The CCCA provides that it is an affirmative defense to all federal crimes that, at the time of the offense, "the defendant, as a result of a severe mental disease or defect, was unable to appreciate the nature and quality of the wrongfulness of his acts. Mental disease does not otherwise constitute a defense" (18 USC, § 20[a]). A number of states have adopted similar language.

Retrospective determinations of cognitive capacity (knowing right from wrong and/or knowing the nature of the act) are difficult enough. However, when a test of insanity contains both cognitive and volitional prongs, as in the case of the American Law Institute (ALI) test, disagreements among forensic examiners abound. Although the defendant knew right from wrong, can the examiner determine whether the defendant was operating under an irresistible impulse or merely did not resist the impulse to commit a crime (American Psychiatric Association 1983)?

The trial of serial killer Jeffrey Dahmer exposed the wide disagreements that can occur among psychiatrists (Simon 1996). In Wisconsin, to be relieved of criminal responsibility, the accused must suffer from a mental disease or defect that substantially interferes with the accused's ability to distinguish right from wrong or to conform his or her conduct to the requirements of the law. Respected forensic psychiatrists testified for both sides. The forensic psychiatrists at Dahmer's trial found some degree of mental disorder in the defendant but differed on whether he had been able to control himself. The prosecution experts found that Dahmer was not suffering from a mental disease that prevented him from distinguishing right from wrong. Moreover, clear evidence existed that he could plan and control his behavior. The defense experts disagreed, saying that Dahmer could not stop killing because he was indeed seriously mentally ill. His paraphilia, in their opinion, approached psychotic proportions. Furthermore, he could not control his murderous impulses even when he wanted to do so. Dahmer's attorney described his client as "a steam rolling killing machine" on the track of madness (Simon 1996, p. 8).

What can be determined in criminal responsibility evaluations such as those for the Dahmer case? The experts in that case disagreed not on the *absence* but on the *presence* of a psychiatric disorder that would prevent Dahmer from knowing right from wrong, as well as from controlling his murderous impulses. Thus the examiner may be able to make a diagnosis, provided that sufficient, credible information is available. But retrospectively evaluating the defendant's ability to distinguish right from wrong, and to know what he was doing, is more difficult than determining the presence or absence of a mental disorder. For example, did the defendant think he was cutting a carrot when he stabbed his wife? Is there corroborating evidence that the defendant did not know that he was killing his wife and thus did not know what he did was wrong? Or is the examiner relying only on the subjective reporting of the defendant?

The defendant's ability to conform his or her conduct to the requirements of the law remains the most opaque to retrospective analysis. In the clinical context, practitioners assess impulse control by a number of behaviors common among those with borderline and antisocial personalities, such as irresponsible spending, sexual promiscuity, reckless driving, and violent actions toward oneself or others. These behaviors can be evaluated continually in treatment by the clinician to gauge a patient's ability to inhibit destructive actions as treatment goes forward. In the evaluation of criminal responsibility, however, guilt or innocence of a defendant is a one-time determination, in contrast to the revisions in clinical opinion permitted by the ongoing treatment of a patient.

Volitional capacity is a matter of degree, rarely fitting all-or-none legal categories. Some element of choice is usually present. Whether a defendant's mental disorder interfered with his or her ability to conform conduct to the requirements of the law is a judgment call. Examiners' theoretical orientations may influence their opinions on the degree of control associated with a particular diagnosis (American Psychiatric Association 1992). In contrast to psychosocial theories of behavior, biological theories of mental disorders may lead to assumptions that the affected individual has less control. Unfortunately, empirical clinical approaches do not provide a reliable basis for psychiatrists to evaluate volition accurately.

For the conviction of a crime, there must be not only a criminal state of mind (mens rea) but also the commission of a prohibited act (actus reus). The physical movement required to satisfy actus reus must be conscious and volitional. The automatism (or unconscious) legal defense recognizes that some criminal acts may be committed involuntarily. The example most often given is the individual who commits an offense while sleepwalking. Other mental or physical conditions that may apply include head injury, seizures, involuntary intoxication by drugs or alcohol, hypoxia, hypoglycemia, and dissociative disorders (Simon 1997).

Claims of involuntary behavior have been made by individuals who allegedly have identified with an aggressor. The classic example occurs in hostage-terrorist situations—the "Stockholm Syndrome." After the terrorist incident is over, hostages may attempt to intercede on behalf of the terrorist or even proffer marriage proposals (Simon 2000). Criminal acts committed by individuals because of these disorders or conditions may be alleged to be involuntary. The best-known case is that of newspaper heiress Patty Hearst. The defense that she involuntarily participated in a bank robbery because of her kidnapping and prolonged captivity failed.

Courts have been skeptical of involuntary behavior claims. In *Johnson v. Metropolitan Life Insurance Company* (1967), the court noted "If anything, modern psychology and psychiatry particularly has counseled that the line between volition and irresistible impulse, conscious and unconscious motive is a murky and uneven one." This complexity is illustrated by the individual who holds the delusional belief that his neighbor is poisoning his water. He has the recurrent impulse to kill the neighbor but resists because he knows it is wrong to kill. One day, he argues with the neighbor about the latter's dog constantly barking. The argument becomes heated. The delusional individual runs into his house, retrieves a loaded pistol, and kills the neighbor. Was the delusional individual's ability to continue to resist the impulse to kill undermined by his ongoing mental illness, ready to be triggered by an occasion such as an argument, or was the argument an occasion where the delusional individual chose not to resist the impulse to kill? Bonnie (1983) has argued for the elimination of the volitional or control elements of the insanity defense except in cases of psychotic disorders. He believes that the combination of the voluntary prong and the vague definitions of "mental disease" beget speculative opinions about the "causes" of criminal behavior.

Thus the assessment of volition is highly uncertain. There is no science of volition (American Psychiatric Association 1992; Beahrs 1991). Retrospective assessment of volitional behavior is unsupported by scientific knowledge. In addition, relatively little systematic research exists on the reliability, and even less research on the validity, of criminal responsibility evaluations generally (Melton 1997). In recognition of these limitations, DSM-IV makes the following cautionary statement about behavioral control: "Moreover, the fact that an individual's presentation meets the criteria for a DSM-IV diagnosis does not carry any necessary implication regarding the individual's degree of control over the behaviors that may be associated with the disorder. Even when diminished control over one's behavior is a feature of the disorder, having the diagnosis in itself does not demonstrate that a particular individual is (or was) unable to control his or her behavior at a particular time" (American Psychiatric Association 1994, p. xxiii).

Assessment of Suicide Intent

The retrospective assessment of suicide intent arises when the cause of a person's death is in question, particularly in insurance and employment litigation or in malpractice and criminal investigations. Was the person murdered, or did he or she die of natural causes, by accident, or by suicide? (See Chapter 6 on "Murder, Suicide, Accident, or Natural Death?" in this volume.)

On August 5, 1962, Marilyn Monroe was found lying nude, face down, with a sheet pulled over her body. No suicide note was found. No disturbance was heard or observed by her neighbors the night before her death. On the morning after her death, an autopsy was conducted by Deputy Coroner Thomas Noguchi, M.D. Five days later, the Los Angeles coroner rendered a preliminary judgment that Marilyn Monroe died of acute barbiturate poisoning from an overdose. On August 17 the judgment was amended to probable suicide. Ten days later the coroner issued his final judgment stating that Marilyn Monroe died of acute barbiturate poisoning from an overdose. Decades later controversy remains over the cause of her death. Was it suicide? Was it an accidental overdose? Or was it, as some have hinted darkly, a murder staged as a suicide (Simon 1996)?

Psychiatrists and psychologists are increasingly called on to consult in cases suspected of being "suicide by cop" or unwitting police-assisted suicides. Some persons intentionally create and escalate life-threatening situations for the police or general public or both that provoke and force the police to unwittingly assist in those persons' suicides (Hutson et al. 1998; Wilson et al. 1998). Criteria are proposed for the retrospective determination of the individual's mental state and intent that also apply to these cases.

Standard suicide risk assessment methods have been used beneficially in clinical settings for many years. However, attempting to reconstruct the mental state or intention of the deceased is less knowable than retrospectively assessing the presence or absence of suicide risk factors alone at the time of death. Although the jurist Oliver Wendell Holmes (Keeton et al. 1984) noted that "even a dog knows the difference between being tripped over and being kicked" (p. 34), psychiatrists and psychologists do not often achieve that level of clarity in evaluating suicide intent. Retrospectively assessing the presence or absence of suicide risk factors may help clarify the question of suicide intent. However, determining a deceased individual's suicide intent and motives can be a daunting task (Simon 1998). A patient's intentions or subjective mental state can be very difficult—sometimes impossible—to discern, even by direct examination.

Psychiatric and psychological definitions of intentional behavior vary considerably from the legal definition. Psychiatric concepts of human behavior are largely deterministic, whereas the law envisions man as possessing free will (Simon 1990). The usefulness of the psychiatric or psychological expert to the court is based on the ability to bridge these two differing views of human motivation. If permitted by the court, psychiatrists and psychologists can testify about intent in suicide cases when given sufficient information. However, testifying about suicide risk factors helps the expert avoid wandering into the definitional thicket of intent.

In *Kumho* (1999) the United States Supreme Court held that the specific *Daubert* criteria do not constitute a definitive checklist. Federal Rule of Evidence 702 does not distinguish between "scientific" knowledge and "technical" or "other specialized" knowledge. The performance of suicide risk assessments is a standard procedure among mental health clinicians. The *Kumho* court admonished the expert witness to approach her or his opinion with "the same intellectual rigor that characterizes the practice of an expert in the relevant field." Testimony about a deceased's mental state or the presence or absence of suicide risk factors should satisfy this *Kumho* requirement.

Assessment of Duress and Undue Influence

Allegations of duress and coercion mainly arise in litigation about testamentary capacity and contractual capacity. According to Rohwer and Schaber (1997):

> An apparent manifestation of assent may be defeated and the resulting contract avoided if assent was obtained by coercion which constitutes duress. A finding of duress requires an improper threat of sufficient gravity to induce the other party to manifest assent to an agreement and assent must have in fact been induced. The threat may be express or implied from words or conduct and must communicate an intention to cause harm or loss to the other party. (p. 203)

Generally, *duress* is defined as a threat to do something unlawful or wrongful (Rohwer and Schaber 1997). Duress is defined by state statute, case law, or both. In assessing the gravity of the threat, one should consider the personality, experience, and sophistication of the person claiming that his or her free will was overborne. A major issue that confounds determinations of duress, especially in retrospect, is the fact that some degree of coercion exists in all relationships.

In the clinical context, practitioners usually draw a subtle but important distinction between *persuasion* and *coercion* (Malcolm 1992). Persuasion is defined as the clinician's aim to use the patient's reasoning capacity to arrive at a desired result. It is an expression of fiducial concern for the patient. In contrast, coercion occurs when the clinician manipulates the patient by introducing extraneous elements that undermine the patient's ability to reason. Coercion usually exploits the patient. The following fictional case examples illustrate these principles.

Case Example 1: The Prenuptial Agreement

A couple is making preparations to marry. Both have been married before and have grown children. Mr. Jones has been psychologically abusive. Ms.

Smith is increasingly worried about going through with the marriage. She refuses to sign a prenuptial agreement on the advice of her attorney because of its "manifest unfairness." While they are in Mr. Jones's library, he pulls a gun from his desk drawer and places it against her head. He presents her with a copy of the prenuptial agreement and warns her to "sign it or else." As Ms. Smith signs under great protest and fear, the transaction is inadvertently witnessed by the housekeeper in the hall. Mr. Jones later destroys the prenuptial agreement after Ms. Smith's attorney calls to advise him that a witness exists to the signing of the prenuptial agreement under duress.

This case example dramatically illustrates the total overcoming of one person's free will by another. In most cases, however, it is more difficult to show that the person claiming duress had no choice.

Undue influence occurs when "the victim was prevented from exercising free choice in the transaction due to the other party taking conscious advantage of a weakened mental state" (Rohwer and Schaber 1997, p. 202). Undue influence also has been defined as influence obtained by improper means (*In Estate of Weir* 1973), and as influence that destroys a testator's free agency and substitutes that of another (*Fischer v. Heckerman* 1989). In other words, the person exerting the influence stands in for the person assenting to a contract or making a will. Claims of undue influence involve either a fiduciary relationship between the parties or a person taking unfair advantage of another person's impaired mental functioning ("a weakened mind"), or a combination of both factors. Thus, to constitute undue influence, the situation must involve a person taking advantage of a fiduciary relationship or mental infirmity. Although the victim may not be sufficiently lacking in mental capacity to assert a defense on that basis alone, the combination of the victim's "mental weakness" and the other party's attempt to consciously take advantage of the victim's vulnerability may be enough to support a claim of undue influence. For example, psychiatrists who have accepted large bequests from patients have been accused of exerting undue influence (Simon 1992). The position of power, trust, and confidence that the psychiatrist possesses in relation to the patient and the patient's transference to the psychiatrist are often the basis of undue influence claims.

Case Example 2: The Bequest

A psychiatrist treats a wealthy widow for recurrent depression over a period of 15 years. She is very grateful for the good care she received. She tells friends that she "adores" her psychiatrist. On a few occasions, she mentions during treatment that her will contains a bequest for the psychiatrist's research on affective disorders. The psychiatrist thanks her. On her death, the psychiatrist receives $15 million. The family brings a suit alleging that the psychiatrist exerted undue influence through his position of power and the "patient's transference idealizing the psychiatrist." The case attracts much publicity before being settled out of court. In the settlement, the psychiatrist receives $500,000 to be used only for research.

Mental impairment is central to cases alleging undue influence. Individuals who voluntarily drink alcohol or take nonprescribed drugs and lose cognitive ability or motivational control may be permitted to void their contracts only if the other party knew or had reason to know of the degree of impairment (Rohwer and Schaber 1997). Individuals who are taking prescribed medications or who are involuntarily drugged or intoxicated are treated the same as individuals with mental defects or disorders, as described earlier.

Psychiatric diagnosis is key to retrospective assessment of testamentary and contractual capacity. However, the presence of a diagnosis does not automatically establish an impaired mental capacity susceptible to undue influence. Although not easy to prove, undue influence can be demonstrated by physical evidence, circumstantial evidence, and the testimony of witnesses (Walsh et al. 1994). Undue influence usually involves a course of conduct rather than a single event. In addition to some impairment, a finding of undue influence requires suspicious circumstances in regard to the behavior of others and additional evidence from collateral sources (Perr 1981). Documentation of the relevant facts about the event in question is rarely recorded. Physical evidence pertinent to the determination of an individual's mental state may exist (e.g., medical examination, computed tomography [CT] scan, magnetic resonance imaging [MRI]).

Assessment of Ability to Enter Into Contracts

Prior to *Faber v. Sweet Style Mfg. Corp.* (1963), most courts considered cognitive capacity as the standard in assessing an individual's ability to enter into a contract. In *Faber* the court rescinded a land purchase transaction because the plaintiff's decision was driven by a manic-depressive psychosis. The court noted that traditional legal standards of measuring competence to contract did not adequately consider the effects of mental disorders. In *Ortelere v. Teachers Retirement Board* (1969), the appellate court ruled that a contract may be rescinded if the executing party was laboring under a mental defect that prevented acting in a reasonable manner and the other party knew of the defect. The plaintiff was being treated for involutional psychosis and cerebrovascular disease. Thus the law makes a distinction between mental disorders that impair an individual's cognitive ability (understanding the nature and consequences of a proposed transaction) and mental disorders that impair an individual's motivation or ability to act reasonably

(Rohwer and Schaber 1984). If an individual lacks cognitive ability, the contract is voidable even if the other party was unaware of the mental impairment. The contract of an individual with impaired motivational control or ability to act reasonably is voidable only if the other party had knowledge of the mental impairment. The law seeks to resolve the tension between protecting individuals with mental disorders and preserving contract transactions.

Cognitive impairments are commonly observed with psychotic disorders, especially schizophrenia, dementia, and delirium, as well as with natural aging. Motivational impairments are seen with affective illnesses, particularly bipolar disorder. Individuals who are either manic, depressed, or both (mixed states) may manifest severely impaired judgment, even though they understand the nature of a transaction.

Some states provide gradations of mental capacity for the recision of contracts, such as individuals with "lesser weakness" of mind in the presence of undue influence (*Smalley v. Baker* 1968). The level of mental capacity required to contract will vary with the nature of the contract. For example, one of life's most important contracts—marriage—requires the least mental competency. A much higher degree of mental competency is required to purchase a home. However, anything that overcomes the individual's freedom of volition invalidates a will or contract.

Case Example 3: The Purchase

Mr. Anderson, a 42-year-old business executive, develops an acute manic episode after promotion to the position of CEO of his company. He purchases a luxury car for $125,000 even though his family has three cars. Mr. Anderson is already in debt and cannot afford to pay for the car. Buying another car is clearly unnecessary and imprudent. He is psychiatrically hospitalized and started on mood-stabilizing medications. After 1 month Mr. Anderson is able to return to work. He brings a legal action to rescind the car purchase agreement. The treating psychiatrist testifies that Mr. Anderson's judgment was severely impaired because he was acutely manic. The salesman at the car dealership admits that Mr. Anderson appeared hyperactive and talkative. He observed that Mr. Anderson paid the full sticker price for the luxury car and signed the purchase agreement without reviewing it. The salesman acknowledged that this was unusual behavior. The court voids the contract on the basis of the medical evidence that Mr. Anderson was unable to act reasonably and that the salesman was aware that Mr. Anderson was not behaving appropriately.

Motivational impairment has been referred to as "affective incompetence" in the clinical context (Simon 1992, p. 123). The ability of psychiatrists to assess motivational impairment in litigation, like volition discussed earlier, has not been subject to scientific research.

Assessment of Testamentary Capacity

The presence of a mental disorder alone does not mean that the afflicted individual lacked the mental capacity to make a will or enter into a contract. Indeed, bad—even foolish—decisions are made everyday by people who do not have a diagnosable mental disorder. In fact, if individuals have testamentary capacity, they can be as capricious as they desire in their wills. Idiosyncratic conduct, by itself, is not conclusive evidence of testamentary incapacity (Shuman 1994). Unless substantial corroborative evidence is present, motivational impairment can remain indiscernible to retrospective psychiatric assessment.

In the retrospective assessment of testamentary capacity, diagnosis is very important in anchoring clinical judgment while also allowing attorneys, as well as opposing experts, to test the individual's reasoning and knowledge (American Psychiatric Association 1992). When no diagnosis is made or the individual does not have a diagnosable mental disorder, expert opinion may fall back on untestable intuition or "clinical judgment." Circumstantial evidence may assume greater importance in the examiner's opinion. This is not to say that the conscientious expert is unable to provide useful information to the court in the absence of a diagnostic formulation. However, the limitations on testability of such testimony should be acknowledged by the expert. For example, publication in a reputable scientific journal requires that the researcher demonstrate that the reported results would occur by chance less than 5% of the time (Shuman and Greenberg 1998). Yet, in both civil and criminal litigation, the expert offers opinions with confidence only to a reasonable degree of medical or scientific certainty (usually more likely than not).

A brief digression on the topic of "reasonable certainty" is pertinent here. The phrase "reasonable medical certainty" is largely sacramental, exacted from experts by lawyers to discourage speculation. It does not further inform but merely casts a spell of pseudoscientific certitude on the court. Rappeport (1985) notes "that reasonable medical certainty does not mean a clear or positive certainty. It means whatever the court, lawyers, or witness seem to want it to mean. One should express opinions with as clear a degree of certainty as is possible, with supporting evidence and not be confused by a scientific concept of certainty" (p. 15). Nor does reasonable medical certainty have a direct relationship with the preponderance of the evidence, which is a jury determination. When asked to give an opinion to a reasonable medical certainty, the forensic examiner should first ask for a definition.

The legal standard takes an absolute rather than a relative approach to the cognitive and motivational capacity to enter a contract or make a will.

Although mental states exist on a continuum, mental capacity is dichotomous—either it is present or absent in regard to a specific legal contract. If an individual has the mental capacity to understand that one is making a will and the nature and extent of one's property but not the objects of one's bounty, then testamentary capacity is absent. Testamentary capacity may not necessarily correspond to the presence or absence of a psychiatric diagnosis. Gradations of testamentary capacity do not exist except that undue influence may invalidate a will or contract, depending on the degree of cognitive or motivational impairment (Perr 1981).

Even when the examiner makes a retrospective diagnosis of psychotic disorder, can he or she know that a person's free will was completely overcome by another person in respect to a specific legal act? This is a difficult enough determination to make for the examiner who conducts a direct examination of the patient or litigant. Individuals with a mental disorder or defect have varying degrees of impairment that rarely eliminate choice.

A useful role for psychiatrists and psychologists in will contests is to explain the effects of a mental disorder on the testator's cognitive process, the effects on cognition of any drugs used in treatment, and the nature of the relationships between the testator and beneficiaries. This testimony permits an exploration of the decision-making capacity of the testator (Shuman 1994).

Case Example 4: The Will

Mr. Boyd, 76 years old, has a diagnosis of multi-infarct dementia. He exhibits symptoms of fluctuating confusion, disorientation, and angry outbursts. An MRI and a CT scan show punctate areas of infarction, primarily in the frontal lobes of the brain. One month prior to his death, after a heated argument with his wife, Mr. Boyd has the nursing home director call his lawyer. Mr. Boyd wants to create a codicil to his will, increasing the amount of money left to his favorite charity. After interviewing his client, the lawyer requests a psychiatric consult. The psychiatrist finds the patient to be in a lucid period. Mr. Boyd understands that he is creating a codicil, understands the extent of his property, and understands the "natural objects of his bounty." After his death his wife and children contest the amended will, based on lack of testamentary capacity. Nursing home records indicate that the patient was fully oriented, "mentally focused," and free of aggressive behavior at the time the codicil was created. Opposing counsel argues that the codicil was an inappropriate, impetuous, angry act that was symptomatic of his demented condition. Moreover, documented evidence exists that the husband was so confused and disoriented that he required care in a nursing home. The court holds that testamentary capacity was demonstrated during a "lucid interval" by the psychiatric examination and the nursing home records at the time the will was amended.

Conclusion

An individual's past mental state may remain opaque to the lens of retrospective psychiatric assessment. Limitations in information, the passage of time, the vagueness of legal definitions, the disjunction between legal and scientific evidence, the personal biases of the examiner, and the absence of reliability and validity research on the retrospective psychiatric assessment of mental states make it mandatory for psychiatric opinions to be carefully constructed on a foundation of supportable fact. Reconstruction of prior mental states demands that the psychiatrist adhere to the principle of honesty and strive for objectivity (American Academy of Psychiatry and the Law 1995).

References

American Academy of Psychiatry and the Law: American Academy of Psychiatry and the Law Ethical Guidelines for the Practice of Forensic Psychiatry. Bloomfield, CT, American Academy of Psychiatry and the Law, 1995

American Psychiatric Association: Diagnostic and Statistical Manual of Mental Disorders, 3rd Edition, Revised. Washington, DC, American Psychiatric Association, 1987

American Psychiatric Association: Diagnostic and Statistical Manual of Mental Disorders, 4th Edition, Text Revision. Washington, DC, American Psychiatric Association, 2000

American Psychiatric Association: Position statement on the insanity defense. Am J Psychiatry 140:681–688, 1983

American Psychiatric Association: The Use of Psychiatric Diagnosis in the Legal Process: Task Force Report 32. Washington, DC, American Psychiatric Association, 1992

American Psychiatric Association: Diagnostic and Statistical Manual of Mental Disorders, 4th Edition. Washington, DC, American Psychiatric Association, 1994

American Psychiatric Association: Diagnostic and Statistical Manual of Mental Disorders, 4th Edition, Text Revision. Washington, DC, American Psychiatric Association, 2000

American Psychiatric Association resource document on peer review of expert testimony. J Am Acad Psychiatry Law 25:359–373, 1997

Beahrs JO: Volition, deception, and the evolution of justice. Bull Am Acad Psychiatry Law 19:81–93, 1991

Bonnie RJ: The moral basis of the insanity defense. American Bar Association Journal 69:194–197, 1983

Butler v Harrison, 578 A2d 1098 (DC 1990)

Comprehensive Crime Control Act, 18 USC, § 20 (1984)

Comprehensive Crime Control Act, 18 USC, § 20(a) (1984)

Daubert v Merrell Dow Pharmaceuticals, Inc., 509 US 579 (1993)

Drewry v Drewry, 8 Va App 460, 383 SE 2d 12 (1989)

Faber v Sweet Style Mfg. Corp., 40 Misc 2d 212, 242 NYS 2d 763 (1963)

Fischer v Heckerman, 772 SW 2d 642 (Ky Ct App 1989)

Frye v United States 293 F 1013 (DC Cir 1923)

Halleck SL: Clinical assessment of the voluntariness of behavior. Bull Am Acad Psychiatry Law 20:221–236, 1992

Hutson HR, Anglin D, Yarbrough J, et al: Suicide by cop. Ann Emerg Med 32(6):665–669, 1998

In Estate of Weir, 154 US App DC 404, 475 F2d 988 (DC Cir 1973)

Johnson v Metropolitan Life Insurance Company, 273 F Supp 589, 594 (D NJ 1967), aff'd, 404 F2d 1202 (3d Cir 1968)

Keeton W, Dobbs D, Keeton R, et al: Intentional interference with the person, in Prosser and Keeton on Torts, 5th Edition. St. Paul, MN, West Publishing, 1984, ch. 2, § 8 at 34

Kumho Tire Co. v Carmichael, 526 US 137 (1999)

Magee B: Confessions of a Philosopher. New York, Random House, 1997

Malcolm JG: Informed consent in the practice of psychiatry, in American Psychiatric Press Review of Clinical Psychiatry and the Law, Vol 3. Edited by Simon RI. Washington, DC, American Psychiatric Press, 1992, pp 223–281

Melton GB, Petrila J, Poythress NG, et al: Psychological Evaluations for the Courts, 2nd Edition. New York, Guilford, 1997

Monahan J, Steadman HJ: Mentally Disordered Offenders. New York, Plenum, 1983

Ortelere v Teachers Retirement Board, 25 NY 2d 196, 303 NYS 2d 362, 250 NE 2d 460 (1969)

Perr IN: Wills, testamentary capacity and undue influence. Bull Am Acad Psychiatry Law 9:15–22, 1981

Rappeport JR: Reasonable medical certainty. Bull Am Acad Psychiatry Law 13:5–15, 1985

Rohwer CD, Schaber GD: Contracts in a Nutshell, 2nd Edition. St. Paul, MN, West Publishing, 1984

Rohwer CD, Schaber GD: Contracts in a Nutshell, 4th Edition. St. Paul, MN, West Publishing, 1997

Shuman DW: Psychiatric and Psychological Evidence, 2nd Edition. St. Paul, MN, West Publishing, 1994, § 15.08

Shuman DW, Greenberg SA: The role of ethical norms in the admissibility of expert testimony. The Judge's Journal 37:5–9, 42–43, 1998

Simon RI: You only die once—but did you intend it? psychiatric assessment of suicide intent in insurance litigation. Tort and Insurance Law Journal 25:650–662, 1990

Simon RI: Clinical Psychiatry and the Law, 2nd Edition. Washington, DC, American Psychiatric Press, 1992

Simon RI: Toward the development of guidelines in the forensic psychiatric examination of posttraumatic stress disorder claimants, in Posttraumatic Stress Disorder in Litigation: Guidelines for Forensic Assessment. Edited by Simon RI. Washington, DC, American Psychiatric Press, 1995, pp 31–84

Simon RI: Bad Men Do What Good Men Dream: A Forensic Psychiatrist Illuminates the Darker Side of Human Behavior. Washington, DC, American Psychiatric Press, 1996

Simon RI: Ethical and legal issues in neuropsychiatry, in American Psychiatric Press Textbook of Neuropsychiatry, 3rd Edition. Edited by Hales RE, Yudofsky SC. Washington, DC, American Psychiatric Press, 1997, pp 1037–1072

Simon RI: Murder masquerading as suicide: postmortem assessment of suicide risk factors at the time of death. J Forensic Sci 43(6):1119–1123, 1998

Simon RI: Legal issues in psychiatry, in Comprehensive Textbook of Psychiatry, 7th Edition. Edited by Kaplan HI, Sadock BJ. Baltimore, MD, Williams & Wilkins, 2000, pp 3272–3289

Simon RI, Wettstein RM: Toward the development of guidelines for the conduct of forensic psychiatric examinations. J Am Acad Psychiatry Law 25:17–30, 1997

Slovenko R: Psychiatry and Criminal Culpability. New York, Wiley, 1995

Smalley v Baker, 262 Cal App 2d 824, 69 Cal Rptr 521 (Cal Ct App 1968)

Spencer v General Electric Co., 688 F Supp 1072 (ED Va 1988)

Walsh AC, Brown BB, Kay EK, et al: Mental Capacity: Legal and Medical Aspects of Assessment and Treatment. Colorado Springs, CO, Shepard's/McGraw-Hill, 1994, section 301

Wilson EF, Davis JH, Bloom JD, et al: Homicide or suicide: the killing of suicidal persons by law enforcement officers. J Forensic Sci 43(1):46–52, 1998

Retrospective Assessment of Mental States and the Law

Daniel W. Shuman, J.D.

$\mathbb{S}$ubstantive legal standards determine the relevance of litigants' mental states. For example, although the criminal law has long recognized an insanity defense that makes relevant the defendant's mental state at the time of the offense, the civil law has long refused to recognize an insanity defense to tort claims for equivalent conduct (Shuman 1992). Because only relevant evidence is admissible, the admissibility of evidence of mental states is determined, in the first instance, by substantive legal standards. The decision, reflected in these substantive legal standards, to make a party's mental state exculpatory or inculpatory is driven by theoretical as well as practical considerations. Theoretical considerations, such as fairness and responsibility, play an important role in the law's decision. Consider, for example, the United States Supreme Court's decision in *Penry v. Lynaugh* (1989). The Court refused to find that capital punishment of a mentally retarded defendant constituted cruel and unusual punishment proscribed by the Eighth Amendment to the United States Constitution but did find that the ban on cruel and unusual punishment required the jury to be instructed that it could consider evidence of mental retardation in mitigation of punishment. The decision reflects a normative judgment about fairness and responsibility that determined the relevance of evidence of a mentally retarded defendant's mental state. "In this case, in the absence of instructions informing the jury that it could consider and give effect to the mitigating evidence of Penry's mental retardation and abused background by declining to impose the death penalty, we conclude that the jury was not provided with a vehicle for expressing its 'reasoned moral response' to that evidence in rendering its sentencing decision" (*Penry v. Lynaugh* 1989, at 328).

In addition to theoretical considerations that determine the relevance of a party's mental state, practical considerations also drive the decision. The law recognizes the practical difficulties in discovering what someone was thinking before performing a particular act and therefore permits an inference to be drawn about mental state from the context of the act. Consider, for example, the following statement of the Illinois supreme court in reviewing a challenge to the sufficiency of evidence to support a conviction for assault: "The gist or essence of the crime of assault with intent to murder is a specific intent to take life and such intent must be proved as charged beyond a reasonable doubt. However, since intent is a state of mind, and, if not admitted, can be shown only by surrounding circumstances, it has come to be recognized that an intent to take life may be inferred from the character of the assault, the use of a deadly weapon and other circumstances" (*People v. Coolidge* 1963, at 536). The first part of this chapter analyzes substantive legal standards that make past mental states relevant in civil and criminal litigation and explores alternate legal standards to address mental states in civil and criminal litigation that might avoid or redefine the necessity for retrospective assessments of mental state in these proceedings.

Once substantive legal standards determine the relevance of the mental state of parties or witnesses, procedural law determines the sources of supporting proof that may be adduced. In particular, the rules of evidence articulate the rigor with which trial courts are required to scrutinize proffered expert testimony before juries or judges are permitted to rely on this expertise. For a panoply of different reasons, the formal threshold articulated by the rules of evidence has recently risen, although in practice it has not been applied consistently across classes of cases or experts. To date, there have been few cases addressing whether a mental health professional's methods and procedures in addressing retrospective assessment satisfy the rigorous standards that appellate courts have articulated to scrutinize the admissibility of expert testimony. However, decisions requiring rigorous scrutiny of all types of expert testimony appear to demand that courts must ultimately address mental health professionals' methods and procedures for retrospective assessment of mental states as one of the core unexamined forensic activities of psychiatrists and psychologists. The second part of this chapter explores the application of these procedural rules to expert testimony about past mental states.

In addition to clinical opinions about past mental states, experts frequently present evidence that a party or witness meets the diagnostic criteria for a mental disorder or syndrome as a way of ascertaining a past mental state. For example, the prosecution in a rape case might offer evidence that the complaining witness suffers from rape trauma syndrome (RST), a cluster of behaviors said to be characteristic of women who have been sexually assaulted, to persuade the fact-finder that it is unlikely that she then consented to have sexual intercourse with the defendant as he now claims. Therefore this chapter also examines the use to which syndrome evidence has been put into assessing retrospective mental states and whether that use is legally sufficient.

Substantive Legal Standards That Make Past Mental States Relevant

The law rarely holds people strictly accountable for their acts. Neither does the law hold people strictly accountable for their thoughts. Rather, most substantive legal standards rest on the assumption that it is fair and appropriate to consider both the actor's conduct and the actor's accompanying mental state or condition in determining legal consequences. Thus, for example, we would not regard as valid a contract signed by a party threatened with death as an alternative to signing, nor would we find a will valid that was signed by someone who understood it to be a rental lease agreement. The law typically assesses the legal effect of acts in conjunction with the accompanying mental state. Therefore legal rules often require an assessment of mental states accompanying acts as an element of a claim or defense. The decision not to hold people strictly accountable for their actions and to take account of their accompanying mental state may ameliorate certain normative problems, but it raises certain practical problems. How are judges or juries to learn, with any degree of confidence, of a person's unexpressed contemporaneous thoughts?

Recognizing the inherent problems of ascertaining unexpressed thoughts, legal decisions often employ "objective" standards that turn on the commonly understood meaning of what is expressed rather than on unexpressed thoughts. Consider the objective rules that apply to contract formation. According to these rules, it is the generally understood meaning of a party's spoken words that is legally relevant and controlling, and not the individual unexpressed thoughts about the meaning of those spoken words. "[U]nder the prevailing 'objective' theory of contract, parties who do not consciously consent to be subject to contractual duties nevertheless are bound so long as their conduct reasonably manifests assent" (Shell 1993, p. 438). Legal rules, such as the objective theory of contract formation, help to avoid the problems of having outcomes turn on ascertaining a party's past private thoughts. In many instances, however, courts and legislatures have not chosen to or have been unable to formulate legal rules of decision that turn on objective considerations. Rules that do not turn on objective considerations require the fact-finder to assess not what a reasonable person might understand such conduct to communicate but instead what a particular actor was actually thinking. These determinations of what a party was actually thinking or feeling become even more complex when the retrospective context is added.

Some legal standards, such as those material to civil commitment and guardianship proceedings, competence to stand trial or be executed, and child custody and visitation, call for assessments of a party's concurrent mental state. Although the past is obviously relevant in assessing current mental state or condition, assessing what a party was thinking at a particular time in the past is not the goal of these assessments. Other legal standards specifically call for the fact-finder to address a party's mental state at some point in the past. In these instances the goal of the assessment is to assist the courts to ascertain what a party was thinking on a particular occasion. The insanity defense makes relevant the defendant's actual mental state at the time of the offense, the requirements for a valid will or contract make the testator's actual mental state at the time of the undertaking relevant, and standard language in life and accident insurance policies excluding coverage for self-inflicted harm makes relevant the insured's actual mental state at the time of his death or injury. Given the apparent practical difficulties posed by such an inquiry, why does the law choose to frame these questions in a manner that predictably presents such difficult factual determinations, and are there alternative legal approaches that avoid these impracticable determinations?

Violations of the Criminal Law

Perhaps the most visible and controversial arena for determinations of past mental state is responsibility for violations of the criminal law. In contrast with most behavioral and social science explanations of behavior, the criminal law proceeds on the assumption that free will exists and that most criminal behavior is the result of a choice for which it is fair to hold the actor accountable. The criminal law deems it appropriate to punish violations committed by individuals who are capable of exercising free will, but not those acts committed by the subset of individuals who are incapable of exercising free will. The law does not bother with empirical proof to support the assumption that free will exists or that mental illness deprives some persons of the opportunity to exercise it; these are fundamental articles of faith for the criminal law. The adoption of these articles of faith, however, does require a vehicle to sort out those to whom the free will assumption should apply and those to whom it should not. The standards for assessing criminal responsibility represent society's effort to distinguish those persons whose mental or emotional condition at the time of the offense justifies punishment from those who do not (Rogers and Shuman 2000).

> The insanity defense reflects the fundamental moral principles of our criminal law. An adjudication of guilt is more than a factual determination that the defendant pulled a trigger, took a bicycle, or sold heroin. It is a moral judgment that the individual is blameworthy. "Our collective conscience does not allow punishment where it cannot impose blame." Our concept of blameworthiness rests on assumptions that are older than the Republic: "man is naturally endowed with these two great faculties, understanding and liberty of will." "Historically, our substantive criminal law is based on a theory of punishing the vicious will. It postulates a free agent confronted with a choice between doing right and wrong, and choosing freely to do wrong." Central, therefore, to a verdict of guilty is the concept of responsibility. Recognition of the insanity defense rests on the conclusion that "it is unjust to punish a person who because of mental illness is without understanding of the nature or quality of his conduct and lacks the capacity to conform his behavior." An acquittal by reason of insanity is a judgment that the defendant is not guilty because, as a result of his mental condition, he is unable to make an effective choice regarding his behavior. (*United States v. Lyons* 1984, at 994)

There are several prevailing current formulations of the insanity defense. The (1843) standard exculpates a defendant who, at the time of the offense, was "laboring under such a defect of reason, from disease of mind as not to know the nature and quality of the act he was doing; or if he did, that he did not know what he was doing was wrong" (at 720). The American Law Institute standard provides that "A person is not responsible for criminal conduct, if at the time of such conduct as the result of a mental disease or defect, he lacks substantial capacity either to appreciate the criminality (wrongfulness) of his conduct or to conform his conduct to the requirements of law. As used in this article, the terms 'mental disease or defect' do not include an abnormality manifested only by repeated criminal or otherwise antisocial conduct" (American Law Institute 1962, § 4.01(1)). And the federal Insanity Defense Reform Act exculpates a defendant when "as a result of a severe mental disease or defect, he was unable to appreciate the nature and quality or wrongfulness of his act" (Insanity Defense Reform Act of 1984 [P.L. 98-473]).

These formulations vary in their scope and willingness to exculpate for volitional impairments as well as the range of impairments that qualify under these standards. However, they all address the defendant's actual mental state accompanying the act charged. Thus they all require the parties to address the defendant's mental state in the past, presenting—at least in this regard—similar problems of retrospective assessment of mental state. Particularly when the defendant had not seen a mental health professional at some time proximate to the act charged, a retrospective assessment of the defendant's mental state at the time of the act under any of these tests is equally demanding (Rogers and Shuman 2000; see also Chapters 4 and 5 in this volume).

Is there an alternative to this demanding inquiry? Might the courts assess criminal responsibility under a standard that does not require retrospective assessments of mental states? One obvious alternative to assessing criminal responsibility without a retrospective assessment of mental states would be to abolish the insanity defense, which several states (Montana, Idaho, Kansas, and Utah) have done (Perlin 1996). However, abolition raises a number of troubling moral and constitutional questions about the punishment of mentally disordered offenders. Even if these questions were conclusively resolved in favor of abolition, what of the practical consequences of abolition? In particular, does abolition of the insanity defense avoid the necessity for retrospective assessments of defendant's mental states at the time of the offense? Some abolition proposals have urged a strict liability approach in which the defendant's mental state is ignored completely, leaving courts to focus only on the defendant's actions. However, in those states that have abolished an insanity defense, the defendant's mental condition at the time of the offense remains an issue in the case, albeit subsumed under mens rea as an element of the offense (Rogers and Shuman 2000). Thus when the crime charged is not a strict liability offense and includes an intent requirement (i.e., knowing, purposeful, negligent), this mental state is an element of the crime charged that the state must prove to convict and the defendant can avoid punishment by negating (Steadman at al. 1993).

Abolition has not removed the issue of the defendant's mental state at the time of the offense from criminal responsibility determinations. In Utah defendants with mental disorders that would have resulted in a not guilty by reason of insanity (NGRI) acquittal but who did not meet the more limited mens rea criteria have been found not to meet the postabolition mens rea requirement to impose criminal responsibility (Steadman et al. 1993). In Montana abolition "did not substantially diminish the frequency with which the issue of mental disease was raised in criminal proceedings," nor the age, diagnosis, or offense charged, although it dramatically reduced the number of acquittals for mental disease (Steadman et al. 1993, p. 127).

Although mental state remains an issue in the case under mens rea, the relevance of the defendant's mental condition is, at least in theory, far more limited than under the prevailing insanity defense standards, as illustrated by the following remark from the state supreme court of Utah's decision upholding that state legislature's abolition of the insanity defense.

> If A kills B, thinking that he is merely squeezing a grapefruit, A does not have the requisite mens rea for murder and would be acquitted under both the prior and the new law....However, if A kills B, thinking that B is an enemy soldier and that the killing is justified as self-defense, then A has the requisite mens rea for murder and could be convicted under the new law but not under the prior law, because he knowingly and intentionally took another's life. Under the amended provision, it does not matter whether A understood that the act was wrong. (State v. Herrera 1995, at 361)

However, as one review of the Idaho decision upholding the constitutionality of its abolition of the insanity defense noted, the changes in the admissibility of past mental states that abolition portends for forensic practice remain ambiguous:

> In upholding the constitutionality of section 18–207, the Searcy court granted broad discretion to the legislature in reforming and even abolishing the insanity defense. As a result of such deference, however, the court conspicuously avoided any attempt to articulate the relationship between mens rea and mental illness. The court's silence leaves this relationship open to two conflicting interpretations. On one hand, trial courts may interpret mens rea broadly so as to encompass all considerations of mental illness, rendering abolition of the insanity defense ineffective. On the other hand, courts and legislatures may define mens rea narrowly so as to exclude all considerations of mental illness, raising due process concerns unaddressed in *Searcy*. ("Note, recent development" 1991, p. 1135)

Thus the ultimate impact of abolition on the evidence of the defendant's mental condition at the time of the offense that could have been adduced under an insanity defense but is not now admissible under mens rea remains to be seen.

There are, of course, strict liability criminal law offenses. For example, laws that criminalize overtime parking do not require proof of a culpable mental state in addition to proof of the proscribed act, and in this regard are not generally seen as controversial. Beyond this category of strict liability crimes, however, criminalizing behavior without proof of a culpable mental state is morally and constitutionally problematic (Green 1997; Perkins 1983). Although punishing overtime parking or speeding without regard to intent may not be troubling, punishing murder or assault without consideration of intent is troubling. For sensible reasons, our society has avoided punishing individuals for serious criminal wrongdoing, without regard to intent, accident, or mistake. "When the law begins to permit conviction for serious offenses of men who are morally innocent and free from fault, who may even be respected and useful members of the community, its restraining power becomes undermined. Once it becomes respectable to be convicted, the vitality of the criminal law has been sapped" (Sayre 1933, pp. 79–80). Our sense of morality and accountability recoils at the thought of holding criminally responsible those whose ability to make responsible choices was seriously impaired by a mental disorder. Thus retrospective assessment of a defendant's mental state remains a problematic but necessary component of a meaningful appraisal of criminal responsibility for serious offenses.

Competence to Execute a Will

A less visible and somewhat less controversial substantive legal standard calling for retrospective assessments of mental state is competence to execute a will. Every jurisdiction denies legal effect to a will or other testamentary instrument executed by someone who lacked the requisite mental capacity. The standard for testamentary capacity is surprisingly similar from state to state, and no state has abolished its testamentary capacity requirement as some states have abolished their insanity defense.

Testamentary capacity to execute a will requires that its author, the testator (M) or testatrix (F), be of *sound mind* at the time the will is executed. The factors generally recognized as necessary to meet this requirement are that, at the time of the making of the will, the testator know that he is making a will, know the nature and extent of his property subject to distribution by the will, know how the will would distribute that property, and know those blood relatives and others who would normally be expected to benefit from the distribution (*Banks v. Goodfellow* 1870). Although these requirements may appear daunting for many elderly individuals, "the courts guard jealously the rights of all rational people, including the aged, the infirm, the forgetful and the queer, to make wills sufficient to withstand the attacks of those left out and those dissatisfied with the expressed desires of the departed...." (*Kentucky Trust Co. v. Gore* 1946, at 752). Thus "[a]dvanced age, senility, confusion, and ill health are insufficient to justify denying probate of a will if the testator possessed testamentary capacity at the time of execution" (*In re Estate of Bracken* 1970, at 380). Sorting out these cases often entails piecing together the testimony of lay and nonmental health care professionals who observed the testator. Although this is perhaps more information than available in many other kinds of cases in which retrospective assessment of mental condition is concerned, in will contests, by definition, the person whose mental capacity is at issue is currently unavailable for assessment. These cases are also unique in another regard.

Unlike criminal acts, which are often impulsive, unplanned, and secretive, execution of a will is normally carefully planned with the benefit of counsel. Therefore it permits a degree of lawyer-client planning not possible by ethical criminal lawyers. There are several strategies available to a lawyer counseling a client whose competence is likely to be challenged because of questions about the client's mental or physical health or the unique nature of the client's asset distribution. One strategy is the use of nonprobate transfers such as inter vivos trusts, joint ownership, and gifts, although they also hold open the possibility of challenges for fraud, undue influence, or lack of capacity, as do self-proved wills (Leopold and Beyer 1990). Another approach that has been recommended when a challenge to the testator's competence is expected is obtaining a videotaped psychiatric or psychological examination and report on the testator's competence contemporaneous with the execution of the will (Shuman 1994). The partisanship of the expert who is selected will, of course, be scrutinized, thus careful selection of the expert and the conditions for preparation of a report are crucial.

A novel approach that avoids retrospective assessments of testamentary capacity is premortem or *living* probate (Beyer 1993; Leopold and Beyer 1990). Premortem probate permits a person who has authored a will or other testamentary instrument to seek a concurrent ruling on its validity, including the issue of testamentary capacity, in a formal judicial proceeding in which the heirs and beneficiaries of the will are notified and permitted to participate. Unlike postmortem probate proceedings, which ironically demand that the person whose mental capacity is at issue be unavailable for assessment, premortem probate is designed so that the person whose mental capacity is at issue is available for assessment. Although premortem probate offers to resolve many of the problems surrounding retrospective assessment of testamentary capacity, it has been criticized as impracticable for reasons of cost (i.e., the possibility of multiple judicial proceedings for multiple wills made during the testator's life), forcing embarrassing disclosure of the details of the will during the testator's life or confrontation of the testator by disgruntled heirs or beneficiaries, and inefficiency (spending time and money adjudicating the validity of a will that the testator may change repeatedly). Thus it has not been widely embraced by states, with the exception of Arkansas, North Dakota, and Ohio (Leopold and Beyer 1990).

A challenge to testamentary capacity addresses the abilities of the testator. A challenge for undue influence addresses the influence that others may have over the testator, notwithstanding the fact that testamentary capacity exists. Thus, even if the testator has the capacity to execute a will, "influence gained by improper means, or influence such that the testator's free agency is destroyed" results in invalidation of the will (Walsh et al. 1994, p. 3-11). Although proof of these circumstances is determined on a case-by-case basis, courts have noted sets of suspicious fact patterns:

> There have been listed certain so-called "badges" of undue influence. They include a physically weak and mentally impaired testator, a will unnatural in its provisions, a lately developed and comparatively short period of close relationship between the testator and the principal beneficiary, participation by the beneficiary in the physical preparation of the will, the possession of the will by the beneficiary after it was written, efforts by the beneficiary to restrict contacts between the testator and the natural objects of his bounty and absolute control of testator's business affairs by a beneficiary. (*Fischer v. Heckerman* 1989, at 645)

Execution and Enforcement of Contracts

Unlike wills, which rely on the approval of the courts for their validation and enforcement, the execution and enforcement of contracts normally takes place outside the courtroom unless the parties reach a disagreement they are not capable of resolving. When a party resorts to the courts to enforce a contract, proof of the competence of the parties to the contract is not a prerequisite to the court's enforcement of the contract. Rather, incapacity is an affirmative defense to the enforcement of a contract that must be raised and proved by the party challenging enforcement of the contract. That affirmative defense requires a party to the contract to prove that, as the result of a mental disorder, she or he did not understand the nature or consequence of the transaction. In the majority of courts the test focuses on cognitive capacity.

> The test of competency to contract is whether the powers of a person's mind have been so affected as to destroy the ability to understand the nature of the act in which he is engaged, its scope and effect or its nature and consequences.…If a person, at the time of entering into a contract, understands the nature, extent and scope of the business he is about to transact, and possesses that degree of mental strength which would enable him to transact ordinary business, he is in law considered a person of sound mind

and memory....Furthermore, a party who has not been adjudicated as mentally incompetent in a court of law is presumed to be competent. However, the presumption of competency is rebuttable. If the presumption of competency is rebutted, then the contract entered into by the mentally incompetent individual is voidable....By contrast, a formal adjudication of incompetency and appointment of a guardian divests the individual of any contractual capacity, thus making any contract entered into by the mentally incompetent person void....(*Davis v. Marshall* 1994, at 6)

However, a minority of jurisdictions have added a volitional component to this test. In those jurisdictions "capacity to understand is not, in fact, the sole criterion. Incompetence to contract also exists when a contract is entered into under the compulsion of a mental disease or disorder but for which the contract would not have been made" (*Faber v. Sweet Style Mfg. Corp.* 1963, at 767–768)

Life or Accident Insurance Contracts

One specific type of contract that often raises the issue of a party's past mental state is a contract for life or accident insurance. Insurance companies selling coverage for accidental death or injury commonly include exclusionary language in their policies for self-inflicted injuries that occur within a certain period of time (Freedman 1990). Their reasons are economic: "While it is possible to compute actuarially the percentage of loss from ordinary mortality, this becomes somewhat more difficult where an insured voluntarily brings about the maturing event" (Appleman and Appleman 1981, p. 346). As a matter of law, however, it is generally recognized that there is no reason they could not agree to do so (Appleman and Appleman 1981). Because suicide is not a rare event,[1] the question of whether an insured committed suicide and its legal consequences is an issue that regularly besets insurance companies, policy beneficiaries, and the courts (Schuman 1993).

Although varying from policy to policy, the exclusionary language typically states that the policy does not cover death "by his own hand," "by suicide," or "by self-destruction" within some set period after the effective date of the policy (Freedman 1990, p. 413). Were the determination to turn solely on the physical act that resulted in the insured's death, matters would be simpler. However, because the impact of this exclusion falls on innocent

---

[1]"Suicide is the eighth leading case of death in the United States, claiming about 30,000 lives in 1997, compared to fewer than 19,000 homicides" (Meckler 1999, p. Z-16).

beneficiaries, courts have tempered the impact of this exclusionary language by reading into it an intent requirement. In the absence of policy language providing that the exclusion applies whether the insured was "sane or insane," courts have not prevented recovery under language excluding suicide "unless the deceased was able to form a conscious intention to kill himself or herself and to carry out that act, realizing its physical—and moral—consequences" (Schuman 1993, p. 757). This standard requires that psychiatric and psychological experts retained by the parties address the mental state of the insured at the time of his or her death, similar to the cognitive assessment required by the *M'Naghten* standard for criminal responsibility, with all the problems associated with this retrospective assessment.

In a minority of jurisdictions, courts construing policies that contain the additional exclusionary language that they apply whether the death by the insured's own hand occurred while "sane or insane" have held that the language does not to apply to instances when the insured was so mentally disordered as not to understand that his act would result in death or that the act was committed under an insane impulse. In a majority of jurisdictions, however, courts construing policies that contain suicide exclusions that apply whether the insured was "sane or insane" have held that the insured is not obligated to pay unless the death was accidental (Freedman 1990). "The majority view is that for an act to be 'suicide, sane or insane,' it is not necessary for the decedent to have realized the physical nature or consequences of his act, nor that he have a conscious purpose to take his life. If the act is one which would be regarded as suicide in a sane person, the loss occasioned thereby would come within the exclusion, regardless of whether the insured decedent realized or was capable of realizing that such an act would cause his death...." (*Aetna Life Ins. Co. v. McLaughlin* 1964, at 102). In policies containing this language, in the majority of jurisdictions, the task of psychiatric and psychological experts is narrowed. It is not to consider cognitively what the decedent was capable of intending or morally appreciated, rather it is a normative decision as to whether the act would be regarded as suicide in a "sane" person.

In the majority of states, an insurance company wishing to exclude coverage for suicide has the capacity to avoid or severely narrow the scope of retrospective assessments by addition of the "sane or insane" policy language. Approaching the same question from an opposing perspective, state legislatures also have the capacity to avoid or severely narrow the scope of retrospective assessment by proscribing limitations on coverage for suicide.

The substantive law of criminal law, torts, wills, and contracts discussed above defines the relevance of a party's past mental states. Relevance is a necessary, although not a sufficient, condition of admissibility of evidence of a party's mental state. The law of evidence imposes an additional set of admissibility requirements. It is to these requirements that we now turn.

The Law of Evidence and Past Mental States

The law permits parties to prove past mental states through the testimony of expert or lay witnesses. Thus, for example, the state may choose to challenge an insanity defense with the testimony of an expert witness, a psychiatrist who examined the defendant several weeks after the crime charged; the testimony of a lay witness, the defendant's spouse who observed his behavior the morning of the murder; or both (Shuman 1994). Although the lay witness may lack the psychiatrist's training in observation skills, the fact testimony of the lay witness may permit the judge or jury to receive a description of the defendant's behavior proximate to the crime charged, which the psychiatrist's testimony may lack. As long as the lay witness confines testimony to descriptive data and does not attempt to draw inferences from it that exceed lay competence (e.g., diagnosis of a mental disorder), the rules of evidence impose few barriers to its receipt. Thus, for example, in one insanity defense, the defendant's cellmate was permitted to offer his observation of the defendant's behavior (standing nude in the cell with toilet paper stuffed in his nostrils) and to summarize it thus: "'he ain't got good sense, he's crazy" (*Stacy v. Love* 1982, at 1214). Because experts may do more than report their observations and instead may express opinions about behavior or actions they did not even observe or may offer an opinion on an ultimate issue for the fact-finder to decide, the rules of evidence governing the receipt of expert testimony purport to impose greater restrictions.

Although novel expert testimony has often invoked rigorous threshold judicial scrutiny, most expert testimony, particularly most psychiatric and psychological expert testimony, has not. As long as the psychiatric or psychological expert has offered only clinical opinion testimony, lawyers and judges addressing admissibility have focused on the qualifications of the witness and left scrutiny of the validity and reliability of the expert's methods and procedures to an adversary presentation before the fact-finder. Only when the expert offered testimony purportedly based in research, for example, by describing the problems of an identification raised by eyewitness identification research or what the research on battered woman's syndrome revealed about the typical behavior of battered woman, did courts purport to scrutinize the science underlying this evidence. However, when psychiatrists and psychologists and other behavioral and social scientists offered clinical opinions that did not explicitly invoke science, courts did not ask as a threshold question of admissibility whether a behavioral or social scientist can provide reliable information to the courts if it is not based in science (Shuman and Sales 1998). Thus, although there are many decisions addressing the admissibility of syndrome evidence or expert testimony about eyewitness testimony research, there are no reported decisions addressing the validity of clinical retrospective assessments of the defendant's mental state in an insanity defense in the context of challenge to its admissibility. Nor are there reported decisions addressing the validity of clinical retrospective assessments of the testator's mental state in a will contest or contract action in the context of a challenge to its admissibility. This may change.

Expert Testimony in the Age of *Daubert*

Prior to the codification of the Federal Rules of Evidence, no uniform standard or rule existed in federal court for the admission of scientific expert testimony. One standard that enjoyed support in many federal courts was the "general acceptance" standard described by the District of Columbia Court of Appeals in *Frye v. United States* (1923) in the course of addressing the admissibility of an early version of the polygraph:

> Just when a scientific principle or discovery crosses the line between the experimental and demonstrable stages is difficult to define. Somewhere in this twilight zone the evidential force of the principle must be recognized, and while courts will go a long way in admitting expert testimony deduced from a well-recognized scientific principle or discovery, the thing from which the deduction is made must be sufficiently established to have gained general acceptance in the particular field to which it belongs. (at 1014)

Although *Frye* was not widely adopted by other courts shortly after the decision, by the 1960s it was more broadly applied.

> As *Frye* was more broadly applied, however, the voices of its critics grew louder. They complained that, in addition to problems of practicability (i.e., problems of determining what must be accepted—the theory, the methodology, the data, its general application or specific application in this technique or procedure, etc.; from which field acceptance must be sought; what is sufficient to determine general acceptance; and how acceptance may be proven), *Frye* failed to address directly the quality of science and excluded important new research. Despite these concerns, many judges seemed to like *Frye* for the same reason some critics disliked it: it allowed judges to pass the buck and avoid making rigorous determinations about scientific reliability and validity. In the face of this heated debate, the Federal Rules of Evidence, promulgated in 1975, the culmination of half a century of debate by leading jurists, practitioners, and academics,

did not contain a single reference to *Frye* or its test. Instead, the Federal Rules of Evidence permitted expert testimony by a qualified expert if it "will assist the trier of fact to understand the evidence or to determine a fact in issue." (Shuman and Sales 1998, p. 1237)

In *Daubert v. Merrell Dow Pharmaceuticals, Inc.* (1993), the United States Supreme Court answered the question about *Frye* and the Federal Rules of Evidence by rejecting the general acceptance test of *Frye* as the standard for the admissibility of scientific evidence under the Federal Rules of Evidence. The standard prescribed by the Supreme Court in *Daubert* requires federal trial courts to engage in a "preliminary assessment of whether the reasoning or methodology underlying the testimony is scientifically valid and of whether that reasoning or methodology properly can be applied to the facts in issue" (at 593). Trial courts were charged to consider whether the underlying theory or technique can be and has been tested, whether it has been subjected to scrutiny by others in the field through peer review and publication, whether the error rate and standards for controlling it are acceptable, and what the degree of acceptance for it is within the scientific community. The Federal Rule of Evidence 702, which *Daubert* interpreted, applies to all expert testimony, whether grounded in scientific, technical, or other specialized knowledge.[2] Although the Supreme Court's pronouncement in *Daubert* only bound the federal courts, it has been widely adopted by many, but not all, state courts.

The Court's decision in *General Electric Co. v. Joiner* (1997) articulated the standard of review that appellate courts should apply when reviewing claims of error in the admissibility of expert testimony under *Daubert*. The Court held in *Joiner* that the abuse of discretion standard, which is the standard generally applied to review trial court evidentiary rulings, applies to review of trial court decisions to admit or exclude scientific evidence under *Daubert*:

> Thus, while the Federal Rules of Evidence allow district courts to admit a somewhat broader range of scientific testimony than would have been admissible under *Frye*, they leave in place the "gatekeeper" role of the trial judge in screening such evidence. A court of appeals applying "abuse of discretion" review to such rulings may not categorically distinguish between rulings allowing expert testimony and rulings which disallow it. (at 142)

---

[2] If scientific, technical, or other specialized knowledge will assist the trier of fact to understand the evidence or to determine a fact in issue, a witness qualified as an expert by knowledge, skill, experience, training, or education may testify thereto in the form of an opinion or otherwise.

Because *Daubert* (as well as *Joiner*) arose within the context of natural science evidence, the federal courts, and the many state courts that chose to follow *Daubert*, disagreed over its application to expert testimony grounded in technical or other specialized knowledge, as well as its application to the behavioral and social sciences. One argument that *Daubert* should not be applied to behavioral and social science evidence, which simplified both the scope of the field as well as failing to account for the creativity of its researchers, was that the questions it examines are often not falsifiable (Richardson et al. 1995). Without directly addressing the differences in natural science and the behavioral and social sciences, the Supreme Court resolved the scope of *Daubert's* application in *Kumho Tire Co. v. Carmichael* (1999), which held that *Daubert* applies to all proffers of expert testimony under the rules of evidence.

> In *Daubert*, this Court held that Federal Rule of Evidence 702 imposes a special obligation upon a trial judge to "ensure that any and all scientific testimony…is not only relevant, but reliable" (509 US, at 589). The initial question before us is whether this basic gatekeeping obligation applies only to "scientific" testimony or to all expert testimony. We, like the parties, believe that it applies to all expert testimony. (*Kumho Tire Co. v. Carmichael* 1999, at 147)

Judges and lawyers accustomed to examining the validity and reliability of what other experts proffer as a condition of admissibility may, in the fullness of time, be less likely to ignore mental health professionals' expert testimony. Thus there is good reason to expect that the reliability of retrospective assessments of mental states may be raised as a threshold issue of admissibility. Indeed, if this enhanced scrutiny increases the emphasis on the role of science in lawmaking, there is good reason to expect more demanding scrutiny by courts and legislatures of the science that underlies the formulation of substantive legal rules, such as the insanity defense. With *Kumho* we seem poised on the edge of a new generation of legal scrutiny in which all expert testimony will be required, as a condition of admissibility, to convince the courts of the reliability of the underlying methods and procedures. The question, of course, is how these criteria will be applied. After resolving the applicability of *Daubert* to all expert testimony in *Kumho*, the Court proceeded to address how its criteria of falsifiability, peer review, error rates, and acceptance within the relevant community should apply to nonscientific expert testimony.

> The petitioners ask more specifically whether a trial judge determining the "admissibility of an engineering expert's testimony" *may* consider several more specific factors that *Daubert* said might "bear on" a judge's gate-

keeping determination....Emphasizing the word "may" in the question, we answer that question yes. Engineering testimony rests upon scientific foundations, the reliability of which will be at issue in some cases....In other cases, the relevant reliability concerns may focus upon personal knowledge or experience....Our emphasis on the word "may" thus reflects *Daubert's* description of the Rule 702 inquiry as "a flexible one." 509 U.S. at 594. *Daubert* makes clear that the factors it mentions do *not* constitute a "definitive checklist or test." Id. at 593. And *Daubert* adds that the gatekeeping inquiry must be "'tied to the facts'" of a particular "case." Id. at 591....We agree with the Solicitor General that "the factors identified in *Daubert* may or may not be pertinent in assessing reliability, depending on the nature of the issue, the expert's particular expertise, and the subject of his testimony...." The conclusion, in our view, is that we can neither rule out, nor rule in, for all cases and for all time the applicability of the factors mentioned in *Daubert*, nor can we now do so for subsets of cases categorized by category of expert or by kind of evidence. Too much depends upon the particular circumstances of the particular case at issue. (*Kumho Tire Co. v. Carmichael* 1999, at 150)

The adoption of a flexible set of considerations to be applied by the trial courts subject to review only for an abuse of discretion leaves much uncertainty about the application of these criteria to psychiatric and psychological evidence. Some gleefully predict that courts will rigidly apply *Daubert* scrutiny to psychiatric and psychological evidence, resulting in the exclusion of most psychiatric and psychological evidence, which they assert is personal opinion devoid of any scientific validity (Grove and Barden 1999). Others fear that rigid adherence to scientific thresholds will have untoward consequences, including depriving parties of the opportunity to tell their stories as required by fundamental constitutional considerations (Slobogin 1999). And still others observe that after all is said and done, it is unclear how much will have changed (Shuman and Sales 1999).

In assessing the impact of the Supreme Court trilogy—*Daubert, Joiner,* and *Kumho*—it is easy to lose sight of the fundamental shift in approach to the admissibility of expert testimony it has triggered. This shift is captured in language from *Joiner,* reemphasized in *Kumho:* "[A]s we pointed out in *Joiner,* 'nothing in either *Daubert* or the Federal Rules of Evidence requires a district court to admit opinion evidence that is connected to existing data only by the *ipse dixit* of the expert'" (*Kumho Tire Co. v. Carmichael* 1999, at 157). This same sense of the shift in approach is captured in another opinion, which notes that an expert's assertion is "not admissible just because somebody with a diploma says it is so" (*United States v. Ingham* 1995, at 226). An expert's qualifications are a necessary but not sufficient condition of the admissibility of the expert's testimony. In the face of an appropriate objection, the trial court must assess, as a threshold question, the validity and reliability of the methods and procedures relied on by the expert to reach any proffered opinions.

Daubert and Retrospective Assessment

How can a psychiatrist or psychologist conducting a retrospective assessment of a party's mental state satisfy this threshold requirement? As Rogers explains (Chapter 10 in this volume), psychiatrists and psychologists conducting retrospective assessments of mental states in civil and criminal litigation are not invariably required to choose between using unproven methods of assessment and failing to participate in forensic assessments. For example, there is a body of research addressing the corroborative model, for which the primary focus is "the collection of independent sources to confirm or disconfirm retrospective accounts by the evaluatee" (p. 290) and the analogue model, which is "used in retrospective studies to address how specific factors may influence the recall or reporting of clinically relevant data" (p. 295), as well as the time-lapse model, which "is an adaptation of test-retest reliability that is applied to the reproducibility of retrospective diagnosis and symptoms" (p. 293) and the biological-marker model, which is a "retrospective account...confirmed by an established biological marker" (p. 299). Reviewing these models, Rogers concludes that:

1. The corroborative model has the broadest clinical applicability and parallels forensic practice. However, care must be taken to use standardized measures that systematically assess the same clinical construct and minimize method variance.
2. The time-lapse model is especially useful for the retrospective measurement of symptoms and associated features, which often form the bedrock of forensic evaluations. For prior episodes or occurrences, time-lapse comparisons provide a rigorous methodology for studying the effects of time on recall. An elegant study would combine the time-lapse model for both evaluatees and informants; this model would allow direct comparisons of time-lapse and corroborative designs. Although easily adapted to clinical research (e.g., first psychiatric hospitalizations), the time-lapse model is more challenging to implement in forensic cases (e.g., personal-injury claims).
3. The analogue model is noteworthy for its experimental rigor, which is often accomplished at the expense of its clinical applicability. For forensic purposes, the analogue model's clinical applicability could be greatly improved if this method were practical for use with persons who are mentally ill. Despite obvious ethical concerns, the retrospective nature of personal-injury evaluations might be better understood with 1) the

use of persons with mood or posttraumatic stress disorders and 2) the simulation of a realistic accident/trauma.

4. The biological-marker model has exceptional experimental rigor and clinical applicability. With reference to forensic practice, its current application appears limited to the retrospective assessment of substance abuse. Within this circumscribed application, the biological-marker model has the remarkable potential to revolutionize the validation of retrospective self-report and psychometric methods.

Clearly, where there is a body of research addressing the subject matter of the psychiatrist's or psychologist's testimony and whether the testimony is couched in scientific or clinical opinion, the entirety of the *Daubert* criteria should be applied and the expert's methods and procedures judged against the research (Shuman and Sales 1998). The more difficult, and as yet unanswered, question is what the courts can or should do when there is no research addressing the subject matter of the expert's testimony or when the inferential leap from the research to the issue in the case is significant. How, for example, should courts that apply *Daubert* assess the admissibility of psychiatric/psychological autopsies, an evaluation of the decedent's past mental state conducted without an examination? (See Chapter 9 in this volume.) Which *Daubert* criteria are left for the courts to apply when there is no research addressing the subject matter of the expert's testimony other than the resuscitated *Frye* test criteria—general acceptance within the relevant community? How does general acceptance help the court assess validity in contrast to reliability? This is the troubling question for clinical opinion testimony that remains after *Kumho*.

In the arena of clinical medicine, the federal courts have been divided on the issue of the admissibility of this testimony on the question of medical causation. Although some courts have concluded that "[n]othing in Rules 702 and 703 or in *Daubert* prohibits an expert witness from testifying to confirmatory data, gained through his own clinical experience, on the origin of a disease or the consequences of exposure to certain conditions" (*Cantrell v. GAF Corp.* 1993, at 1014), others have concluded that "a clinical medical expert cannot express an opinion as to a causal relationship between a chemical compound and a plaintiff's disease, although the opinion is based on the sound application of generally accepted clinical medical methodology, unless the causal link is confirmed by hard scientific methodology as per the *Daubert* factors...." (*Moore v. Ashland Chem. Inc.* 1998, at 280). Not only are the issues of causation in clinical medicine in these toxic tort cases unresolved in the federal courts but also it is far from clear whether the question of causation in these cases should be resolved in the same fashion for psychiatric and psychological assessments of mental status. When and how the Supreme Court will resolve these issues remains uncertain. In the meantime, psychiatrists and psychologists who stay current with the scientific knowledge in their fields and do not venture beyond what this research supports in their opinions will satisfy both the evidentiary and the ethical requirements for presentation of reliable information to the courts (American Academy of Psychiatry and the Law 1995; Committee on Ethical Guidelines for Forensic Psychologists 1991).

In an effort to ground their testimony in a body of research, many psychiatrists and psychologists have addressed retrospective mental states in court through the use of a diagnostic category or syndrome evidence. Much diagnostic category or syndrome evidence used to address past mental states consists of evidence of or derivative of posttraumatic stress disorder (PTSD) (Stone 1993). Elsewhere others have exerted much effort to address the relevant research on PTSD and related syndrome evidence and its sufficiency to survive evidentiary validity and reliability thresholds (e.g., Faigman and Wright 1997; McCord 1985; Schacht 1985). The question addressed here is related to but different from the issues of validity and reliability of the diagnostic classification system, as well as particular diagnoses and syndromes. Assuming that this research meets the evidentiary threshold of *Daubert* and its alternative formulations, is it appropriate to use syndrome evidence to make retrospective assessments of mental state? In the parlance of *Daubert*, the question addressed here is one of fit— "whether the reasoning or methodology properly can be applied to the facts in issue" (*Daubert v. Merrell Dow Pharmaceuticals, Inc.* 1993, at 593). Even if syndrome or diagnostic categories are valid and useful for treatment or prognosis, for example, the question remains as to whether they are a valid and useful tool for forensic retrospective assessment.

PTSD is unique, the only disorder categorized in DSM-IV (American Psychiatric Association 1994) that purports to address causation or etiology. A diagnosis of depression does not purport to explain what causes depression or whether some particular causative element resulted in that condition. Similarly a diagnosis of obsessive-compulsive disorder does not purport to explain anything about what caused it. PTSD, however, explicitly assumes that it results from trauma, and a diagnosis of PTSD requires the presence of a traumatic event in the subject's life. Thus it is understandably tempting to conclude that a PTSD diagnosis will assist in the retrospective assessment of the stressor that caused the PTSD, that is, that if PTSD exists, then the stressor claimed to have caused it did indeed occur.

Although the diagnosis of PTSD assumes the presence of a traumatic stressor, reasoning backward from a diagnosis of PTSD to the occurrence of a particular event that served as the stressor is problematic (Simon 1995). PTSD was not created for the purpose of validating the occurrence of past events but rather for understanding current mental and emotional problems. Nothing in DSM-IV's diagnostic criteria purport to identify differences in those PTSD symptoms that result from natural disasters, military combat, or violent assaults (Shuman 1989). Indeed the research reveals that how a person will respond to a particular stressor is determined in part by unique individual variables. For example, one study of PTSD in Vietnam veterans found that the strongest risk factor was combat experience but that childhood socioeconomic status, prior psychiatric symptoms, and childhood abuse were also shown to predict which veterans would develop PTSD (Green 1995). A diagnosis of PTSD thus does not provide the basis for inferring the occurrence of a particular event that precipitated it. Moreover, the use of a PTSD diagnosis to support a particular syndrome, such as rape trauma syndrome (RTS), and the inference that a particular stressor (i.e., nonconsensual sex) must have occurred, resulting in RTS, confounds the problem.

> Because PTSD was originally constructed with war veterans in mind…the use of the PTSD diagnosis with rape survivors can be problematic. PTSD only accounts for some (not all) of the postrape symptoms identified by researchers and has been criticized for failing to acknowledge the complexity of women's responses to trauma (Koss et al. 1994). Although many of the symptoms associated with rape trauma overlap with the diagnostic criteria of PTSD, RTS cannot be considered synonymous with it.
>
> The PTSD criteria…cover the intense fear that many rape survivors experience, as well as the desire to avoid situations that are reminders of the rape experience. However, the PTSD criteria do not account for the depression, anger, sexual dysfunction, guilt, humiliation, and disruption in core belief systems about the self and others that are also common symptoms among rape survivors (e.g., Atkeson et al.1982; Becker et al. 1982; Janoff-Bulman and Frieze 1983; Kilpatrick et al. 1985; McCann and Pearlman 1990). The National Women's Study indicated that there are a number of rape survivors who meet the criteria for depression, for example, but who do not meet the criteria for PTSD (Acierno et al. 1996; Boeschen et al. 1998, pp. 417–418)

Some courts have understood this distinction between the presence of PTSD symptoms and the occurrence of a particular event that served as the stressor and have limited the use of PTSD to prove the occurrence of the stressor (*Hutton v. State* 1995; *People v. Beldose* 1984; *People v. Pullins* 1985; *Spencer v. General Electric Co.* 1988). For example, in *Spencer* the court rejected the use of RTS, thought to describe the course of PTSD in women who have been sexually assaulted, to prove that the plaintiff was raped on the job by a supervisor. The court reasoned:

> Evidence of PTSD occasioned by rape (or RTS) is not a scientifically reliable means of proving that a rape occurred. PTSD is simply a diagnostic category created by psychiatrists; it is a human construct, an artificial classification of certain behavioral patterns. RTS was developed by rape counselors as a therapeutic tool to help identify, predict, and treat emotional problems experienced by the counselor's clients or patients. It was not developed or devised as a tool for ferreting out the truth in cases where it is hotly disputed whether the rape occurred. (*Spencer v. General Electric Co.* 1988, at 1075)

Other courts have, seemingly, not grasped this distinction between diagnosis and validation of the occurrence of a particular traumatic stressor, and have admitted evidence of PTSD to prove that the traumatic event occurred (*Jensen v. Eveleth Taconite Co.* 1997; *State v. Liddell* 1984; *State v. McQuillen* 1984). The *Jensen* court's reasoning typifies the approach of courts permitting this evidence to be admitted:

> [T]he plaintiffs' expert witnesses was [sic] thorough and meticulously presented. The methodology for arriving at their opinions was laid out clearly by each witness. The key question in this damages phase of the trial was the link between the actions of the defendants and the claimed emotional injuries of the plaintiffs. The expert testimony was therefore without doubt relevant to the issue before the court. (*Jensen v. Eveleth Taconite Co.* 1997, at 1297)

These two quoted opinions stand in stark contrast. The opinion in *Jensen* is typical of pre-*Daubert* opinions applying minimal scrutiny to the reliability of the expert's methods and procedures, leaving rigorous scrutiny of them to an adversary presentation before the fact-finder, in deference to the jury's role in our democratic tradition. The opinion in *Spencer*, more faithful to the subsequent *Daubert, Joiner*, and *Kumho* trilogy's model of gatekeeping, assumes that it is the responsibility of the court to examine carefully the reliability of the expert's methods and procedures and its fit for the issues presented in the case before permitting the expert to offer an opinion before the jury. As courts embrace *Daubert*, however, their application of its considerations often reflect a reticence to abandon the primacy of the jury's role as fact-finder.

Conclusion

The law demands that parties seeking to prevail on numerous claims and defenses present evidence of a party's past mental state. The law also demands that expert testimony offered to support or defeat these claims or defenses meet a validity/reliability threshold as a condition of admissibility.

The chapters that follow offer guidance to psychiatrists and psychologists as providers of this testimony, and to lawyers and judges as consumers of this testimony, with the goal of improving the quality of the information presented in the courts.

References

Aetna Life Ins. Co. v McLaughlin, 380 SW 2d 101, 102 (Tex 1964)

American Academy of Psychiatry and Law: American Academy of Psychiatry and the Law Ethical Guidelines for the Practice of Forensic Psychiatry. Bloomfield, CT, American Academy of Psychiatry and the Law, 1995

American Law Institute: Model Penal Code (1962)

American Psychiatric Association: Diagnostic and Statistical Manual of Mental Disorders, 4th Edition. Washington, DC, American Psychiatric Association, 1994

Appleman JA, Appleman J: Insurance Law and Practice. St. Paul, MN, West Publishing Company, 1981

Banks v Goodfellow, 5 LR 5 QB 549 (1870)

Beyer GW: Pre-mortem probate. Probate and Property 71:6, 1993

Boeschen LE, Sales BD, Koss MK: Rape trauma experts in the courtroom. Psychology, Public Policy, and Law 4:414–432, 1998

Cantrell v GAF Corp., 999 F2d 1007 (6th Cir 1993)

Committee on Ethical Guidelines for Forensic Psychologists: Specialty guidelines for forensic psychologists. Law and Human Behavior 15:655–665, 1991

Daubert v Merrell Dow Pharmaceuticals, Inc., 509 US 579 (1993)

Davis v Marshall, Ohio App LEXIS 3538 (1994)

Faigman DL, Wright AJ: The battered woman syndrome in the age of science. Arizona Law Review 39:67–115, 1997

Faber v. Sweet Style Mfg. Corp., 40 Misc 2d 212, 242 NYS 2d 763 (1963)

Fischer v Heckerman, 772 SW 2d 642 (Ky Ct App 1989)

Freedman W: Freedman's Richards on the Law of Insurance, 6th Edition. Rochester, NY, Lawyers Cooperative Publishing, 1990

Frye v United States, 293 F 1013 (DC Cir) (1923)

General Electric Co. v Joiner, 522 US 136 (1997)

Green BL: Recent research findings on the diagnosis of posttraumatic stress disorder: prevalence, course, comorbidity, and risk. Posttraumatic Stress Disorder in Litigation: Guidelines for Forensic Assessment. Edited by Simon R. Washington, DC, American Psychiatric Press, 1995, pp 13–29

Green, SP: Why it's a crime to tear the tag off a mattress: overcriminalization and the moral content of regulatory offenses. Emory Law Journal 46:1533–1614, 1997

Grove WM, Barden RC: Protecting the integrity of the legal system: the admissibility of testimony from mental health experts under Daubert/Kumho analyses. Psychology, Public Policy, and Law 5:224–242, 1999

Hutton v State, 663 A2d 1289 (Md 1995)

In re Estate of Bracken, 475 P2d 377 (Okla 1970)

Insanity Defense Reform Act of 1984, 18 USC § 4241–4247

Jensen v Eveleth Taconite Co., 130 F3d 1287 (8th Cir 1997)

Kentucky Trust Co. v Gore, 192 SW 2d 749 (Ky 1946)

Kumho Tire Co. v Carmichael, 526 US 137 (1999)

Leopold AL, Beyer GW: Ante-mortem probate: a viable alternative. Arkansas Law Review 43:131–199, 1990

McCord D: The admissibility of expert testimony regarding rape trauma syndrome in rape prosecutions. Boston College Law Review 26:1143–1213, 1985

Meckler L: Surgeon General begins drive against suicide, The Washington Post, August 10, 1999, p. Z-17

M'Naghten, 8 Eng Rep 718 (1843)

Moore v Ashland Chem Inc, 151 F3d 269 (5th Cir 1998)

Note, recent development: due process—insanity defense—Idaho Supreme Court upholds abolition of insanity defense against state and federal constitutional challenges. State v Searcy, 118 Idaho 632, 798 P2d 914 (1990). Harvard Law Review 104:1132–1137, 1991

Penry v Lynaugh, 492 US 302 (1989)

People v Beldose, 681 P2d 291 (Cal 1984)

People v Coolidge, 187 NE 2d 694 (Ill 1963)

People v Pullins, 378 NW 2d 502 (Mich App 1985)

Perkins RM: Criminal liability without fault: a disquieting trend. Iowa Law Review 68:1067–1081, 1983

Perlin ML: The insanity defense: deconstructing the myths and reconstructing the jurisprudence, in Law, Mental Health, and Mental Disorder. Edited by Sales BD, Shuman DW. Pacific Grove, CA, Brooks/Cole, 1996, pp 314-359

Richardson JT, Ginsberg GP, Gatowski S, et al: The problems of applying Daubert to psychological syndrome evidence. Judicature 79:10–16, 1995

Rogers R, Shuman DW: Conducting Insanity Evaluations, 2nd Edition. New York, Guilford, 2000

Sayre FB: Public welfare offenses. Columbia Law Review 33:55–84, 1933

Schacht TE: DSM-III and the politics of truth. Am Psychol 40:513–521, 1985

Schuman G: Suicide and the life insurance contract: was the insured sane or insane? That is the question or is it? Tort and Insurance Law Journal 28:745–777, 1993

Shell GR: Contracts in the modern Supreme Court. California Law Review 81:431–527, 1993

Shuman DW: The Diagnostic and Statistical Manual of Mental Disorders in the courts. Bull Am Acad Psychiatry Law 17:25–32, 1989

Shuman DW: Psychiatric and Psychological Evidence, 2nd Edition. Colorado Springs, CO, Shepard's/McGraw-Hill, 1994

Shuman DW: Therapeutic jurisprudence and tort law: a limited subjective standard of care. Southern Methodist University Law Review 46:409–432, 1992

Shuman DW, Sales BD: The admissibility of expert testimony based upon clinical judgment and scientific research. Psychology, Public Policy, and Law 4:1226–1252, 1998

Shuman DW, Sales BD: The impact of Daubert and its progeny on the admissibility of behavioral and social science evidence. Psychology, Public Policy, and Law 5:3–15, 1999

Simon RI: Toward the development of guidelines in the forensic examination of posttraumatic stress disorder claims, in Posttraumatic Stress Disorder in Litigation: Guidelines for Forensic Assessment. Edited by Simon RI. Washington, DC, American Psychiatric Press, 1995, pp 31–84

Slobogin C: The admissibility of behavioral science information in criminal trials: from primitivism to Daubert to voice. Psychology, Public Policy, and Law 5:100–119, 1999

Spencer v General Electric Co., 688 F Supp 1072 (ED Va 1988)

Stacy v Love, 679 F2d 1209 (6th Cir 1982)

State v Herrera, 895 P2d 359 (Utah 1995)

State v Liddell, 685 P2d 918 (Mont 1984)

State v McQuillen, 681 P2d 822 (Kan 1984

Steadman HJ, McGreevy MA, Morrissey JP, et al: Before and After Hinckley: Evaluating Insanity Defense Reform. New York, Guilford, 1993

Stone A: Post-traumatic stress disorder and the law: critical review of the new frontier. Bull Am Acad Psychiatry Law 21:23–36, 1993

United States v Ingham, 42 MJ 218 (1995), cert. denied, 516 US 1063 (1996)

United States v Lyons, 739 F2d 994 (5th Cir 1984)

Walsh AC, Brown BB, Kaye K, et al: Mental Capacity: Legal and Medical Aspects of Assessment and Treatment. Colorado Springs, CO, Shepard's/McGraw-Hill, 1994

What Can We Ever Know About the Past?

A Philosophical Consideration of the Assessment of Retrospective Mental States

John Z. Sadler, M.D.

On March 30, 1981, a young man from Texas, John W. Hinckley Jr., attempted to assassinate then-President Ronald Reagan. Hinckley nonfatally wounded Reagan and three other people as they emerged from the Washington Hilton and walked toward their waiting limousine. The well-publicized, perhaps sensational, trial of Hinckley was characterized by significant disagreement among clinical expert witnesses about the defendant's state of mind, motivations, and intentions preceding and at the time of the shootings.

A fundamental problem faced by the expert witnesses at that time is the same problem addressed in this book, which is how to assess, in the forensic setting, the past mental states of people. What was going through Hinckley's mind in the days prior to the shooting? What were the intentions and goals behind his murderous behavior? How can we make claims about another person's intentions, goals, motivations, and mental processes, particularly when they have occurred in the past? On what evidence and reason can we make claims about such states of mind? What causal power do such mental contents exert?

The goals of this chapter are several. One is to illustrate the relationship between the problem of retrospective mental states (RMS) and a set of long-standing philosophical problems. The second is to provide a philosophical background for the considerations presented in subsequent chapters of this book. A third is to indicate actual or potential "weak links" in the chain of reasoning, procedures, and policies binding the court and the clinic on the retrospective mental state issue. Although philosophical arguments alone rarely, if ever, sway attorneys, judges, clinicians, or the lay public, a basic philosophical understanding of RMS may give attorneys and clinicians a means to critically evaluate their reasoning, strategy, or methods.

What kind of philosophical problem is posed by the assessment of RMS? Rather than a single philosophical problem, RMS present a whole slew of them. Although the facets of RMS are many, they are philosophically centered (as will be discussed later) on the question of knowledge in philosophy, that is, in epistemology. Where does knowledge come from? What must we believe to obtain knowledge? Does knowledge have a nature that we can secure or master? How can we be certain of the truth of our claims to knowing? How can we secure genuine knowledge? These are the questions posed by epistemology, and their bearing on RMS is straightforward: How can we make claims to know something about another person's past state of mind? How can we know if our claims are true? What kinds of knowledge claims are claims about RMS? At its core, the epistemological problem of RMS could be stated as "How can we differentiate mere opinion from truths about RMS?" This is a tall order philosophically, particularly because of the *situation* of RMS—a seeking to gain knowledge about another person's past intentions and motivations.

In this chapter I use the *Hinckley* case (Low et al. 1983) as an exemplar and reference point for the problems associated with RMS. The widespread publicity, public outcry, and social discussion surrounding the Hinckley trial and acquittal by reason of insanity perhaps poses a risk of overfamiliarity. On the other hand, the familiarity of this case serves the purpose of example well; many readers will have substantial background knowledge from which to think through the case once again. In the first part of this chapter, I discuss the philosophical problems of epistemology in general terms, showing perhaps obvious ways how they could apply to the *Hinckley* case. In the second part of the chapter, I delve more deeply into the epistemological network of assumptions, methods, and standards that lie beneath the discussion of RMS. In the third part, and really interwoven into the second, I point toward a few samples of philosophical ideas and methods that have been applied to the classic epistemological problems, and which could be (and in some indirect sense have been) brought to bear on the assessment of RMS.

Epistemology and Its Problems

Often attributed to the witty and articulate British philosopher A.J. Ayer (1977), the *standard account* of knowledge has a particular logical form. By standard account I mean a discussion that has, through the test of time with countless skeptics, emerged as a significant reference point of consideration on the theory of knowledge, one which, if not universally accepted, is the treatment that must be contended with. Anglo-American (analytical) philosophy presents the standard account of knowledge through the simple phrase *justified true belief*—that is, *knowledge is justified true belief*. In its logical form:

> *X* knows that *p* if and only if:

1. *X* believes that *p*;
2. it is true that *p*; and
3. *X* is justified in believing that *p* (if *X* does).

Here *X* refers to the knowing subject, the person wanting knowledge, while *p* stands for any given state of affairs. As one might imagine, however, knowledge claims and the theory of knowledge can quickly run afoul—indeed, at each of these three steps. Consider the standard account applied to a particular "factoid" in the case of *Hinckley*:

> Dr. *X* knows that *John Hinckley shot Reagan in order to impress Jodie Foster* because:

1. Dr. *X* believes that *John Hinckley shot Reagan in order to impress Jodie Foster*;
2. it is true that *John Hinckley shot Reagan in order to impress Jodie Foster*; and
3. Dr. *X* is justified in believing that *John Hinckley shot Reagan in order to impress Jodie Foster* (if Dr. X does).

At a superficial glance, the skeptic notices a number of potential problems:
Problems with the first line of reasoning:

Dr. *X* may not believe *p*, but views this claim instead as a legal strategy to aid his side. Therefore, Dr. *X* would not have knowledge, because knowledge requires belief, that is, conviction, commitment, or faith about the state of affairs being considered. Dr. X's claim about the source of Hinckley's behavior may be a clever bit of rhetoric, but it is not a fact on which Dr. X would base important personal, clinical, or social decisions.

Problems with the second line of reasoning:

Dr. X could be mistaken, or:

Dr. X could be isolating a component of a more complicated truth: that Hinckley shot Reagan in part because of his wish to impress Jodie Foster, but also for other reasons, such as his wish to be killed by Secret Service agents, or because he wished for personal notoriety, or because he believed Reagan to be a threat to America's welfare, etc. That is, the view articulated by Dr. X may not correspond to, or be coherent with, the network of facts or evidence presented. So Dr. X's belief, however sincere, may not be true, and therefore is not knowledge. Dr. X may also believe that the sun revolves around the earth, but this is not true, and therefore it also is not knowledge.

Problems with the third line of reasoning:

Dr. X may have an inadequate amount of evidence to support his conclusion that *John Hinckley shot Reagan in order to impress Jodie Foster.* Furthermore, he may have used faulty reasoning in interpreting the evidence.

Dr. X may have failed to take into consideration the evidence collected by all witnesses, and thereby is not justified in claiming *John Hinckley shot Reagan in order to impress Jodie Foster.* Although Dr. X holds this belief about Hinckley, and it might very well be true, Dr. X's true belief may not be *justified by* the available evidence—his true belief may be based on faulty reasoning or on "dumb luck," so to speak. So although Dr. X may possess and believe in the facts, he does not have knowledge, because knowledge is embedded in a network of evidence that points toward a fact and justifies true belief.

Epistemological matters, however, are much worse than what is suggested by these simple challenges. As simple and facile a structure as the standard account is, it masks many more philosophical problems, which can be approached when one begins to apply the treatment and to ask particular questions of the key elements: justification, truth, and belief. Let us consider some particular philosophical problems relevant to RMS, with reference to these three key terms. In the space of this chapter, I will not be able to discuss all the ramifications but can perhaps present an indicative sample.

Key Epistemological Problems Related to RMS

In this section I discuss three main epistemological problems that are particularly relevant to the practical issue of determining RMS: the location, objectivity, and justification of truth. Other selections, of course, are possible. Furthermore, the conceptual direction from which I approach each problem is only one of many, much like the numerous starting directions that can be used to attack a scientific question.

The Location of Truth

Where is the location of the truth of RMS? Consider our exemplar thesis that Hinckley shot Reagan to impress Jodie Foster. The truth or falsity of such a claim, under the standard account of knowledge, must have some benchmark or source to adjudicate whether such a claim is true or false. That is, the knower must have some reference point, a reality checkpoint, from which to decide whether such a claim is true. What is this reference point, or where is this *location* of the truth? Is the truth encoded, like information on a computer hard drive, in John Hinckley's brain? Might it instead reside in the scientific machinations of the examining clinician's psyche? Does the truth emerge from the consensus-building discussions of all holders of evidence (e.g., clinicians, family, friends, employers, attorneys)? Does the truth reside in the court process and the jury's verdict? Where might the truth be found?

For Plato the truth resided in mentalistic and ideal forms—we might say today that for Plato truth had a particular cognitive architecture. Prior to, and often including, the modern period of Western philosophy (eighteenth and nineteenth centuries), appeals to the location of the truth of claims resided in appeals to God's omniscience—the great puzzles of the world were often resolved by exclaiming, "Only God knows!" However, with the rise of science and other secular methods of knowing, holding God as the location of the truth fell into disfavor. Furthermore, given the pluralism of our shrinking planetary culture, God as the location of the truth was impractical and befuddling, since 1) only a portion of the people of the world make such appeals, and even between them, there are 2) different deities to appeal to, in addition to 3) the differing opinions from various godheads, not to mention 4) the differing interpretations of their wisdom! Moreover, God as the location of the truth only begged the philosophical question, which, now restated, still persists: Where can we locate God's truth?

Today the location of the truth, divine or secular, is still a relevant question. During the early and mid-twentieth century, the dominant strand in the philosophy of science, logical positivism (and later logical empiricism), viewed the location of the truth as residing in relationships between observation statements (statements about observable events) and the logical properties of theoretical statements that link such observations to theory. For logical positivists and the later logical empiricists, the methods of science paved the way to certain truths; the problem was in developing strict relations between observation statements and theoretical statements. Intellectual history, though, has shown that such strict logical relations were not to be found, nor were they derivable. Thomas Kuhn, among others (see Salmon and Kitcher 1989 for a good philosophical review), showed that scientific knowledge was bound by history, training, and values; scientific knowledge held to no particular deductive logic. Still later, and moving into contemporary epistemology, a host of other viewpoints about the location of the truth, including truth being an illusion on the one hand or a mere convention on the other, emerged from various stripes of postmodern thought (for good reviews, see Bernstein 1985; Phillips 1996).

The *Hinckley* trial provides a fine example of the problem of the location of the truth. During the trial the defense called Dr. William Carpenter to testify regarding Hinckley's ability to "appreciate" the wrongfulness of his conduct at the time of the shootings (Low et al. 1983). It was clear before Carpenter testified that he had a then-contemporary psychiatric conception of what constituted *appreciation.* For Carpenter, Hinckley could have understood and stated that the shootings were "wrong," as in illegal or immoral, but he did not appreciate their wrongfulness because of his emotional state of desperation, his identification with the Travis Bickle movie character, his longing for the actress Jodie Foster, and his wish for death, all of which interfered with his *ability to act* morally. For Carpenter, appreciation was a complex cognitive-emotional-conative (motivational) concept that could not be teased apart into simpler components. This situation prompted a substantial amount of discussion among the prosecution, the defense, and the court, as illustrated by this short passage from the transcription, in which Mr. Adelman argues for the prosecution:

> Mr. Adelman:.....[I]f the court will instruct the jury that appreciation is limited to cognition, then to have this man testify that it is more than that is quite misleading and really undermines the Court instruction.
>
> Now, we are not asking Dr. Carpenter to say one word less about anything he has to say, except that he should testify within the framework of what the law means by appreciate. If he can do that, fine, but to have him go on and talk about emotional appreciation, which is his theory maybe, he then invades the province of the Court. He becomes the definer of the law.

> The Court: Well, I can make it clear tomorrow. I can make it clear to him. I don't want to be in a position of just cutting them off at the knees. However, I will indicate to them, Mr.

Fuller, that the instructions—you are attempting to develop more out of the concept of appreciation in *Brawner* than what is in the four corners. You advance the notion that *Brawner* is an advanced approach to this whole field of psychiatry and the defense of insanity, and *Brawner* must be read within the liberal context that you view it and as others view it, but until the Court of Appeals or some authoritative source speaks and embraces and extends the concept to the extent that you want to extend it, I am not willing to do it. At the same time, I am not willing to just summarily cut your witness off.

I can indicate in no uncertain terms to the jurors that what they are to follow, that they may hear concepts, that the ultimate, that the ultimate ruling guidelines that they are to follow are given by the Court in the instructions of law....(Low et al. 1983, p. 35)

The problem (among others) of the location of the truth undergirds this discussion amidst the witnesses, the prosecution, the defense, the court, and, implicitly, the jury. For the witnesses (the clinicians), the truth is (presumably) a relevant concept from which their methods of science and professional training are built—scientists seek truths, medicine and psychiatry are built on the truths of science, the role of the psychiatric expert witness is to state those truths to the degree they are known. For the court, truth is a more problematic concept—does the court see the legal process as a locator of truth, so that the location of truth is in the process and adjudication of the law, or is the truth peripheral to the court's interests, with a concept like justice being the prevailing ethos? Certainly, the judge is troubled by the conflict between what might be called Dr. Carpenter's conception of the truth about appreciation and by the precedents that have constrained the court's understanding of the concept of appreciation, namely, the rule that the appreciation concept is a strictly cognitive one. For the respective attorneys, the location of the truth is also obscure: torn by the pronouncements of precedent, the need for client advocacy, the polarizations of the adversarial model, and the requirement to interpret and anticipate the outcomes of expert testimony, the truth may be far in the periphery. The jury may be more sanguine but no less distant from the truth. From the jury's perspective, they may very well assume that the court is the location of the truth, that their job is to find out the truth, and that their verdict will realize that truth. After all, the witness swears to tell the truth, the whole truth, and nothing but the truth.

So from this limited consideration, I propose several potential positions about the issue of the location of the truth: truth from the findings of science and expert application, truth from the precedent of law, truth from the conduct of law, and truth as peripheral to justice. It is possible, moreover, to pinpoint more precisely these putative locations of the truth for their components and to find still more puzzles. For instance, taking the *truth as peripheral to justice* generalization, how does one justify such a conclusion without making an appeal to still more truths, which in turn need locating and justifying? This problem, often called the "infinite regress of the justification of knowledge" (Dancy 1995, p. 246), refers to the difficulty in building truths that stand on their own; ones that do not depend on an infinite regress of other truths, each in turn requiring its own justification.

Truth and Objectivity

A second issue relevant to RMS assessment has to do with the concept of *objective* truth. Objectivity in regard to science and other human endeavors has a cluster of meanings, all relevant here. Most commonly, it means freedom from bias; an objective claim neither tacitly nor overtly favors one viewpoint, perspective, or method. In nineteenth- and early twentieth-century science, it has often meant a claim free from value judgments or evaluative interests; objectivity is a just-the-facts claim (Proctor 1991). In philosophy, objectivity has had a number of meanings; perhaps more recently it has come to be used as the opposite of relativism: the idea that an objective claim, if not the truth, is at least the best approximation available. The problem with objectivity as a bootstrap for science, ethics, the law, or other claim-making endeavors is that it suffers the same difficulty that truth itself suffers, that of the problem of justification. The problem of justification, however, will be discussed later.

Accepting, for the moment, the concept of objectivity in regard to the truth, I might ask, who are the objective parties in the *Hinckley* courtroom? Mr. Hinckley, his counsel, and his experts, as well as the prosecution's counsel and witness, all have sources of impressive bias, so impressive we need not particularize them—profit, freedom, and reputation all spring to mind. Do the judge and jury enjoy objectivity? Perhaps more so, but they too are subject to selection biases and political pressures. Perhaps we could claim that no single individual is objective, but the court process ensures objectivity. However, we know this is unreliable because we know innocent people have been convicted and guilty people exonerated. How can an objective process result in such heinous error?

The philosophy of history offers a parallel set of concerns. One question about the making of historical claims is whether the historian can be objective. The historian, like the clinician or the attorney, has access to a limited set of materials, traces, and personal contacts with which to make intelligible (at the least) and preferably explanatory discussions of an historical event. To accomplish such a task, the explainer must *select* and *order* the priority, importance, or salience of such materials, a core task of history-writing, lawyering, or doctoring that is inherently subjective. In this context, subjectivity carries the conservative meaning that there are no universally accepted methods, procedures, and techniques for selecting and ordering the historical materials. So does this mean that the historical, clinical, or legal claim exists simply at the whim of the author?

Not necessarily. To say that the explainers (historians, clinicians, attorneys) must be selective in their attention to and manipulation of concepts and events, and that there are no universally accepted criteria for this process, is not the same as saying the process is arbitrary or whimsical. Indeed, the procedures of law, medical practice, and historiography impose practical, regulatory, and epistemological standards to which credible, competent practitioners must adhere. For instance, prosecutors cannot withhold evidence, psychiatrists must examine their patients, and historians must disclose their reference materials.

What can be concluded on this point about objectivity is that each field—medicine, law, history—has methods that perhaps *delimit* a range of conclusions but do not determine them, and whose conventions within the discipline underdetermine the outcome. From this standpoint, objectivity emerges from constraints imposed by the discipline; not just *any* conclusions about cases can be drawn, but more than one set of potential conclusions may exist within the discipline's set of methodological constraints. When considering these latter points in regard to recent changes governing expert witnesses, it is apparent how recent American law has moved toward particular conventions in clinical expert testimony that might be cast as intended to diminish the underdetermination of outcome or, stated differently, to move to a narrower, more demanding epistemological standard for expert witnesses.

I am referring here to the recent appearance of the *Daubert* and *Kumho* standards (*Daubert v. Merrell Dow Pharmaceuticals, Inc.* 1993; *Kumho Tire Co. v. Carmichael* 1999). These United States Supreme Court decisions are discussed thoroughly elsewhere in this book; for our purposes here, let me just summarize the particulars by noting their philosophical importance. *Daubert* upped the epistemological ante for the admissibility of scientific evidence in trials, and *Kumho* generalized this ante for any expert testimony, scientific or otherwise. Prior to *Daubert*, admissibility of expert testimony was determined by the *general acceptance* of the evidence in the relevant scientific field. *Daubert* added four criteria for trial judges to apply (as they deem relevant, so the standard is flexible) in admitting expert scientific testimony. The first may confound two distinct but related concepts: that of a claim's *testability* and whether such a claim has in fact *been tested*. In the literature this criterion is often simply listed as *testing*. The second criterion suggests that a scientific claim has been subject to *peer review* and publication in the relevant scientific literature. The third criterion to consider is the *known or potential rate of error* about scientific claims or generalizations. The fourth and last criterion points back to the older *Frye* (*Frye v. United States* 1923) standard, that of general acceptance within the relevant scientific community.

The testability/tested standard (TT) has explicit philosopher credentials in Justice Blackmun's opinion for the Court, wherein he cited the distinguished philosophers of science Carl Hempel (1966) and Karl Popper (1992). The testability part of this standard means that a scientific claim must be logically capable of being put to an empirical test (e.g., that the claim must be subject to consensually verifiable observations that either do or do not support the hypothetical claim). (An interesting question regarding the *Hinckley* case is whether Dr. Carpenter's claim about Hinckley's emotional appreciation could be falsified with the available evidence, because Carpenter was referring to the defendant's psychologically conflicted inner motivational state.) A related concept for Popper was that scientific claims must be falsifiable, that is, capable of being disconfirmed by empirical testing. (Popper's ideas around falsifiability and *falsificationism* will reappear later in this chapter when I discuss the justifiability of knowledge claims.) The main philosophical objection to Popperian falsificationism is that many, perhaps most, generally accepted scientific theories and facts have a research history containing disconfirmatory evidence or negative evidence (Jacob 1995; Wallace 1988). The testing portion of the TT standard means that the scientific claims in question have actually been tested in an empirical setting. In the *Daubert* case, testimony was made that the bulk of the scientifically refereed empirical studies supported the defendant's claim of no drug teratogenicity; the falsifying testimony from the plaintiff's side was based on animal and test-tube studies that were not comparably peer reviewed. Regarding falsifiability, however, it would be easy to imagine and document cases where opposing expert claims have comparable amounts of supportive and refuting evidence. Then what?

It is presumably intended that trial judges decide about the application of testibility versus actual testing in cases of expert scientific testimony; that is, depending on circumstances, evidence can be admitted that is only potentially capable of testing or has as yet not been tested. This will be particularly acute in psychiatric testimony, where many of the standards of practice, however testable, are based on individualistic judgments rather than on cumulative generalizations based on population data. (See following section in this chapter on justifying true belief.)

The second criterion, that of qualified peer review and publication in relevant scientific journals, deserves some philosophical reference as well. For many contemporary philosophers of science (e.g., Grinnell 1992; Longino 1990), whatever objectivity science has resides in a communitarian-evaluative character, that is, methods and techniques constitute science less than other qualities involved with science's social process: qualities such as the open availability of scientific methods and data, the encouragement of rigorous critique of others' work, the equal opportunity for scientific accomplishment for anyone willing to do the work (the interchangeability of the investigator), and the disclosure of biasing interests. These qualities, embodied in procedures such as journal peer review, may not render science immune from bias and ideology but may enable scientific consumers to draw their own conclusions and may also permit a more nuanced, flexible, and representative view of scientific objectivity than that provided by a strictly falsificationist doctrine.

The third and fourth criteria support the conclusions that are a practical necessity in the courtroom situation, where a final decision is required and there is little tolerance for the never-ending flux of science. Error rates will pose a problem for psychiatric/psychological expert witnesses, because the extant literature about their margins of error in clinical judgments is not very flattering (Garb 1998). General acceptability, in combination with the other criteria, will extend the *Frye* (1923) standard to a higher level. Historically, *Frye* often rendered the expert's opinion as an appeal to authority, although such an epistemological criterion is not taken seriously in philosophical literature or the philosophy classroom, for many of the same reasons noted earlier concerning the retreat from divine authority. The *Daubert* standards permit a more respectable epistemology for scientific testimony, albeit one whose application to particular cases, as noted by Chief Justice Rehnquist in his concur/dissent article (*Daubert* 1993), will be difficult and variable.

Justification of Truth

Earlier in this chapter, I noted that the third criterion of the standard treatment of knowledge was that true beliefs must be justified (i.e., I cannot just possess the facts and believe in them, I must have good reasons to possess and believe them). Indeed, much critical argument in science, medicine, law, and history (not to mention philosophy) revolves around whether one claim is better than another. Because the justification of truth and belief (the other two components of the standard account of knowledge, heretofore referred to as *true belief*) logically require a judgment of value (the *good* in *good reasons*), all knowledge has an evaluative, normative, or value-judging component. In the scientific arena, justification of knowledge involves such value-related questions as 1) which theory better explains the data, 2) what constitutes an adequate (good) scientific explanation, 3) what kinds of data or evidence are deemed relevant to the question asked, 4) what constitutes an apropos interpretation of the evidence, and 5) what conclusions are warranted by the evidence, to name just a few of the justificatory elements of knowledge. The acceptance that knowledge, including scientific knowledge, has valuational elements is a later–twentieth-century phenomenon; surely Thomas Kuhn's work on the history of science (Kuhn 1970; Salmon and Kitcher 1989), as well as his description of the values involved in scientific theory choice (Kuhn 1977), were important landmarks in convincing scientists and the public alike of the normative nature of our most esteemed kind of knowledge, science.

As a philosophical domain, the justification of true belief is also a rich vein to mine regarding RMS. This domain houses a collection of serious philosophical questions faced by virtually all participants in the judicial process. I would imagine that these philosophical questions are experienced as practical problems in some cases, some are not experienced at all but approaches to them are simply acted on in other cases, and still others are recognized as conceptual/philosophical problems in still other settings. Some of these questions as they pertain to RMS include how to

1. reconcile the four traditional sources of knowledge: sensation, introspection, memory, and reason;
2. choose and apply salient scientific data to particular cases;
3. justify knowledge about others (intersubjectivity);
4. make inductions based on true premises;
5. choose among competing theories and explanations; and
6. credibly justify causal claims about motivations and intentions.

Sources of Knowledge

Perhaps the most important of these conceptual/philosophical problems is the question of how to reconcile the four traditional sources of knowledge: sensation, introspection, memory, and reason (Dancy 1995). The justification angle is the need to justify the scheme one has used in integrating the four sources of knowledge. Even without a detailed discussion of these sources of knowledge, they can serve to introduce the following issues. The clinical-forensic situation poses an opportunity for all four sources to be drawn on: the clinician, jury, and attorney all directly observe testimony, the defendant, witnesses, and lawyers. The clinician is asked to render expert opinion about the state of mind of the defendant in the past. Such an assignment requires the clinician to rely on personal observations, introspect about the significance of such observations, and remember the salient material for testimony and other purposes, as well as reason through the application of such material to the charges and trial circumstances. Similar tasks occupy the attorney, although in the form of legal strategies. The defendant can provide only limited, directly observable (sensible) information about himself or herself as it pertains to the charges; most of the salient information will be supplied in the form of a narrative or story about his or her past motivations, thoughts, and intentions (e.g., memory as a source of knowledge). Most defendants or plaintiffs will devote significant reflection to what is revealed to examining clinicians and attorneys (introspection) and will, in concert with their attorneys, reason through the significance of particular revelations. That each of these sources of knowledge can fail or mislead is a banality, as are the differing perspectives for each of the "knowers" in the forensic setting. What is philosophically more interesting is the relation of interpreting the discrepant perspectives of the knowers. For instance, how much weight should be given reason as opposed to memory? Another example might be the question of a moving story being more persuasive than a salient application of legal precedent, clinical reasoning, and scientific data.

In this latter situation, an example from the *Hinckley* case is again instructive. Consider this sample of testimony from Park Elliott Dietz, the prosecution's expert, concerning Hinckley's ability to conform his conduct to the law (i.e., not attempt to shoot the President).

> A.　(Dietz) That on March 30, 1981, as a result of mental disease or defect, Mr. Hinckley did not lack substantial capacity to conform his conduct to the requirements of the law.
> 　　...Now, specific examples of evidence:
> 　　First of all, his decisionmaking ability itself was [intact] on March 30th. He was able to make other decisions on that date. He decided where to go for breakfast, what to eat....He was not a man incapable of making decisions about his life, about which of these relatively minor things to do.
> 　　He deliberated and made a decision to survey the scene a[t] the Hilton Hotel. There was no voice commanding him to do that. There was no drive within him pushing him to do that. He decided, as he tells us, to go to the Hilton to check out the scene....
> 　　We know from the facts that he chose his bullets, that he loaded his revolver. He has never said that a voice commanded him to choose the shiniest bullets or that he had, for some other reason, to choose...the exploding Devastator bullets. This reflects decision-making and choice....He is...taking the time to write the "Jodie letter" to explain

that one of his goals for the assassination attempt, and to explain that he had a deliberate reason for carrying it out. A man driven by passion, by uncontrollable forces, is not often inclined to take the time to write a letter to explain.... (excerpted from Low et al. 1983, pp. 64–66, my correction of "a" to "at")

Dietz goes on to further itemize Hinckley's deliberations, his choice of site, his waiting for a clear shot, and so forth.

Consider, in contrast, the style of William Carpenter's defense testimony in the face of a related question about Hinckley's ability to "appreciate" (i.e., differentiate) right from wrong:

Q.   Mr. Adelman [for the prosecution]: Can't you infer that he knew on that day that carrying a gun out on the streets of Dayton was wrong? Yes or no.

A.   He in that purely intellectual sense has always known that carrying a gun like that was wrong, was illegal. But what I'm saying is it is not because of that consideration that he left the gun behind. He left the gun behind for other reasons, not because he was mindful. I don't think he was concerned with the legality of it one way or the other. He was concerned with other things....

...He wanted—he had on his mind...the despair he felt as he left New Haven and his inability to make a simple and successful encounter of Jodie Foster. He was now trying to get himself back into a frame of mind where he felt more competent, more able, more effective in life [and he] found himself doing this by taking on the Travis Bickle parallel.

He felt he could accomplish this—and he did have suicidal thoughts at the time—through the stalking of President Carter. In that context he then is trying to psych himself up to be able to take action on them, so that he had, if you will the mental scenario in place.

There was not the intensive impulsivity that could lead to his taking action and he was hoping things to increase the likelihood.... (excerpted from Low et al. 1983, p. 41, my specification of Adelman for prosecution)

What is remarkable about this contrasting testimony is not the differences about the particulars; indeed, there is a lot of agreement. Both experts admit to mental abnormalities for Hinckley; both admit that he knew right from wrong in a least one sense (cognitive). Both agree that Hinckley lacked substantive impulsivity in his actions. What is remarkable is their contrasting styles of testimony. Dietz is razor sharp, lucid, polished, systematic, authoritative—the embodiment of rational expertise. Carpenter, however, tells a much better story—Carpenter's testimony has the lifeblood of narrative—there is drama, romance, pathos, even a hint of tragedy in this short passage. That Carpenter "won" (Hinckley was found not guilty by reason of insanity) is just a footnote, but a conceptually provocative one.

The philosophical significance of this point is that at least one of the decisive factors in the use of expert testimony could be the tacit models of truth-justification used by the various parties, including the jury. Was the jury won over by a better story? How should we weight the various domains and styles of truth-claims? What style fits the problem of RMS? Would Dietz have prevailed if the expert's burden was to *predict* the future behavior of the defendant?

Salient Scientific Data

Determining how to choose and apply salient scientific data to particular cases is a problem at least as old as modern science itself (von Wright 1971). As often occurs today, nineteenth-century intellectual life cast the so-called natural sciences (physics, chemistry) and the so-called social sciences (sociology, anthropology, history, economics) as rivals in terms of their scientific rigor. In contrast, the neo-Kantian philosopher Wilhelm Windelband (1980) saw a complementary relationship between the natural and the "human" sciences. For Windelband natural science sought to understand the world in terms of laws, prediction, and causal explanation. Furthermore, natural science casts such understanding in the form of generalizations about groups of individuals. We see this characterization today in medical science, where people are not studied as individuals but rather as exemplars of diseases or disorders. Psychiatric (natural) science makes claims about the similarities of people with major depression or schizophrenia and seeks knowledge that ideally holds true for all people with schizophrenia. Windelband characterized this kind of law-driven, universalized scientific knowledge as *nomothetic*, meaning law-governed.

In contrast to nomothetic knowledge, Windelband saw social sciences such as history not as characterizing the world in terms of universal laws but rather as singular understandings of particular events or individuals in their uniqueness. Although for natural science the individual is ideally interchangeable (all individuals with schizophrenia should be alike in schizophrenia-salient ways), for the human sciences the individual is the unique focus of explanation. In history the development of an historical event is such a charge; in psychiatry the intensive study of the individual patient (as in psychoanalysis) is an example. Such knowledge of unique events and individuals Windelband called *idiographic* science.

Such perspectives are particularly complementary for disciplines like psychology, where both elements may be applied. Indeed, the implementation of nomothetic and idiographic science can be seen in contemporary psychiatry and psychology when, for instance, researchers study the molecular/genetic mechanisms of serious mental disorders (nomothetic science) and when therapists develop psychotherapeutic understandings of a particular patient's problems and life situation (idiographic science). The German philosopher and psychiatrist Karl Jaspers (1883–1969) cast analogous ideas as the difference between *Erklären* (explanation) and *Verstehen* (understanding), with explanation being suited to the natural sciences and understanding suited to the social and historical sciences (Jaspers 1997).

The dilemma in the courtroom is that these approaches may not be complementary at all but, rather, may even be contradictory. One can readily recognize the epistemological tension between the carefully wrought nomothetic science of Elizabeth Loftus's memory studies (Loftus 1996) and the patients' and therapists' personal, moving idiographic narratives of alleged sexual abuse in false memory syndrome cases. In the adversarial forensic setting, the polarities of nomothetic and idiographic science can become caricatures, two relatively independent, self-sufficient, arguably scientific perspectives pitted against each other.

As McHugh (1995) and McHugh and Slavney (1998) point out, the conceptual grasp of narrative understandings are so deep, as is the explanatory power of causal explanation, that knowers often feel the need to commit to one or the other to resolve the cognitive dissonance. These sorts of intellectual alliances may be made explicit and strategic in the courtroom. Is narrative the salient data? Are controlled studies related to courtroom case themes salient data? How should we choose? This nomothetic/idiographic science split is but one obvious example of the dilemma of choosing salient findings and applying them credibly.

Intersubjectivity

At the core of the determination of RMS, and perhaps the least explicitly appreciated by the practitioner, lies the philosophical question of *intersubjectivity*, or the problem of justifying knowledge about others. Intersubjectivity is really a cluster of problems: How is it that I can understand so vividly and readily other people's mental lives? Indeed, I can often experience other people's emotional experiences almost as vividly as I experience my own. How is it, in face of such a remarkable accomplishment, that my understanding fails so miserably at times? This latter question raises the critical methodological puzzle of intersubjectivity: How can I possess reliable knowledge of other people? How does my understanding of other people go astray?

Few thinkers can claim to have made more direct contributions to the intersubjectivity question for psychiatry than did Karl Jaspers. For him intersubjectivity was a critical issue not just for the philosopher but also for the psychiatrist. The psychiatrist's work, after all, depends on rigorous, reliable, and valid understanding of the mental life of other people. If psychiatrists do not have this capacity, what do they have to offer?

Doing full justice to Jaspers's discussions about intersubjectivity and the methods of the psychiatrist is far beyond the scope of this chapter (see Wiggins and Schwartz 1997a, 1997b for fine reviews, from which much of this discussion is derived). However, a few comments can be made that are indicative of Jaspers's thought in this area.

Jaspers believed that the ordinary understanding of other people, which characterizes our everyday living, involves roughly two kinds: *shallow* and *deeper*. The shallow type of understanding occurs when we understand other people as being significantly different from us. This kind of understanding of John Hinckley might result in statements like "Somebody who would do that (attempt assassination) has to be crazy." In this more shallow understanding, the other person is viewed as an object. In contrast, the deeper understanding to which Jaspers believed psychiatrists must aspire is characterized by strong, compelling experiences of the world similar to those of the person (patient) himself or herself.

The term "self-transposal" (Wiggins and Schwartz 1997b, p. 23) conveys Jaspers's sense of the knower transposing herself into the patient's shoes. A brief, nonclinical example vividly illustrates this distinction. Have you ever walked into a movie theater late or joined a group of people watching television where the people there were already involved with the show, the story, and the characters? In these situations the viewers will often exhibit signs of being moved emotionally: they will be tearful at the tragic parts or excited and aggressive during the action scenes. When an outsider walks into such a situation and witnesses both the show and the viewers' responses, the show may seem banal and cartoonish, even silly. The outsider understands, yes, that someone important has just died on the screen, which makes the viewers feel sad, but the outsider is not moved to tears at all. Indeed, his understanding is of Jaspers's first, shallow type, while the engaged viewers are experiencing Jaspers' second, deeper understanding. The psychiatrist, according to Jaspers, must become immersed in this deeper, more engaged, more empathic way of experiencing the patient. This immersion into the phenomenal world of the patient is apparent even in the short excerpts of testimony by Park Dietz and William Carpenter that were presented earlier.

But what exactly is scientific, or rigorous, about such deeper *Verstehen?* Wiggins and Schwartz (1997a) describe it briefly:

In order to become scientific knowledge, understanding must become communicable (*mittelbar*), debatable (*diskutierbar*), and testable (*nachprüfbar*). And the only way that this can occur is for such understanding to achieve formulation in fixed, rule-governed concepts (*feste regelmässige Begriffe*) and particular assertions (*einselne Behauptungen*). (p. 24)

Evidence for understanding was also an important concept for Jaspers. It is how, to use this chapter's terms, the Jaspersian psychiatrist justifies his knowledge claims. The clinician's ways of obtaining this kind of primal evidence were through clinical observation of the patient's expressions, conduct, and behavior, through interviewing and attending to the patient's talk, and through reading the patient's written expressions. However, the question of *how much* evidence is necessary to justify one's knowledge claims is a problematic one, not just for Jaspers, but for the whole of modern philosophy.

Induction

Whether guided by the teachings of Jaspers or by philosophy or science, one can approach the question of adequacy of evidence through the particular logic of *induction* versus *deduction*. To make a *deductive* inference, such as a mathematical claim, one simply must have true premises, and the conclusion then follows irrevocably:

1. Triangles are three-sided, closed geometric figures.
2. This geometric figure is three-sided and closed.
3. Therefore this geometric figure is a triangle.

In contrast, consider this sort of claim:

1. The turkey has been fed corn every morning for the past six months.
2. Today is Thanksgiving morning.
3. Therefore the turkey will be fed corn today.

Instead, what in fact happens "today" is that the turkey becomes the feast for the farmer's family. This kind of inference is an *inductive* inference, and although it suits everyday reasoning, and certainly medical practice most of the time, the logic does not permit the certainty of a deductive inference. This is the problem of induction, which the Scottish philosopher David Hume is usually credited for articulating (Hume 1748/1999). Translated into the forensic/clinical arena, no amount of evidence is conclusive, and logic does not permit a more certain conclusion after 100 or even 10,000 occurrences of the same event. Past behavior may predict future behavior but not necessarily so in a particular case. Furthermore, in the case of the turkey, the morning is not the *cause* of the corn being issued, although there is a close temporal relationship between each new day and the feeding of corn. So the problem of induction extends to claims about causes as well: two events occurring in close proximity, although often related causally, are not necessarily so. The problem with induction is that it encompasses not only the history of probabilistic prediction in science but also the struggle with probable causes in the law. How shall we justify this thread of evidence as the cause of the defendant's behavior? This problem with causes will be addressed further in the following discussion.

Interpretation

The "conflict of interpretations," a popular phrase attributed to Paul Ricoeur (1974), involves choosing among competing theories and explanations. It refers in our setting to the different ways of explaining or understanding RMS, ways that may often not be compatible with each other. In reviewing the Hinckley case, one can see uses of narrative understanding or *Verstehen*, as well as causal/empirical explanatory concepts like *impulsivity*, often in the same testimony. How compatible are the ways of making sense of RMS? Often, not very, as suggested earlier by the reference to recovered memories of abuse. Whose interpretation—whose reconstruction—of this past mental state should we choose?

An ancient tradition in philosophy has occupied itself with precisely this type of question: "How shall we interpret our texts, our sciences, our lives?" Named for Hermes, the messenger, *hermeneutics* originally aimed to develop methods for interpreting religious texts; the church fathers were concerned that the Bible was being interpreted, not within the context in which it was written, but through the eyes, so to speak, of people in a different historical era (Seebohm 1997). How could such skewed readings of the Scriptures be trusted?

Since then, hermeneutics itself has been shaped by different historical eras, cultural concerns, and social challenges (Palmer 1969). It has been claimed as the basis of literary theory, the organizing thread of the human sciences, the lever to understanding the deepest metaphysical questions of human existence, and, most recently, the springboard of "cultural studies." It could be argued that every clinician uses his or her own hermeneutic, just as it could be argued that every person possesses a philosophy, however tacit or assumed. The question in the forensic setting is what hermeneutics (what principles of interpretation) are being used in reaching an understanding of any psychiatric patient.

There is a strong interest, reflected in threads of the psychiatric literature, in hermeneutical questions, although the literature seldom addresses them as such. For instance, there is much discussion about models of medicine and their importance to psychiatric practice. Such models attempt to answer the hermeneutical question "Which theory, method, or science do I use to understand this patient?" The psychiatric practitioner often deals with the ambiguity of the complex psychiatric patient by applying, in rote fashion, one scientific perspective—a particular hermeneutic—when another might be more apt to the patient and the situation (McHugh and Slavney 1998). In contrast, there are those who advocate the use of multiple or pluralistic scientific perspectives to understand the complex human animal—a different hermeneutic. Similarly, those who believe that only psychoanalytic theory (or only biological/descriptive theory) is needed to understand psychiatric patients have adopted a particular hermeneutic. Even psychiatrists who say they practice biopsychosocial psychiatry (Engel 1977, 1980) are guided by a particular hermeneutic. Throughout the clinical literature, articles and books present various unifying theories to govern the complex practice of medicine or psychiatry (e.g., Goodman 1991; Guze 1992; Sabelli and Carlson-Sabelli 1989; Sadler and Hulgus 1989, 1992). These too are works concerned with hermeneutic tasks.

The appraisal of psychiatric hermeneutics lies outside the scope of this work. For a brief but illuminating review of hermeneutic applications in psychiatry, see Phillips (1996).

Justification

The introduction of causes into a discourse about RMS (e.g., "What mental state caused Hinckley to attempt to assassinate Reagan?") is philosophically suspect from the beginning. The concepts of cause, causation, and causal relations regarding motivations and intentions are a great puzzle in the history of philosophy. For instance, Hume's response to the question of the knowability of causal relations was that all we can ever really know are "constant conjunctions" between events, and that from those we can derive general laws to guide us about the world (Hume 1748/1999). But we have already seen the limits of such constant conjunctions from the earlier discussion about the difficulties inherent in induction. Be this as it may, if we admit the concept of causes, causal laws, and causal relations into clinical psychology and psychiatry (and the law seems to want this), we are left with philosophy's riddles.

The philosophical knots concerning the concept of cause are arcane and technical. A few simple points can be made, however, to indicate some of the ways clinicians and attorneys can be at cross-purposes about causes in the forensic setting. About 35 years ago, John Mackie (1965, 1974) first articulated a model of causal relations that attempted to circumvent many of the classical problems of causal reasoning and causal relations. Mackie's formulation has since become known as the *insufficient but necessary part of an unnecessary but sufficient* (INUS) condition model of causality. It is particularly appealing to clinicians for reasons that are readily apparent. Conventional medical statements of single causes are misleading, and clinicians, when pressed, will admit that virtually all maladies, including psychiatric disorders, are *multifactorial*, meaning they have multiple causes. Even the ideal model of medical monocausation, that of infectious disease, where the *germ* is the single *cause* of the infection, does not hold up to the briefest analysis. As Henrik Wulff (1984) notes in his study of cause and medical classification, even an infectious disease like pneumococcal meningitis (PM) does not necessarily occur in the presence of the bug unless other permissive factors are also present, such as a splenectomy or the failure to vaccinate. Even if the possible causes were limited to these three, it would be difficult to defend one as the sole cause, because all three conditions must occur in conjunction for the disease to appear.

To deal with this sort of ambiguity about causation, Mackie, and later Wulff, invoked the INUS condition, which would claim that a condition like splenectomy or the presence of pneumococcus would be an *insufficient but necessary part of an unnecessary but sufficient* complex of causes. This simply means that the splenectomy is essential for the development of PM but is not in itself adequate to cause it—other conditions are needed as well, none of which are in themselves adequate to cause the disease either. Also note that the combination of conditions are *only* sufficient, that is, they *may* cause the disease state but do not *have* to—other conditions may cause the disease instead. The appeal of this kind of causal reasoning in the medical setting is that it permits the assimilation of causally relevant conditions as a group and also (just as importantly) permits the "fudge" factor of other, nonspecified conditions to be discovered later and added to the INUS condition set to enrich the causes. So if, for instance, it was found in the future that a sleep debt was also necessary but not in itself sufficient to cause PM, it could be added and assimilated into the evolving causal formulation of that disorder.

For Wulff and other theorists of medical causality (e.g., Engelhardt 1981, 1984), the INUS condition is attractive to clinicians because it has a particular pragmatic appeal; that is, it permits viewing causes as *targets of therapy:* if absence of vaccination is an INUS condition (risk factor) for meningitis, then vaccinating people will preclude PM. Moreover, in this particular case, the failure to vaccinate is an atypical condition for a physician (the standard of care is to vaccinate after splenectomy), so the INUS model also permits a concept of negligent cause; that is, if the doctor failed to vaccinate the patient, then the cause of the PM was the doctor's inaction on the INUS condition of vaccination.

Herein lies the connection and the similar appeal of INUS-style reasoning to the law (Engelhardt 1981, 1984; Hart and Honoré 1985). The law also has specific practical interests in causality, one of which is the determination of responsibility and guilt. What is significant here is not so much the differences in causal reasoning, which are not so large, but rather the *practical interests* that frame the causal attribution. To the court, the failure to vaccinate meets legal criteria for cause because the law deals with human culpability, not bacterial or splenic culpability. However, to the clinician, to say the failure to vaccinate is the cause of PM rankles, because the clinician's practical interest in causes lies with the possibility of therapy and prevention. Remember, the "US" in INUS refers to the three conditions being only permissive, not determinative. But to the court, there is a good chance that giving the vaccine would have prevented the PM, whereas not giving the vaccine was an abnormal act, and the court is, after all, focused on personal responsibility. To the clinician, seizing on the failure to vaccinate seems simply a move to single out one factor and distort it into being solely determinative; thus it seems to pick on the doctor unfairly, because, after all, the various factors are all of equal *causal* weight in the INUS condition.

But the court may say that they are not all of the same *moral* weight. In an analogous fashion, this interpretation pertains to RMS and the *Hinckley* case. I could propose (purely theoretically) that the causes of John Hinckley's assassination attempt were based on three INUS conditions: 1) his disregard for what he knew to be wrong, 2) his wish to attract Jodie Foster's attention, and 3) his wish to be killed by Secret Service agents. At the risk of appearing to speak for the examining clinicians, I would like to suggest that it is plausible for a forensic specialist like Park Dietz to seize the salient legal point in terms of causes. That point is the INUS condition of Hinckley's disregard for right, because this INUS condition is the one of pragmatic interest to the court. On the other hand, it is also understandable that William Carpenter, a researcher committed to elaborating the pluralistic causes of schizophrenia, might instead insist on the multifactorial equality of these three INUS conditions. Thus there exists not a clash of *sciences* but rather a clash of *interests*.

I have endeavored to indicate only a sample of the philosophical issues involved in the assessment of RMS in the forensic setting. In so doing, I have intentionally raised more questions than provided answers. With such daunting conceptual knots, it is a wonder that any claims about RMS are considered credible, much less true knowledge. Perhaps this chapter and this book overall will contribute to the unraveling of some of these knots.

References

Ayer AJ: Language, Truth, and Logic, 2nd Edition. New York, Dover, 1977

Bernstein RJ: Beyond Objectivism and Relativism: Science, Hermeneutics, and Praxis. Philadelphia, PA, University of Pennsylvania Press, 1985

Dancy J: Problems in epistemology, in The Oxford Companion to Philosophy. Edited by Honderich T. New York, Oxford University Press, 1995, pp 245–248

Daubert v Merrell Dow Pharmaceuticals, Inc., 509 US 579 (1993)

Engel GL: The need for a new medical model: a challenge for biomedicine. Science 196:129–136, 1977

Engel GL: The clinical application of the biopsychosocial model. Am J Psychiatry 137:535–544, 1980

Engelhardt HT: Relevant causes: their designation in medicine and law, in The Law–Medicine Relation: A Philosophical Exploration. Edited by Spicker SF, Healey JM, Engelhardt HT. Boston, MA, D. Reidel, 1981, pp 123–127

Engelhardt HT: Comments on Wulff's "The causal basis of the current disease classification," in Health, Disease, and Causal Explanations in Medicine. Edited by Nordenfelt L, Lindahl BIB. Boston, MA, D. Reidel, 1984, pp 179–182

Frye v United States, 54 App DC 46, 47, 293 F 1013, 1014 (1923)

Garb HN: Studying the Clinician: Judgment Research and Psychological Assessment. Washington, DC, American Psychological Association, 1998

Goodman A: Organic unity theory: the mind-body problem revisited. Am J Psychiatry 48:553–563, 1991

Grinnell F: The Scientific Attitude, 2nd Edition. New York, Guilford, 1992

Guze SB: Why Psychiatry Is a Branch of Medicine. New York, Oxford University Press, 1992

Hart HLA, Honoré T: Causation in the Law, 2nd Edition. New York, Oxford University Press, 1985

Hempel CG: Philosophy of Natural Science. Englewood Cliffs, NJ, Prentice-Hall, 1966

Hume D: An Enquiry Concerning Human Understanding (1748). Edited by Beauchamp TL. New York, Oxford University Press, 1999

Jacob F: The Statue Within: An Autobiography. Translated by Philip F. Plainview, NY, Cold Spring Harbor Laboratory Press, 1995

Jaspers K: General Psychopathology, Vols 1 and 2. Translated by Hoenig J, Hamilton MW; foreword by McHugh PR. Baltimore, MD, Johns Hopkins University Press, 1997

Kuhn TS: The Structure of Scientific Revolutions, 2nd Edition. Chicago, IL, University of Chicago Press, 1970

Kuhn TS: Objectivity, value judgment, and theory choice, in The Essential Tension. Chicago, IL, University of Chicago Press, 1977, pp 320–329

Kumho Tire Co. v Carmichael, 119 S Ct 1167 (1999)

Loftus E: The myth of repressed memory and the realities of science. Clinical Psychology: Science and Practice 3(4):356–362, 1996

Longino HE: Science as Social Knowledge: Values and Objectivity in Scientific Inquiry. Princeton, NJ, Princeton University Press, 1990

Low PW, Jeffries JC, Bonnie RJ: 1983 Supplement to Criminal Law: Cases and Materials. Mineola, NY, The Foundation Press, 1983

Mackie J: Causes and conditions. American Philosophical Quarterly 2:245–264, 1965

Mackie J: The Cement of the Universe: A Study of Causation. Oxford, Clarendon Press, 1974

McHugh PR: What's the story? The American Scholar 64(2):191–203, 1995

McHugh PR, Slavney PR: The Perspectives of Psychiatry, 2nd Edition. Baltimore, MD, Johns Hopkins University Press, 1998

Palmer RE: Hermeneutics: Interpretation Theory in Schleiermacher, Dilthey, Heidegger, and Gadamer. Evanston, IL, Northwestern University Press, 1969

Phillips J: Key concepts: hermeneutics. Philosophy, Psychiatry, and Psychology 3(1):61–69, 1996

Popper K: Conjectures and Refutations: The Growth of Scientific Knowledge, 5th Edition, Rev. London, Routledge, 1992

Proctor RN: Value-Free Science? Purity and Power in Modern Knowledge. Cambridge, MA, Harvard University Press, 1991

Ricoeur P: The Conflict of Interpretations: Essays in Hermeneutics. Evanston, IL, Northwestern University Press, 1974

Sabelli HC, Carlson-Sabelli L: Biological priority and psychological supremacy: a new integrative paradigm derived from process theory. Am J Psychiatry 146:1541–1551, 1989

Sadler JZ, Hulgus YF: Hypothesizing and evidence-gathering: the nexus of understanding. Family Process 26(3):255–267, 1989

Sadler JZ, Hulgus YF: Clinical problem-solving and the biopsychosocial model. Am J Psychiatry 149(10):1315–1323, 1992

Salmon W, Kitcher P (eds.): Four Decades of Scientific Explanation. Minneapolis, MN, University of Minnesota Press, 1989

Seebohm T: Hermeneutics, in Encyclopedia of Phenomenology. Edited by Embree L, Behnke EA, Carr D, et al. Boston, MA, Kluwer Academic, 1997, pp 308–312

von Wright GH: Explanation and Understanding. Ithaca, NY, Cornell University Press, 1971

Wallace E: What is truth? some philosophical contributions to psychiatric issues. Am J Psychiatry 145:137–147, 1988

Wiggins OP, Schwartz MA: Edmund Husserl's influence on Karl Jaspers's phenomenology. Philosophy, Psychiatry, and Psychology 4(1):15–36, 1997a

Wiggins OP, Schwartz MA: Karl Jaspers, in Encyclopedia of Phenomenology. Edited by Embree L, Behnke EA, Carr D, et al. Boston, MA, Kluwer Academic, 1997b, pp 371–376

Windelband W: History and natural science. Introduced and translated by Oakes G. History and Theory 19:165–185, 1980

Wulff HR: The causal basis of the current disease classification, in Health, Disease, and Causal Explanations in Medicine. Edited by Nordenfelt L, Lindahl BIB. Boston, MA, D. Reidel, 1984, pp 169–177

Assessment of Mental State at the Time of the Criminal Offense

The Forensic Examination

Thomas G. Gutheil, M.D.

> [Clinicians] are expected, as a result of interviews which take place long after the event, and often with a defendant who has benefitted [sic] from treatment (not to mention legal advice), to tell the court exactly what went through a defendant's mind when he or she was doing what they [sic] did. (N. Walker, in Slovenko 1995, p. 239)

The insanity defense is one of the most colorful, controversial, and fascinating issues at the interface of law and medicine. To improve our grasp of this complex issue, a case example may aid us in bringing out the facets of the subject.

The author thanks H. Bursztajn, M.D., Robert I. Simon, M.D., Daniel Shuman, J.D., and anonymous reviewers for useful suggestions.

Case Example: The Insanity Defense

The forensic psychiatrist is called by a defense attorney to visit the state forensic hospital to evaluate Mr. Jones, a 55-year-old divorced father of two who allegedly killed his estranged ex-wife 4 months earlier. The attorney wants to investigate the feasibility of an insanity defense for the crime. The previous 4 months of Mr. Jones's hospitalization have been spent in the active treatment and often in the physical restraint of Mr. Jones, who has been wildly psychotic. He has refused most evaluative efforts and denies having any knowledge of the crime; in fact, he insists on being allowed to call his ex-wife to explain where he is being held and why he is late in sending alimony. Antipsychotic and mood-stabilizing treatments have recently resulted in considerable clinical improvement.

Now that he has calmed down, Mr. Jones is reasonably cooperative with the interview. Over many hours he describes his growing distraction and preoccupation with what he calls "spiritual concerns about electronic bodies"—concerns that began to interfere with his successful career as a Web site developer for a large Internet company. He grew progressively isolated from his few friends, lost weight, and spent increasing time online in Internet chat rooms devoted to religious and New Age themes.

Over the weeks prior to the crime, Mr. Jones developed the notion of disembodied "rogue intelligences" loose on the Internet in "cyberspace" that were capable of "possessing"—taking over and controlling—human beings who were exposed to them. Mr. Jones further began to believe that his ex-wife, who used the Internet extensively in her real estate business, had been taken over in this manner; he concluded this from some of her remarks and a certain expression on her face of "machine-like vacuousness."

Mr. Jones reported that, during an argument over visitation rights, he was seized with fear, rage, and despair at his ex-wife's inhuman state, believing that *he* was now at imminent risk of being "possessed" through her and thus essentially killed or eliminated as a personal identity. Allegedly to defend himself against this terrifying fate, he seized a kitchen knife and stabbed her in the heart—apparently fatally—then proceeded to stab her 32 more times, one for each year of her age. He threw the knife away in the garbage, not wanting to touch the blood on it for fear of "spiritual contamination." However, he left the body on the kitchen floor, where it was later discovered by the milkman, who called the police.

The forensic psychiatrist gathers further data. Autopsy reports reveal that the subsequent stab wounds occurred after the ex-wife was clearly dead. Police reports reveal that the knife was not found, perhaps because the garbage was collected after the crime, and that the defendant was "raving about some computer stuff" at the time of his arrest. The arresting officer cannot recall any clearer version of events. Mr. Jones's teen-age son describes his father as a longtime "cyber-geek" but does not recall any specific details about the father's beliefs, since "we haven't talked much about anything important since the divorce."

Before continuing the investigation, the forensic psychiatrist pauses to reflect on the case up to this point. Mr. Jones's illness appears to be genuine at first assessment, but does it meet insanity *criteria* at the time of the offense? How much credit can be given to Mr. Jones's self-reported depiction of his mental state at the time of the alleged offense—a critical datum, if not *the* critical datum—in this evaluation, given how much he may believe it to be in his interest to be found nonresponsible for the crime? Was the murder weapon simply discarded or effectively concealed, and is the difference meaningful? What is the implication of the body being left at the scene? We will return to this case example later.

Criminal Responsibility and the Insanity Defense

To place into context the forensic examination in this most controversial of forensic topics, the insanity defense, some background information on the issue itself will serve as orientation. Two aspects to be reviewed briefly here are the context of the insanity defense in the legal system and its context in society.

Context in the Legal System

An examination of the context of the insanity defense in the legal system requires a consideration of both 1) the theoretical basis for this line of defense and 2) the public's perception of fairness inherent to our court system.

Theoretical Basis

Is it always a crime to shoot a president? The answer to this question, which is commonly used to test forensic knowledge, is of course "no." For example, the shooting may occur by an unfortunate accident or—admittedly less likely—in self-defense (Gutheil 1983).

These answers reveal a basic fact of criminal justice, namely that actions alone—even quite serious ones—do not constitute crimes in and of themselves. A mental state involving intent must also be present. In legal terms the actus reus (evil or criminal action) must be accompanied by the mens rea (evil intent). To put it differently, a *crime* rather than a mere *act* requires intent on the part of the perpetrator (Appelbaum and Gutheil 1991; Gutheil 1999; Slovenko 1995).

If the sanity of a defendant is questioned, usually by the defense attorney, the essential issue is whether the accused (the defendant) should be held responsible for his or her actions, as should all persons ordinarily; or whether by virtue of a mental illness, the defendant, *according to certain legal criteria*, should not be held responsible for the criminal act. The defense's plea for exoneration on grounds of criminal nonresponsibility is referred to as the *insanity defense*. Note that deciding whether to make this determination is primarily a legal rather than a psychiatric question (Appelbaum and Gutheil 1991; Gutheil 1999; Slovenko 1995).

The Perception of Fairness

Courts in a civilized society must be credible to function and to serve successfully as a viable alternative to vigilante justice. An important aspect of this perception is that persons who should be viewed as nonresponsible for their actions are not treated as though they bore full responsibility for those actions (Appelbaum and Gutheil 1991; Gutheil 1999).

For example, a 3-year-old child who throws a block at a playmate is not charged with assault as would be an adult who performed that same action. Thus the appropriate use of the insanity defense serves the social perception of the court's fairness by attempting to distinguish between those who should be punished and those who should be exonerated.

Context in Society

The societal context of the insanity defense involves both the perceptions of the public at large toward the insanity plea and the patterns of usage of this defense over time.

Public Views

Even the most ostensibly clear legal matters undergo profound alteration when considered by the public. The public has never greeted the use of the insanity defense with anything but scorn and dismay. This defense is viewed not as a moral attempt to preserve the fairness of the legal system but instead as a means whereby, on dubious grounds, dangerous felons are released back into the larger society to do more harm.

Patterns of Usage

The public perception of the insanity defense as being plagued by problems is fed by various forces that cannot be reviewed here in any detail (see Gutheil 1999). One fact most consistently ignored by the public is the rarity of the use of this defense. It is employed in less than 1% of felony cases (Miller 1998), and in only one-fourth of that 1% will it succeed with the jury (Melton et al. 1997). Despite this low frequency of use of the insanity defense, public outcry is the predictable sequel to almost any insanity-based exoneration.

The Forensic Question

The forensic examination for criminal responsibility or insanity consists of two main phases: 1) identification of the mental disorder affecting the defendant at the time of the crime and 2) comparison of the defendant's symptoms and behavior at the time of the crime to the standard criteria for that particular disorder. During the phase when the official criteria for a disorder are considered, the forensic examiner faces a twofold challenge: 1) to complete the assessment in hindsight and 2) to rule out malingering on the part of the defendant. Finally, regardless of the forensic specialist's recorded findings and court testimony, the ultimate determination of insanity is made by the court itself.

Identification of the Mental Disorder

The first part of the forensic examination involves identifying the mental illness, typically a major mental illness such as a psychosis, in the defendant at the time of the criminal act. Theoretically, it is also possible for persons affected by lesser conditions, such as severe personality disorders, to qualify for exculpation. A successful insanity defense involving this type of diagnosis is less common, however, apparently because decision-makers see these conditions as less severe.

Organic conditions (identified by the historically common but now awkward term *mental defect*) also qualify persons for the insanity defense. This category would include mental retardation, effects of brain lesions such as head trauma or tumors, dementing illnesses, and certain seizure disorders (e.g., temporal lobe epilepsy). However, because such conditions are usually but not always chronic and persistent (e.g., mental retardation), assessing them in retrospect is far less challenging than are the more transient psychotic states. In other words, the organically impaired examinee in the present is likely to closely resemble the same examinee in the past. Thus, with rare exceptions (lucid intervals in subdural hematoma), the insanity evaluation of such persons resembles a present-state evaluation.

Comparison to Official Criteria

After a mental disorder has been established, the second and more nearly essential phase of the insanity examination requires comparing the particular mental state of the defendant at the time of the alleged act to the insanity criteria established in statutes and case law in that jurisdiction. Of course, the requisite mental states may also be regarded as part of the official criteria. The historical and legal issues on this point involve a plethora of detail beyond the scope of this chapter, but the most relevant aspects of the subject are summarized here (see Appelbaum and Gutheil 1991; Eigen 1995; Melton et al. 1997; Miller 1998; Rogers and Shuman 2000; Slovenko 1995).

Several major types of insanity criteria exist in the United States, with a common one being the insanity defense standard and its variations as articulated in 1955 by the American Law Institute (ALI) in its Model Penal Code (American Law Institute 1955). This standard held an individual nonresponsible if, at the time of the act in question, he or she possessed a substantial incapacity from mental disease or defect (mental disorder or organic impairment) either to *appreciate* the wrongfulness of the conduct in question or to *conform* that conduct to the requirements of the law. Other standards address presence or absence of an "irresistible impulse," the defendant's knowledge of right and wrong at the time of the act, and whether the act was a product of the person's mental illness (Appelbaum and Gutheil 1991; Gutheil 1999; Melton et al. 1997; Miller 1998).

In contrast to the ALI's substantial incapacity standard, the federal standard requires an "inability" to appreciate wrongfulness. The retrospective assessment of mental states, of course, takes different forms according to whichever standard is being employed. The ideal insanity evaluation takes place immediately after the defendant admits committing the criminal act. But when a defendant denies having committed the act, the retrospective determination of mental state shifts the investigative burden onto other sources of data in a move that may change the role of forensic examiner to that of fact-finder.

Under certain circumstances, intent can be inferred from the act itself, even when the alleged intent is different. A defendant who robs a bank, for example, and claims that it was an act of divine justice has telegraphed another intent by keeping the money.

A different approach is used in some states that grant exculpation only if the defendant's impairment from mental disorder left him or her unable to form even the requisite mental state (mens rea) for the crime. For example, a defendant may have been too impaired to form the specific intent that statutorily defines a particular crime. Only five states (Montana, Idaho, Utah, Nevada, and Kansas) have adopted this approach so far. It is a more extreme test for exculpation, requiring a far greater degree of mental disturbance. For the forensic examiner, such an assessment is comparably difficult, but the retrospective nature of the evaluation remains the same.

The Forensic Challenge

The assessment of insanity presents a twofold challenge for the examiner. First, the examination must be done in hindsight, sometimes long after the criminal act. Second, although malingering is at least a theoretical consideration in every forensic examination for any purpose, rarely is an examinee's interest in feigning mental disturbance so strong as in the insanity context, especially when the crime is serious and the punishment severe.

Indeed, the examination of the insanity claimant sits at the nexus of a marked paradox: no one other than the examinee has potentially as clear and accurate a picture of what was going on inside his or her head. That is, only the examinee can ever really know what his or her mental state was at the time of the offense, and yet no one has as strong a motive for distorting that clarity.

An additional challenge is the distinction between moral and legal wrongfulness. In our earlier case example, Mr. Jones may have believed that killing his "possessed" wife in "self-defense" was not morally wrong, but did he possess awareness of the legal wrongfulness of killing per se? The insanity defense assessment would apply to the latter question.

Finally, the greatest challenge for the forensic examiner may lie in determining whether an act occurred because of "substantial incapacity" (sometimes "inability") to conform conduct to the requirements of the law or, instead, because of some unwillingness or resistance toward maintaining such conforming behavior. Could Mr. Jones have fled or walked away without killing? Mental health professionals are often more comfortable with assessment of the appreciation prong of the defense than with the conforming conduct prong. One reason for this degree of comfort appears to be that the former seems more clinical, while the latter seems more arbitrary and subjective. In any case some clinical states (e.g., mania, deliria, seizure phenomena) may operate more directly to diminish the capacity to conform behavior, and the examiner should investigate this possibility.

The Final Determination

Although the forensic evaluator may testify as to his or her *opinion* about the defendant's mental state at the time of the criminal act (and, in our adversary system, also be challenged by attorneys and their own experts on the other side), the ultimate *finding* that determines exoneration remains the prerogative of the fact-finder, judge, or jury. The expert witness may address the relevant criteria, but the determination of insanity itself belongs to the court.

The Hindsight View

Some [insanity] cases might be analogized to an orgasm: there is excitement, a discharge [of tension], and then relaxation. Examining an individual at the time of relaxation may give no clue that there was a discharge. (Slovenko 1995, p. 244)

The insanity evaluation is locked into the hindsight view because it must occur not only after the crime but also after apprehension of the supposed perpetrator. In some cases the matter is delayed beyond the intrinsic slowness of the law by the need to restore the mentally disordered offender to competence, after which the examination as to insanity may ethically proceed. Surprisingly, the hindsight view offers some advantages in the insanity exam.

Advantages

One formulation comparing the examinations for competence to stand trial to those for insanity holds that competence to stand trial is a snapshot (i.e., a present-state examination), while insanity itself is a movie (Gutheil 1999). This latter image is intended to capture the way in which evaluation for insanity must take into account the defendant's entire life, seen as a longitudinal history, as it may bear on the mental state at the relevant time. Early development, familial interactions, particular traumata, family genetics, and life experiences might all play a role in the assessment.

In a similar sense the hindsight view forces the examiner to look beyond the crime to the defendant's longitudinally viewed psychiatric history. Matters of relevance would include the recognized features and symptoms of the major mental disorder in question, the natural history of that disorder, and the clinical awareness of the various ways that the disorder may impinge on cognition, affect, and behavior.

Disadvantages

Despite these heuristic advantages of the hindsight position, the fundamental problem for the examiner is the re-creation of another person's mental state at a time and under circumstances usually far removed from the critical moment (Appelbaum and Gutheil 1991; Gutheil 1999; Melton et al. 1997; Miller 1998; Slovenko 1995). This constitutes a problem not only for the present interview but also for standard measures such as psychological testing, whose validity decreases in the post-factum setting (Melton et al. 1997). Psychological testing may be useful, however, to measure intelligence level and to document the presence of a major current mental illness that may reinforce (but not prove) determination of a past condition. Many experts suggest that, for just such purposes, psychological testing should be done in all insanity evaluations to provide some standardized data amid the largely clinical-intuitive context required in this case. Such testing may be particularly helpful with personality-disordered examinees. Neuropsychological testing may be similarly helpful for those with organic conditions.

Note that some attorneys will resist these testing procedures out of fear that they will have to live with the results willy-nilly. This decision should be discussed with the attorney; the expert may need to explain to the attorney the weakness of his or her opinion, if any, in the absence of this standard item. Testing may also assist the expert and attorney in meeting a challenge to admissibility based on the *Daubert* criteria, as explained later (*Daubert v. Merrell Dow Pharmaceuticals, Inc.* 1993).

The removal in time of the examination from the act itself has several implications. First, mental conditions may evolve spontaneously over time, so that the person seen today may not be the same person psychologically who was acting at the time of the crime. The passage of more time permits more opportunity for normal forgetting to take place as well. In addition, the period after capture may involve emergency or more sustained psychiatric treatment, sometimes in the service of restoration to competency. Although justified on medical and humane grounds, such interventions inescapably alter and hence "contaminate" the attempt to ascertain by hindsight the defendant's clinical state.

An additional contaminant role is played by adverse events associated with the defendant's pursuit, capture, arrest, charge, and incarceration. These experiences are stressful for anyone (except perhaps hardened psychopaths), and as such they are capable of creating psychiatric symptomatology of their own in a situation that may be difficult to distinguish from conditions present at the time of the act.

Finally, the reality of facing punishment is a significant stressor, whether punishment is likely to be prolonged incarceration under probably noxious conditions or, in some cases, execution. The experience of confronting such a fate is clearly potentially pathogenic in its own right, the results of which must be distinguished from mental states contemporaneous with the crime.

This discussion should make clear that mental illness may follow the crime as well as be a possible element within it. However, the larger point to be drawn is that mental illness may bear a *number* of possible relationships to the criminal act. Dietz (1992) has thoughtfully summarized the interactions among mental illness and criminality in a manner particularly useful for our discussion.

First, *the crime may be caused by a mental disorder* such as a psychosis (Dietz 1992). In our earlier example, if Mr. Jones's delusion is authentic, the murder would have been, at least in part, the result of his delusional distortion of reality. In accordance with the *Durham* test for insanity (*Durham v. US* 1954) used briefly in the Washington, D.C., area and still in use in New Hampshire, nonresponsibility is granted if the criminal act is a *product* of the mental illness; a number of insanity claims certainly fit this model. Thus retrospective evaluation would involve identifying the psychosis and relating it to the requisite criteria.

A second category is *criminality due to a compulsion* (Dietz 1992). A number of possible causes related to mental illness might fit this model; they range from paraphilias, impulse disorders, and Tourette's syndrome to posttraumatic stress disorder (PTSD; e.g., "Vietnam syndrome"). One example, albeit a cliché, would be the combat-scarred veteran who, triggered by a loud noise into a flashback to a combat situation, attacks a bystander. To give such a claim more durable validity, the retrospective evaluation would seek evidence of the particular compulsion predating the actual criminal act.

A third association between disorder and crime is a *criminal act based on the defendant's personality disorder* (Dietz 1992). This is a controversial area, since some scholars believe that exoneration should be reserved for mental disturbances at no less than the psychotic level—although, of course, the fact-finder makes this ultimate determination. Clearly, persons with antisocial personality disorder are commonly involved in criminality, but the power of this finding is diluted by the fact that criminal behavior is an element of the disorder's definition. Patients with borderline personality disorder are also prone to impulsive behavior that may find criminal expression (e.g., assault); these persons may qualify for exoneration if the psychic disturbance is sufficiently severe. However, the hindsight assessment in this population is complicated by the capacity of such patients to recover rapidly from a "micropsychosis" and to appear fully normal and functional shortly after even a severe disturbance.

A fourth pairing of disorder and crime constitutes *criminal conduct with a coincident mental illness* (Dietz 1992)—a situation resembling the old standardized test response to two matched phrases, "True, true, but unrelated." In this situation both the criminal act and the mental disorder are genuine but the disorder is forensically incidental in that it fails to impinge on the requisite criteria. The hindsight challenge is particularly keen because the examiner has evidence for the reality of the illness but must make the finer distinction as to whether its particular manifestations affected, say, appreciation of the wrongfulness of the conduct. The case of Mr. Jones, for example, might theoretically involve a delusional disorder occurring contemporaneously with but not "causing" the crime.

The fifth association is *a mental disorder caused by the crime* (Dietz 1992). As noted earlier, the fact of having murdered someone, for example, coupled with the legal sequelae, may produce a mental illness such as depression or severe dissociation after the fact, so that a genuine illness exists, but its presence confuses the question of earlier illness related to the commission of the crime. A particularly interesting example of this phenomenon occurs when an individual experiences what amounts to PTSD as a result of his or her own criminal act. Although that diagnosis usually results from external traumata, persons who commit especially violent crimes under altered states of mind may well feel all the sequelae of PTSD from the trauma of their own actions (Harry and Resnick 1986).

Finally, *a mental disorder may be malingered after the crime* in an attempt at exoneration (Dietz 1992). This issue constitutes our next topic. Before addressing it, however, two special cases that pose particular problems in this area should be noted: intoxication and amnesia.

Voluntary intoxication is not accepted for almost all insanity claims, although *involuntary* intoxication (the unannounced LSD in the fraternity punch bowl) and so-called *pathological* intoxication may qualify in some cases. Retrospective assessment of these features in the absence of blood levels close in time to the offense and the absence of clear historical data is extremely difficult (Appelbaum and Gutheil 1991; Melton et al. 1997).

Amnesia alone is usually not exonerating and is readily feigned, even by unsophisticated persons. In some situations the clinical picture (e.g., severe dissociation, PTSD) may include an amnesic component and may qualify if the disorder in its entirety meets criteria (Appelbaum and Gutheil 1991; Melton et al. 1997).

Feigning Illness: The Problem of Malingering

Because of the penalties associated with being found guilty of a crime, the defendant may understandably seek exoneration through malingering psychiatric illness in hopes of qualifying for an insanity defense. Not all defendants have such an interest. The more "prison-wise" recidivists may understand that commitment to a forensic hospital for an undetermined period and a lifetime stigmatizing label as a mental patient are not necessarily an improvement on fixed jail time with opportunities for earlier release. In contrast, delusionally depressed persons may actively seek punishment for their feelings of guilt.

Detection of malingering has become a science of its own (Resnick 1998; Rogers 1988, 1997), and the subject is too extensive to review in depth here. The critical point in the present context is that the assessor in the insanity context has the added burden of detecting in the present examination the presumptive feigning of a past illness or mental state at some earlier time, that is, an illness or state not necessarily present (or even being feigned in the present) in the person standing before one now. The matter is further complicated if some genuine illness appears in the present state of the examinee.

Some useful rubrics for assessing malingering may be outlined here, but the reader is referred to Resnick (1998) and Rogers (1988, 1997) for more detail. Rogers (1988) notes that hallmarks of malingering include an overplayed and dramatic presentation; deliberateness and carefulness in communicating to the examiner; a pattern inconsistent with psychiatric diagnoses; an inconsistent self-report; and endorsement by the examinee of obvious symptoms. Resnick (cited in Rogers 1997, p. 48) also notes the presence of an understandable motive to malinger (in the present context, to achieve exoneration); variability of presentation; improbable psychiatric symptoms; and confirmation of malingering, either by admission after confrontation or by strong (external) corroborative information, such as a past history of dissimulation.

The Forensic Evaluation

> Making a retrospective judgment is not like looking in a rear-view mirror. In making a retrospective judgment, the forensic psychiatrist relies not only on a personal examination of the accused, but also on statements of witnesses and police reports. (Slovenko 1995, pp. 242–243)

Laypersons commonly appear to assume that the psychiatric determination of insanity rests on the unsupported statement of the defendant: the suspect whines an exonerating claim ("I just wasn't myself at the time of the crime"), and the only question is whether the forensic evaluator is "fooled." Laypersons, of course, assume the evaluator is fooled with distressingly high frequency.

In reality obtaining the actual database for the forensic evaluator requires casting the widest possible net to gather information that—although taking into account the self-reports of the defendant as to his or her mental state—goes far beyond that individual to less interested and less self-serving sources of information.

The Forensic Interview

The ethical requirement of forensic warnings about nonconfidentiality, potential harms from the interview, and the like is rarely more critical than in the interview phase of the insanity examination, if only because the stakes are often high. Details of forensic warnings will not be addressed in this discussion and can be found elsewhere (Appelbaum and Gutheil 1991; Gutheil 1998).

To structure this description of the evaluator's approach, let us return to the case example that opened this chapter. The accused, Mr. Jones, presents the murder as a kind of delusionally based desperate act of self-defense. We would begin with taking Mr. Jones through the details of the days preceding the crime, with particular attention to the day of the crime itself, beginning with waking up in the morning. Attention would be focused on his inner states along the way; his thoughts, feelings, and fantasies; the presence or absence of particular psychiatric symptoms; and external stimuli or stressors. His perceptions would not be taken simply at face value but rather would be challenged, probed, and explored. Here the forensic evaluator's skeptical inquiry and challenging approach can be seen most clearly to differ from the nonjudgmental acceptance of self-report by the clinical treater.

Attention would also be paid to the presence or absence of altered states of consciousness, including dissociation and intoxication, as well as to claims of complete or partial amnesia for the crime or its context. Note should be taken of the fact that most nonpsychotic persons cannot kill without *some* dissociation at that moment; thus this factor in isolation should perhaps not be seen as exonerative (Porter et al. 2001).

In the present case, Mr. Jones identifies the murder weapon, a knife, as being adventitiously available and impulsively obtained. Of course in a different scenario, deliberately obtaining a weapon and other signs of preparation for the crime would have the effect of challenging a claim of nonresponsibility.

Obviously, the accused's entire relationship with his ex-wife should be explored in meticulous detail from its inception. Particular attention should be paid to the specific argument about visitation that was the proverbial last straw before the murder, as well as to other historical grounds for mere anger, hostility, or aggression toward her on nonpsychotically subjective or "reality" grounds.

The examiner should continue with exploring Mr. Jones's ideas about computer-derived "possessions" and attempt to assess his degree of conviction about them: were they impressions and hunches or convincing beliefs? Inquiry would be made about whether Mr. Jones believed he had any other choice than murder to deal with the fear of being possessed: could he have called police, scientists, or even computer experts? Could he have simply left or fled the scene, and, if so, why did he not do so? Did he know that killing his ex-wife was considered a crime? Did he have awareness or fear of the possibility of capture and punishment? Would he have committed the crime had there been a "policeman standing at his elbow" (a prototypical mental exercise [illegal as a test in some jurisdictions] designed to focus on true absence of awareness of wrongdoing)? Why did he discard the knife, and what did he imagine would happen to it? Why did he do nothing about the dead body? Did he experience guilt or remorse afterward?

Why did Mr. Jones stab his ex-wife exactly 32 times after she was apparently dead? Did he contemplate flight, concealment, evasion of authorities? Would any personal advantages accrue—for example, freedom from alimony payment—if his ex-wife were to die?

Meloy (1992) has suggested a novel approach to the interview, as follows:

> Gathering data about a crime is easier if the clinician employs certain techniques borrowed from cognitive therapy. After taking an ordinary account, consider trying these additional techniques. Ask the defendant to speak in the present tense when recalling the time before, during and after the offense. Let the person free-associate to his thoughts, feelings and behavior, without any initial direct questioning. Have him visually imagine the crime as he describes it; alternatively move him, through suggestive questioning, from external to internal experience and then back. Have him adopt alternative visual perspectives on the crime (e.g., How would you have looked to the victim? What would you be doing? If there had been a camera in the wall, what would it have seen? What would the police see when they first arrived on the scene of the crime?). (p. 51)

A comparable approach, useful when the examinee appears overwhelmed by present affect, is to have him or her describe what happened as if describing a television show on a small screen. This approach sometimes permits a level of useful detachment to establish certain details of the offense.

Although not strictly a part of the interview, the presence of a confession (or comments made early in the legal process) provides an additional source of self-report, as it were, but one that must be viewed with caution. On the one hand, a confession that proffers an explanation for the crime that is not based on mental disorder is highly relevant. A similar case can be made for the suspect who calls 911, who notifies police that a crime has been committed, or who blurts out expressions of remorse or guilt. In our case example, if Mr. Jones had indicated that he killed his ex-wife because "she really pissed me off about visitation," this comment would supply a motive for the crime inconsistent with insanity. On the other hand, mentally disordered individuals may be prone to specious confessions out of delusional guilt and other disturbances of reality testing, factors that should be sought out and ruled out by the examiner (Morse 1982).

Some authorities also suggest videotaping forensic interviews (American Academy of Psychiatry and the Law 1999). Doing so can decrease ambiguity about who said what with what demeanor.

Typical Disorders

As we explore these questions, we compare Mr. Jones's descriptions with those of other mentally ill individuals—in this case, primarily those with delusional disorders—to ascertain whether Mr. Jones's delusions resemble established clinical phenomena. We consider what might be termed ironically the "plausibility" of the delusion itself, that is, whether the properties described do or do not have an internal logical consistency, even if it is "dream logic." For example, there is some consistency to the idea that if one person can be possessed, another could be; moreover, delusions of personal alteration or replacement of objects close to one (Capgras syndrome, delusions of Fregoli) are familiar in psychiatry. Delusions can, of course, be quite original and creative, and thus unique, but we gain some support for the validity of our assessment if dynamically familiar patterns of comprehensible symptoms emerge. This formulation might be balanced or countered by knowledge that the described delusion—rogue intelligences in cyberspace—has been the subject of several science fiction stories over the past 10 years. Did Mr. Jones read these stories or see movies based on them, then conveniently borrow a theme from popular culture in order to malinger an illness?

Life History

The next area of investigation is Mr. Jones's life history. Special attention will be paid to psychiatric symptoms, treatment, any hospitalizations, and the like. Note, however, that some experts recommend *beginning* with the historical exploration, because this subject matter is less emotionally charged than that surrounding the crime itself. As a result, the inquiry may be less threatening and, it is hoped, more self-revelatory and less contaminated by self-serving motivations. This author agrees with this approach.

Concurrent medical conditions should be explored with the additional goal of identifying health professionals who might have cared for the defendant near the relevant time. In the case of Mr. Jones, for example, his recent weight loss is a relatively objective finding that may have been brought to the attention of a physician.

This part of the evaluation most closely resembles the kind of *associative anamnesis* that forms the core of clinical work, where the clinician is attempting to arrive at a diagnosis and a case formulation through the biopsychosocial model. Note, however, that a common pitfall for the amateur assessor is to assume that arriving at a diagnosis is either the main task or the final goal of the insanity evaluation, under reasoning such as, "This man clearly had schizophrenia at the time of the crime, ergo, he is legally insane." The error, of course, is the failure to address the requisite legal criteria that operate independently of the diagnosis. As noted later in this chapter, even the severity of the diagnosis may have little to do with an insanity determination.

Overreliance on diagnosis aside, the insanity claim is obviously better supported if a major mental disorder is identified that long predates the crime, such as a bipolar disorder with a 20-year history. However, many acute states striking someone for the first time without any harbingers may yet be valid bases for exoneration if they meet the requisite legal criteria. The evaluator must remain open to this less common possibility.

From such inquiries and similar lines of questioning, the evaluator attempts to develop a picture of the defendant's mental state regarding choices, perceptions, and alternatives at the time of the crime. But this repository of clinical information is only the starting point of the investigation and arguably the most suspect source of data.

Use of Instruments

Relatively few standardized instruments exist to aid the evaluator in the insanity evaluation. One exception is Rogers Criminal Responsibility Assessment Scales (R-CRAS; Rogers 1984), a test that attempts to measure factors relevant to the insanity determination in a relatively quantitative manner on a series of scales. After the evaluator assigns certain values to the scale elements, which address relevant psychiatric symptoms such as hallucinations, organicity, and possible malingering, a decision tree model produces a final opinion.

A comprehensive critique of the R-CRAS is not possible here but is available elsewhere (Melton et al. 1997). The main advantage of this instrument appears to be its systematic delineation of relevant areas of inquiry in an organized fashion, an approach that will certainly be helpful to the novice evaluator.

Contemporary Observers

In determining whether a defendant is crazy, there is simply no substitute for the fullest possible account from all sources of the defendant's behavior at the time of the alleged crime (Morse 1982). The most essential sources of data in an insanity evaluation are contemporary observers, and the more disinterested, the better: witnesses, victims, bystanders, arresting officers, family members, and health care professionals. All may have noted the defendant's condition during the most forensically meaningful period, that immediately surrounding the crime.

Contact with these important third parties should be arranged through the retaining attorney, who—as experience regrettably teaches—may balk at the request, out of either apathy or financial concerns. This resistance should be managed in the usual manner through education, exhortation, or energetic insistence. The data involved are so essential to the evaluation that an attorney's intransigence in not providing access to third parties may mandate withdrawal from the case. For a helpful outline of third-party sources, see Table 4–1 (Melton et al. 1997).

Table 4–1.   Sources of third-party information

1. **Information regarding evaluation itself**
   a. Referral source
   b. Referral questions
   c. Why evaluation is requested (i.e., what behavior triggered the evaluation?)
   d. Who is report going to?
   e. When is report to be used?

2. **Offense-related information**
   a. From attorney's notes
   b. From witnesses, victim(s)
   c. From confession, preliminary hearing transcript, etc.
   d. Autopsy reports
   e. Newspaper accounts

3. **Developmental/historical information**
   a. Personal data (traumatic life events, unusual habits or fears, places lived)
   b. Early childhood illnesses (if organic deficit suspected)
   c. Family history (especially if young and still living with family)
   d. Marital history (especially in espousal homicide cases)
   e. Educational, employment, and military history
   f. Social relationships
   g. Psychosexual history
   h. Medical and psychiatric records

4. **"Signs of trouble"**
   a. Juvenile and criminal court records
   b. Probation reports

5. **Statistical information (i.e., studies of the behavior of individuals with the defendant's characteristics)**

Source.   Reprinted from Melton GB, Petrila J, Poythress NG, Slobogin C: *Psychological Evaluations for the Courts: A Handbook for Mental Health Professionals and Lawyers,* 2nd Edition. New York, Guilford Press, 1997, p. 235. Copyright © 1997 The Guilford Press. Used with permission.

In the case of Mr. Jones, the family is not particularly helpful, but friends of the deceased wife may be able to report her description of interactions with her ex-husband. The arresting officers, although not clinically savvy, do convey that Mr. Jones appeared to be "raving" about the relevant subject matter at the time of his arrest.

Two important caveats should be invoked here in regard to third-party evaluation. First, laypersons may experience extreme difficulty in recognizing even severe psychiatric disorders, especially conditions such as paranoid disorders that may leave cognition relatively intact. Their descriptions should be scrutinized with this possibility in mind. Questions about the suspect's behavior that deviated from the norm may be more productive than queries about mental disturbance as such.

Second, persons close to the suspect who are interviewed after the crime may deny or minimize their perceptions or descriptions of anything being amiss. This reaction may occur out of their feelings of guilt or embarrassment at their failure to have taken some preventive or remedial action.

Does the retaining attorney (in particular, the criminal defense attorney) count as an "outside observer"? To some degree the answer would be "yes" because disclosures by the defendant—if available within the limits of attorney-client privilege—may provide additional information that may be unavailable from other sources. However, the defense attorney is a far from disinterested observer and may well have an obvious agenda in the matter. The examiner should winnow such data with care.

Do the media offer any useful input? Print media and, to a far greater degree, audiovisual media such as TV reports, although often capturing contemporary experiences and events, must unfortunately be considered to present a usually highly distorted and sensationalized view of both crime and mental disorder, not to mention their possible interaction. However, some data from those sources may provide issues on which to confront the defendant. In a hostage situation evaluated by this author, for example, the defendant's clear negotiating skills with police, which were captured on a news program videotape, challenged the man's claim of totally psychotic functioning.

Behavioral Factors

Behavioral factors are similarly highly relevant to the evaluation. The three most common bases for raising questions about the validity of an insanity claim are flight or comparable efforts to keep from being caught, concealment of the crime itself, and concealment of evidence of the crime. All three reactions on the part of the perpetrator imply some awareness of the wrongfulness of the act in question. In the case of Mr. Jones, the evidence is contradictory: he neither fled nor hid the body, although he did discard the murder weapon, consequently "concealing" it when the garbage was collected. Was this discarding an actual attempt at concealment, or did another motive apply—such as fear of contamination or a wish for neatness? Note that the forensic examiner is not required to resolve definitively all contradictory data or evidence, since that is the task of the fact-finder. The expert's role is to identify the impact on his or her opinion of the diverse elements of the case and to be prepared to explain the basis of the opinion.

Resnick (2000) has provided useful mental checklists of examples of behavioral factors that raise suspicion of knowledge of wrongfulness:[1]

A. Efforts to avoid detection
    Wearing gloves during a crime
    Waiting until cover of darkness
    Taking a victim to an isolated place
    Wearing a mask or disguise
    Concealing a weapon on the way to a crime [as opposed to, or in addition to, concealing it after]
    Falsifying documents (passport or gun permit)
    Giving a false name
    Threatening to kill witnesses
    Giving a false alibi
B. Disposing of evidence
    Wiping off fingerprints
    Washing off blood
    Discarding a murder weapon
    Burying a murder victim secretly
    Destroying incriminating documents
C. Efforts to avoid apprehension
    Fleeing from the crime scene
    Fleeing from the police
    Lying to the police

Note that in our case example, Mr. Jones's behavior fits none of these indices of suspicion except for his disposal of the murder weapon. Even that act has some ambiguous force in shaping the expert opinion, because his stated reason for discarding the knife also related apparently to his delusion.

---

[1]Adapted from Resnick PJ: *American Academy of Psychiatry and the Law Forensic Review Course Syllabus.* Presented at the annual meeting of the American Academy of Psychiatry and the Law, Baltimore, Maryland, 2000. Used with permission.

The Question of Conforming Conduct

In those jurisdictions that employ some version of the ALI standard (American Law Institute 1955), an exonerating alternative to substantial incapacity to appreciate wrongfulness is the substantial incapacity to conform one's conduct to the requirements of the law. During cries for reform after John Hinckley's trial for attempted assassination of President Ronald Reagan, this prong of the insanity defense came under much critical scrutiny. At least one apparent basis was the obvious difficulty in distinguishing the defendant who "could not" conform his behavior from the one who "would not" or "did not." A comparable difficulty faces the distinction between a truly *irresistible* impulse and an impulse merely *unresisted*. Some of the would-be reformists, including the American Psychiatric Association, have argued for the abolition of this prong on the basis that—although psychiatry might have something to offer the courts in determining and proffering evidence for the impact of mental illness on ability to appreciate wrongfulness—the retrospective determination of a person's control of behavior lies outside psychiatry's ability to assess.

Resnick (2000) offers another valuable checklist, paraphrased here, to focus this aspect of the evaluation when required by local statute:[2]

1. Could the defendant defer, if not refrain, from the act (i.e., was there some measure of control present)?
2. Could the defendant refrain from general delusional, hallucinatory, or compulsive pressures versus specific ones?
3. Was ability to conform compromised by mental illness or by concomitant intoxication or rage?
4. What were the defendant's perceived or feared consequences for not following delusional, hallucinatory, or compulsive pressures? What personal weight was given to those consequences?
5. Did alternative choices exist for responding to delusional pressures (as in the case example of Mr. Jones, by calling on computer experts, etc.)?

The retrospective determination of these nuances poses a marked challenge for the forensic examiner.

---

[2]Adapted from Resnick PJ: *American Academy of Psychiatry and the Law Forensic Review Course Syllabus.* Presented at the annual meeting of the American Academy of Psychiatry and the Law, Baltimore, Maryland, 2000. Used with permission.

Alternate Scenarios

Another evaluation factor might be termed the *alternate scenario*. In the case example of Mr. Jones, the murder occurred during an argument about visitation rights, which could have been a sufficient motive for violence by itself. If Mr. Jones became psychotic after the argument on realizing what he had done, then that would represent mental illness *resulting* from the crime as opposed to *causing* it.

Other common alternate scenarios involve the intrinsic value of the crime itself. A rational motive, such as profit or expression of normal anger, should raise the suspicion either of malingering or of mental illness unrelated to the criminal acts. Thus insanity claimed regarding a bank robbery is more suspect because of the intrinsic value of the money than an apparently "purely psychotic" crime without apparent personal gain. In our illustrative case example, was Mr. Jones pressed for alimony payments and thus financially desperate? If so, the crime would have more "value" (and a less convincing insanity aspect) than if no other factors supervened.

Finally, note that simple ignorance of the legal issues as a basis for failing to appreciate wrongfulness does not constitute grounds for an insanity claim ("I didn't know it was against the law to keep a pit bull in my driveway"). The basis of the claim must be a mental disorder.

The Problem of Attorney Coaching

Most attorneys behave ethically as officers of the court, but an occasional attorney will contaminate the evaluation process by supplying the defendant with clinical information or, in some extreme cases, model symptoms consistent with a particular mental disorder for the defendant to emulate and claim as his or her own. This situation is not unlike what occasionally occurs in personal injury litigation when the examinee comes to the evaluation bearing a photocopy of the relevant page from DSM-IV, which has been supplied by the helpful attorney who wants to "help my client focus on the problem."

Examinees usually cannot be asked directly what their lawyers said because of attorney-client privilege, which forensic examiners should generally avoid breaching. Signs of coaching may sometimes be detected, however, in the examinee's use of inappropriately sophisticated terminology or concepts ("Jeez, I dunno, Doc, it was, like, I just coon't conform my conduct to the requirements of the law"), but clear indications of this form of undue influence may be subtle or even invisible. Forensic examiners should be aware of this issue and remain alert for any signs of it.

The Final Opinion

As so concisely stated by Slovenko (1995), formulating an opinion at any point, however close to or distant from the evaluation, can be problematic. "How can a psychiatric expert with a reasonable degree of certainty formulate an opinion as to a defendant's mental state at a time removed from the evaluation by days, weeks, months, and, in some cases, years (Slovenko 1995, p. 244)?"

The examiner must assemble all the foregoing inputs into as coherent a picture as possible of the defendant's mental state at the time of the offence. In presenting, reporting on, or testifying about this opinion, the witness should explain the relationship between the psychiatrically relevant aspects of the database and the relevant legal criteria. The witness should avoid stating the ultimate issue ("Mr. Jones is insane") but should instead present the opinion in operational terms ("Mr. Jones suffered from a delusional disorder that, in my opinion to a reasonable degree of medical certainty, impaired his ability to appreciate the wrongfulness of his conduct in the following manner, etc.").

Finally, as in all forensic evaluations, the examiner should also be psychologically prepared either 1) to arrive at an opinion contrary to that desired by the retaining attorney or 2) to be unable to arrive at a definitive opinion at all, depending on the direction in which the data lead.

New Legal Admissibility Decisions

How forensic experts present their opinions to the court often bears on the reception of those opinions. Melton et al. (1997) emphasize that this process may not always be a comfortable one: "Clinicians involved in the legal process should be careful to think like scientists to give an accurate picture of the probabilistic nature of their facts, even if this stance heightens the discomfort of both the clinician and the court" (p. 12).

Two of the most important United States Supreme Court decisions affecting expert testimony are *Daubert* (1993) and one of its progeny, *Kumho* (*Kumho Tire Co. v. Carmichael* 1999). In terms of their effect on the admissibility of expert testimony, these highly complex decisions are analyzed in detail elsewhere (Grudzinskas and Appelbaum 1998; Gutheil and Stein 2000; Zonana 1994). Their basic premises are summarized here in highly condensed form as they relate to assessment of mental state at the time of the criminal offense.

In *Daubert* the Supreme Court essentially restructured the manner in which the admissibility of scientific testimony would be judged, at least in federal courts but also in those state courts that have adopted this standard. Trial court judges were assigned the task of winnowing valid scientific testimony from "junk science," that is, idiosyncratic, unsupported, or statistically invalid expert claims. Those judges were invited by the Supreme Court to consider such factors as methodological soundness, error rates, experimental reliability, peer review publication, and similar matters in determining whether scientific expert testimony should be heard by the jury without fear that self-styled expertise would influence their opinions inappropriately.

Apparently some courts were treating expertise based on simple training and experience as an exception, as though *Daubert* need not be applied (since such knowledge was not a "laboratory" science that is susceptible, for example, to error rate analysis). In *Kumho* the Supreme Court corrected this erroneous impression by holding that expert testimony based on training and experience must demonstrate the same intellectual rigor as other scientific evidence. This latter issue is particularly applicable to psychiatry (Gutheil and Stein 2000), in which laboratory data play relatively little part in clinical assessments and in which extensive clinical experience is often a critical element in the forensic examiner's conclusions.

For insanity evaluations the forensic examiner is challenged to base on scientific rigor as much of a highly clinical process as possible. Use of validated approaches such as the R-CRAS (Rogers 1984) and others discussed in this chapter (e.g., Rogers and Shuman 2000; Stock and Poythress 1979), use of standardized instruments (with acknowledgment of their limitations), and employment of standardized criteria (but see later caveat) will all be helpful in accomplishing this goal by demonstrating such rigor. The forensic examiner for either side must anticipate being challenged by the opposing side before the actual trial in a "*Daubert* hearing" designed to test the validity and consequent admissibility of that expert's testimony. Experts should thus prepare to be able to state clearly the bases and clinical foundations on which their opinions rest. A list of guidelines for the forensic examination is supplied in Table 4–2 as an aid to the novice.

Diagnostic Problems

The crux of the insanity evaluation is whether the disorder, if present, meets the requisite legal criteria. Disparity between these two factors may take several forms.

One defendant may have a documented, lifelong, serious major mental illness that still does not meet the specific local criteria for exoneration. Another may have a fleeting, transient mental disorder that precisely impinges

Table 4–2.   Guidelines for the essential elements of an insanity evaluation

1. **Review of relevant statutory or other insanity criteria and definitions**

2. **Review of data surrounding alleged crime**
   Police reports
   Witness/victim reports
   Forensic evidence, including autopsy reports, chemistries, toxicology,
       ballistics, fingerprints, results of other forensic examinations
   Personal interview of defendant, including account of the crime and context,
       extensive history, family history, malingering screen, etc.
   Interviews of relevant personnel, including witnesses, family members,
       treaters, corrections personnel, and the like when possible
   Physical examination, if indicated
   Neurological screening; follow-up, including imaging studies, if indicated
   Psychological and/or neuropsychological testing
   Other standardized instruments
   Medical and psychiatric/psychological records
   School, vocational, and other relevant records or collateral data

on the insanity criteria and would thus qualify for exoneration. A third may have a mental disorder that meets criteria but cannot be clearly categorized in our present nomenclature, although individuals with one of the disorders "not otherwise specified" in DSM-IV (American Psychiatric Association 1994) are theoretically as eligible for exoneration as others exactly meeting the diagnostic criteria. The uncertain diagnosis must raise doubts, if not in the evaluator's mind, then in the jury's. The evaluator must draw comfort from the care taken in the evaluation and leave the final decision to the fact-finder.

It is remarkable that, despite the limitations described in this chapter, a relatively high degree of interrater reliability in diagnosis can be achieved (Stock and Poythress 1979), as long as all evaluators have full access to the same database and are at comparable levels of forensic training. Studies also note a fairly high agreement between expert opinion and court finding (Melton et al. 1997), although these results somewhat bypass the usual adversary nature of the proceeding by using single examining psychiatrists rather than one from each side.

Despite these potentially reassuring findings, the expert witness testifying in court in an insanity case must accept the fact that most studies show that juries use an idiosyncratic moral calculus as to who should be punished rather than as being particularly influenced by expert opinion. Rarely is it so true as in insanity testimony that "the expert witness is a hood ornament on the vehicle of litigation, not the engine" (R.I. Simon, personal communication, October 1997). Although this view should encourage appropriate humility in the forensic examiner, it should not deter him or her from the careful performance of this most challenging forensic task.

Conclusion

Despite the inherent problems with retrospective assessment of mental states, the importance of the role played by the forensic examiner in the legal process should not be underestimated. As Slovenko (1995) noted, "Notwithstanding its difficulties, the retrospective psychiatric opinion continues to be employed because it fulfills certain needs....Put another way, the retrospective psychiatric opinion, although not scientific, is used for want of a suitable alternative" (p. 256).

The forensic evaluator performing an assessment for criminal responsibility faces the most challenging and difficult of all forensic investigations. The greatest part of this difficulty lies not only in determining the presence of a mental state in the past but also in simultaneously determining if that past mental state met certain criteria. Only through the painstaking data gathering described earlier can this task be accomplished, but data gathering alone does not suffice. In the final analysis a fusion of hard fact, logic, and inspired intuition must coalesce to produce the final opinion, which in turn is placed before the fact-finder. As with all forensic determinations, the evaluator must also be prepared to fail to come to a conclusion; data may be unavailable, contradictory, or insubstantial. "I do not know" remains an acceptable conclusion, as in all areas of forensic work.

Regardless of the final opinion, the expert witness in insanity cases is still needed by the legal system to aid in resolving its moral conundrum of guilt and exoneration. The challenges inherent in the hindsight assessment of another person's mental state should not deter us from the attempt to participate usefully in this task.

References

American Academy of Psychiatry and the Law Task Force: Videotaping of Forensic Evaluations. J Am Acad Psychiatry Law 27:345–358, 1999

American Law Institute: Model Penal Code, § 410.1(1) (Tentative Draft #4). Philadelphia, PA, American Law Institute, 1955

American Psychiatric Association: Diagnostic and Statistical Manual of Mental Disorders, 4th Edition. Washington, DC, American Psychiatric Association, 1994

Appelbaum PS, Gutheil TG: Clinical Handbook of Psychiatry and the Law, 2nd Edition. Baltimore, MD, Williams & Wilkins, 1991

Daubert v Merrell Dow Pharmaceuticals, Inc., 509 US 579 (1993)

Dietz P: The mentally disordered offender: patterns in the relationship between mental disorder and crime. Psychiatr Clin North Am 15:539–551, 1992

Durham v US 214 F2d 862 (DC Cir 1954)

Eigen JP: Witnessing Insanity: Madness and Mad-Doctors at the English Court. New Haven, CT, Yale University Press, 1995

Grudzinskas AJ Jr, Appelbaum KL: General Electric Co. v. Joiner: Lighting up the post-Daubert landscape? J Am Acad Psychiatry Law 26:497–503, 1998

Gutheil TG: Madness, medicine and justice: a cross-examination of the insanity defense. Harvard Medical Alumni Bulletin 57:32–37, 1983

Gutheil TG: The Psychiatrist as Expert Witness. Washington, DC, American Psychiatric Press, 1998

Gutheil TG: A confusion of tongues: competence, insanity, psychiatry, and the law. Psychiatr Serv 50:767–773, 1999

Gutheil TG, Stein MD: Daubert-based gate-keeping and psychiatric/psychological testimony in court: review and proposal. J Am Acad Psychiatry Law 28:235–251, 2000

Harry B, Resnick PJ: Posttraumatic stress disorder in murderers. J Forensic Sci 31:609–613, 1986

Kumho Tire Co. v Carmichael, 119 S Ct 1167 (1999)

Meloy R: Violent Attachments. New York, Jason Aronson, 1992

Melton GB, Petrila J, Poythress NG, et al: Psychological Evaluations for the Courts: A Handbook for Mental Health Professionals and Lawyers, 2nd Edition. New York, Guilford, 1997

Miller RM: Criminal responsibility, in Principles and Practice of Forensic Psychiatry. Edited by Rosner R. London, Arnold, 1998, pp 198–215

Morse S: Failed explanations and criminal responsibility: experts and the unconscious. Virginia Law Review 68:971–1060, 1982

Porter S, Birt AR, Yuille JC et al: Memory for murder: a psychological perspective on dissociative amnesia in legal contexts. Int J Law Psychiatry 24(1):23–42, 2001(2001)

Resnick PJ: Malingering, in Principles and Practice of Forensic Psychiatry. Edited by Rosner R. London, Arnold, 1998, pp 417–426

Resnick PJ: American Academy of Psychiatry and the Law Forensic Review Course Syllabus. Annual Meeting of the American Academy of Psychiatry and the Law, Baltimore, MD, 2000

Rogers R: Rogers Criminal Responsibility Assessment Scales (R-CRAS). Odessa, FL, Psychological Assessment Resources, 1984

Rogers R (ed): Clinical Assessment of Malingering and Deception. New York, Guilford, 1988

Rogers R (ed): Clinical Assessment of Malingering and Deception, 2nd Edition. New York, Guilford, 1997

Rogers R, Shuman DW: Conducting Insanity Evaluations, 2nd Edition. New York, Guilford, 2000

Slovenko R: Psychiatric postdicting, in Psychiatry and Criminal Culpability. New York, Wiley, 1995, pp 239–257

Stock H, Poythress NG: Psychologists' opinions on competence and sanity: how reliable? Paper presented at the annual meeting of the American Psychological Association, New York, August 1979

Zonana H: Daubert v. Merrell Dow Pharmaceuticals: a new standard for scientific evidence in the courts? Bull Am Acad Psychiatry Law 22:309–325, 1994

CHAPTER

5

Retrospective Assessment of Malingering in Insanity Defense Cases

Phillip J. Resnick, M.D.
Michael R. Harris, M.D.

Malingering is defined in DSM-IV-TR as "the intentional production of false or grossly exaggerated physical or psychological symptoms, motivated by external incentives such as avoiding military duty, avoiding work, obtaining financial compensation, evading criminal prosecution, or obtaining drugs" (American Psychiatric Association 2000, p. 739). This definition explicitly recognizes the motivation to fake psychiatric illness to "beat" a criminal charge.

Concern about defendants faking mental illness to avoid criminal re-

Portions of this chapter are from Resnick P: "The Detection of Malingered Psychosis." *The Psychiatric Clinics of North America* 22:159–172, 1999. Used with permission.

sponsibility dates back to at least the tenth century (Brittain 1966; Collinson 1812; Resnick 1984). By the 1880s, many Americans considered physicians a generally impious, mercenary, and cynical lot who might participate in the "insanity dodge" (Rosenberg 1968). After the Hinckley insanity verdict, columnist Carl Rowan (1982) stated, "It is about time we faced the truth that the 'insanity' defense is mostly last gasp legal maneuvering, often hoaxes, in cases where a person obviously has done something terrible (p. 10B)." Because of the high degree of jury skepticism, a diagnosis of malingering by even one mental health professional is likely to cause an insanity defense to fail.

Numerous authors (Abrahamson 1983; Rosenhan 1973; Yates et al. 1996) have noted that psychiatrists are reluctant to consider the possibility of malingering, even in situations in which a nonprofessional would consider such behavior understandable. Yates et al. (1996) found that although malingering was frequently suspected in an emergency department setting, psychiatric residents rarely "diagnosed" malingering in their final assessments. One reason is that the diagnosis of malingering is a direct accusation that the examinee is a liar. Some clinicians fear being sued; others fear being physically assaulted. Nonetheless, consideration of malingering must be part of every "not guilty by reason of insanity" (NGRI) evaluation. In this chapter, we focus on detecting various types of mental disorders malingered by defendants pleading NGRI.

Legal Definitions of Insanity

Insanity refers to the absence of criminal responsibility because of a mental illness. Legal definitions of insanity vary among different jurisdictions. The two major standards in current use in the United States are the McNaughten standard and some variation of the American Law Institute (ALI) standard.

Under the McNaughten rule, a defendant is not held criminally responsible if he or she did not know the "nature and quality" or the wrongfulness of his or her actions at the time of the crime because of a "defect of reason, from disease of the mind." A dissociative disorder or mental retardation may be malingered to create the illusion that a defendant did not know the nature and quality of his or her act. Another defendant may falsely allege that he or she delusionally believed that he or she was about to be killed and thus killed in misperceived self-defense.

The ALI test states that "A person is not responsible for criminal conduct if, at the time of such conduct, as a result of a mental disease or defect, he lacks substantial capacity either to appreciate the criminality (wrongfulness) of his conduct, or to conform his conduct to the requirement of the law" (American Law Institute 1962, §4.01). Inability to conform conduct is a volitional test, whereas lack of knowledge of wrongfulness is a cognitive test. A mania or a command hallucination to kill may be malingered to suggest that a defendant could not conform his or her conduct to the requirements of the law.

Specialized Interview Techniques to Ascertain Truth

Clinicians have been searching for ways to determine truth for many centuries. Technological advances have not progressed to the level of any truly reliable method.

Sodium Amytal Interviews

The popular notion that sodium amobarbital (Amytal) is a "truth serum" is unsupported by the literature. People's ability to maintain a falsehood under sedation varies significantly (Redlich et al. 1951). The susceptibility of people to leading questions while under the drug's influence has raised concerns about the accuracy of memories and confessions obtained during such interviews (Rogers and Shuman 2000). Most authors recommend that sodium Amytal interviews be used only when other methods fail to recover memories or to clarify the diagnosis in catatonic states (Rogers and Wettstein 1997). Shorter-acting barbiturates are actually safer. Informed consent must be obtained, and the entire interview should be videotaped. If the clinician uses information obtained during a sodium Amytal interview to draw conclusions, the information is generally admissible in court. However, factual information obtained during the interview cannot be used to prove the truth of a specific assertion (Adelman and Howard 1984). For example, a defendant who claims under Amytal that he or she did not commit a crime could not have that information admitted to prove innocence.

Hypnosis

As with sodium Amytal, a popular but unsupported belief persists that memories obtained during hypnosis are accurate. Hypnosis has not been proven to ascertain truth, even though some people have recovered memories of license numbers through hypnosis that were previously unavailable to them. Courts have varied in their approaches to allowing hypnotically refreshed testimony to be admitted as evidence. In a 1979 affidavit to the

United States Supreme Court, the prominent hypnosis expert Martin Orne (1979) recommended that five criteria should be met before information obtained under hypnosis be admitted in court: 1) only a specially trained psychiatrist or psychologist, not otherwise involved in the case, should be used, 2) the examiner should be supplied with as few details about the case as possible, in writing, 3) the examinee should be asked for free recall before being hypnotized, 4) the entire session should be videotaped, and 5) only the subject and examiner should be present. Some courts have endorsed these recommendations (*State v. Hurd* 1980), but others have rejected testimony based on hypnotically refreshed memories (*People v. Shirley* 1982). Clinicians must exercise extreme care in using hypnosis to establish the accuracy of memories, the validity of amnesia, or the genuineness of a dissociative identity disorder.

Polygraphy

The scientific validity of polygraph testing has been widely criticized (Iacono and Lykken 1997). Most courts will not admit polygraphic evidence. Some difficulties result from the various questioning techniques used. The relevant/irrelevant question technique presents the subject with questions relevant to the event in dispute and compares his or her responses with those for questions irrelevant to the event. A larger physiological response to the relevant questions is considered evidence of deception. This technique has a very high false-positive rate in criminal investigations and has been largely abandoned. The most commonly used technique, the control question technique, uses questions that most people would find guilt-provoking (e.g., "Have you ever committed an unusual sex act?") to deliberately elicit a "guilty" response. The technique assumes that an innocent person will have a greater response to the "control" questions, whereas a guilty person will respond more to offense-relevant questions. This technique has been shown to be strongly biased against innocent subjects and can easily be "beaten" by the use of physical and psychological countermeasures. The guilty knowledge test is more reliable than the other two tests but is rarely used because of its complexity and its lack of generalizability to all criminal settings. This technique requires the examiner to construct a series of multiple-choice questions based on the data of the individual case, such that only investigators and the actual perpetrator would know the correct responses. This technique is better at detecting innocence than guilt, and many examiners do not investigate cases fully enough to use this technique. The lack of scientific reliability of polygraph testing and court inadmissibility preclude its use during NGRI evaluations.

Clinical Interviews

No studies to date have reported that clinicians can consistently detect malingering solely on the basis of an unstructured clinical interview. Psychiatrists' ability to detect lies in strangers is little better than chance (Ekman 1985). Numerous authors (Lovinger 1992; Masling 1966; Robins 1985) have shown that the nature and quality of the data obtained during interviews are affected by interviewer bias, use of leading questions, and situational factors. The use of leading questions or symptom checklists allows malingerers unfamiliar with psychiatric disorders to qualify for a diagnosis of major depression and posttraumatic stress disorder (PTSD) (Lees-Haley and Dunn 1994). Examiners' confidence in their ability to detect malingering has no relation to their actual ability (Ekman 1985).

Kucharski et al. (1998) found that when forensic examiners concentrate on specific factors during an interview, rather than on forming a global impression, their ability to detect malingering improves. The presence of uncommon or unusual hallucinations, uncommon or unusual symptom presentation, and a marked difference between currently reported symptoms and preoffense psychosocial functioning were factors that allowed experienced clinicians to differentiate malingerers from honest defendants with 90% accuracy. This study suggests that a systematized approach to interviewing defendants pleading insanity increases the accuracy of detecting malingering.

Clinical Methods for Detecting Malingering

Clinicians should use multiple sources of data, including interviews, collateral sources of information, and psychometric tests, in detecting malingering (Resnick 1997; Ziskin 1995). Reliance on clinical interviews alone will not allow the examiner to diagnose malingering in any but the most obvious cases.

When a defendant is suspected of malingering an insanity defense, the clinician must look carefully for evidence of inconsistency in symptoms:

- There may be inconsistency in the defendant's report itself. For example, a malingerer may articulately explain that he or she is confused and unable to think right.
- There may be inconsistency in what a defendant reports and the symptoms that are observed. For example, a malingerer may state that he or she is hearing voices during the interview but may show no evidence of being distracted.

- There may be inconsistency in observation of the symptoms themselves. For example, a hospitalized defendant may behave in a confused manner with a psychiatrist but then play excellent bridge on the ward with other patients.
- There may be inconsistency between performance on psychological testing and a malingerer's report of his or her level of performance. For example, a defendant may state on an intelligence test that he or she does not know how many legs are on a dog but perform well as an investment banker.
- There may be inconsistency between what the malingerer reports and how genuine symptoms manifest themselves. For example, a defendant may report that visual hallucinations are seen in black and white, whereas genuine visions are seen in color.

Detailed knowledge about actual psychotic symptoms is the clinician's greatest asset in recognizing simulated psychosis. Therefore, the phenomenology of genuine hallucinations, delusions, and other syndromes is reviewed in this chapter.

Approaches to Defendants Pleading Insanity

Before seeing a defendant, the clinician should be equipped with as much background information as possible (e.g., police reports, witness statements, autopsy findings, past psychiatric records, statements of the defendant, and, very important, observations of correctional staff). It is often helpful if a social worker can interview family members before the clinician's examination.

Defendants who may subsequently raise an insanity defense should be seen as soon as possible after the crime. If a clinician is retained by a defense attorney, then the defendant often can be evaluated within a few days of the crime. However, requests from judges and prosecutors usually are not received until at least 2 months after the crime. Early evaluation reduces the likelihood that the defendant will have been coached about the legal criteria for insanity by other prisoners or the occasional unethical attorney. The more quickly defendants are seen, the less time they have to plan deception, work out a consistent story, and rehearse their lies. Normal memory distortions also are less likely to occur. Moreover, prompt examination enhances the clinician's credibility in court.

The farsighted clinician will record in detail the defendant's early account of the crime, even if the defendant is not competent to stand trial. (Prosecution-employed examiners may not do this for ethical reasons.) Once defendants are placed in a maximum-security hospital, they are likely to learn how to modify their story to avoid criminal responsibility. Additionally, the clinician should take a careful history of past psychiatric illnesses, including details of prior hallucinations, before eliciting an account of the current crime. Malingerers are less likely to be on guard because they infrequently fully anticipate the relevance of such information to the current insanity issue. If defendants should subsequently fake psychosis to explain their criminal conduct, it will be too late to falsify past symptoms to lend credence to the deception. Reports of prior hallucinations and delusions should be confirmed in past hospital records.

Clinicians should be particularly careful to ask open-ended questions in suspected malingerers and let defendants tell their complete story with few interruptions. Details can be clarified later with specific questions. Inquiries about hallucinations should be carefully phrased to avoid giving clues about the nature of true hallucinations. The clinician should try to ascertain whether the defendant has ever had the opportunity to observe psychotic persons (e.g., during prior employment). Clinicians may feel irritation at being deceived, but any expression of irritation or incredulity is likely to make the malingerer more defensive (Miller and Cartlidge 1972).

Clinicians may modify their interview style when defendants are suspected of malingering psychosis. The interview may be prolonged because fatigue diminishes the malingerer's ability to maintain a counterfeit account (Anderson et al. 1959). Rapid firing of questions increases the likelihood of getting contradictory replies from malingerers, but it also may create confusion among mentally impaired persons. The clinician may obtain additional clues by asking leading questions that emphasize a different illness than the malingerer is trying to portray (Ossipov 1944). Questions about improbable symptoms may be asked to determine whether the malingerer will endorse them. For example, "Have you ever believed that automobiles are members of organized religion?"(Rogers 1987). Another device is to mention, within earshot of the suspected malingerer, some easily imitated symptom that is not present. The sudden appearance of the symptom suggests malingering.

Psychometric Tests for Malingering

The detection of malingering by standardized psychometric testing has been the focus of considerable research in recent years. Although hundreds of psychometric tests are available to examiners, few have been validated in the detection of malingering. The most important of these tests for NGRI evaluations are discussed. The evaluator should keep in mind that absence of evidence of faking on psychometric testing does not mean that a genuinely psychotic defendant could not still malinger an exculpatory delusion or command hallucination.

Structured Interview of Reported Symptoms

Structured interviews show more reliability in detecting malingering than do unstructured interviews because they reduce the degree of variability between interviewers. The Structured Interview of Reported Symptoms (SIRS) was designed by Rogers et al. (1992) specifically to detect malingered psychiatric illness. The test questions were designed on the basis of eight indicators derived from the empirical literature on malingering, and five indicators were derived intuitively. Eight primary scales on the SIRS provide indices of rare symptoms, uncommon symptom pairing, atypical symptoms, disproportionate numbers of obvious symptoms, excessive reporting of everyday problems as symptoms, abnormally high proportion of psychiatric symptoms, excessive reports of symptom severity, and self-reports discrepant with genuine patients. Administration of the SIRS takes between 30 and 60 minutes. Studies report high interrater reliabilities for all scales (r=0.91–1.00). The SIRS has been tested with inpatient, forensic, and correctional samples with consistently high accuracy in discriminating malingerers from truthful evaluees (Rogers 1997).

Before the SIRS is used in NGRI evaluations, the examiner must be familiar with the test manual and have completed several practice administrations. The manual emphasizes the importance of strict adherence to the wording of the questions and avoidance of nonverbal cues. Although the SIRS can be valuable in detecting malingering, no single test should be used as the sole justification for such a critical determination (Rogers 1997).

Minnesota Multiphasic Personality Inventory—Revised

The Minnesota Multiphasic Personality Inventory—2 (MMPI-2) (Hathaway and MicKinley 1989) is the most validated psychometric test for evaluating suspected malingering of psychopathology. This instrument consists of 567 statements that the subject marks "true" if he or she feels the statement applies to him or her and "false" if not. A wide range of "scales" have been developed for evaluation of MMPI-2 responses; a "scale" consists of a selected subset of the 567 test items. Some scales evaluate the subject's consistency in responding to the test items, whereas others have been correlated through research with certain psychological characteristics or types of psychopathology. Use of this instrument during insanity evaluations is recommended when malingering is suspected.

Greene (1997) recommended that after the defendant has completed the answer sheet, the form should be reviewed carefully for omissions. The consistency of item endorsement then must be evaluated with the built-in inconsistency and infrequency scales of the MMPI-2—the VRIN (Variable Response Inconsistency) scale, the F (Infrequency) scale, and the F_B (Back Infrequency) scale. The VRIN scale measures inconsistent patterns of item endorsement and is not affected by the presence of psychopathology. This contrasts with F and F_B, in which elevated scores may be the result of inconsistent endorsement of test items, the presence of psychopathology, or malingering. All three scales should be scored and evaluated before specific malingering indices are assessed. This will avoid confusion of inconsistent item endorsement with malingering to avoid false-positive findings.

Multiple indices of malingering have been proposed for the MMPI-2. The F (infrequency) scale is the traditional index of malingering, although elevations on this scale may result from causes other than malingering (i.e., random responding, severe psychopathology, and inconsistent responding). No consistent cutting score (i.e., minimum score that differentiates truthful responders from malingering responders) on the F scale is associated with malingering in all studies. Most authors recommend use of the F scale in combination with other scales rather than as a single measure of malingering.

Three other infrequency scales have been developed for the MMPI-2: the Infrequency-Psychopathology [F(p); Arbisi and Ben-Porath 1995] scale, the "Fake Bad" scale (FBS; Lees-Haley et al. 1991), and the Inconsistent Response (IR; Sewell and Rogers 1994) scale. The F(p) scale has the highest intercorrelation with the traditional F and F_B scales and is much less sensitive to the presence of psychopathology. Thus elevation on the F(p) scale is strongly suggestive of malingering when inconsistent responding as assessed by the VRIN scale and indiscriminate responding as assessed by the TRIN (True Response Inconsistency) scale can be ruled out. The F(p) scale has shown high reliability in detecting malingered responses in correctional populations and with coached simulators (Bagby et al. 1997). The IR scale has considerable overlap with F(p) and has shown no advantages over this scale in detection of malingering. The FBS was developed to detect malingering in personal injury cases and has a modest to low correlation with other indices of malingering.

Another traditional indicator of malingering is the F–K index (Gough 1950), in which the raw score of the K (Correction) scale is subtracted from the raw F score. Although this index has been used extensively in research, a review of the research with the MMPI-2 indicates that a fairly high cutting score is required to separate honest responders from malingerers. This may be especially important in persons with severe psychiatric disorders because they will have elevated F scale scores and possibly inflated F–K indices. Greene (1997) noted that an F–K score of 22 is required to accurately identify malingerers in mentally ill populations with 95% accuracy, but in persons without mental disorders, an F–K score of zero will meet the same level of accuracy. Although the F–K score has been effective in distinguishing honest from fake-bad MMPI-2 protocols, most research has indicated that this index is not as effective as the F scale in making the discrimination (Graham et al. 1991; Rogers et al. 1995).

The Wiener and Harmon Obvious and Subtle scales attempt to identify inconsistent responding by measuring the evaluee's response to items that are clearly indicative of mental illness, such as suicidality, as opposed to less obvious items, such as early-morning awakening. The difference in T scores (raw scores normalized to a mean of 50 and standard deviation of 10 points) between Obvious and Subtle scales correlates well with other malingering indicators and may be used as an additional indicator of deception (Greene 1997). Graham (2000) noted that the Obvious and Subtle scales have been deleted from the MMPI-2 because they are less accurate than the other standard validity scales [F, F(p)] in identifying fake-good and fake-bad response sets, especially when attempting to differentiate between exaggerated profiles and severe psychopathology.

In summary, the MMPI-2 may be reliably used to detect malingered psychopathology with acceptable accuracy and low rates of false-positive classification. Clinicians who use the MMPI-2 in this manner should consult the literature to determine appropriate cutting scores for the various scales to be used in their evaluation. The chapter by Greene (1997) and the book by Graham (2000) are especially useful in this regard.

The M Test

The M test was developed as a brief screening instrument for malingered schizophrenia (Beaber et al. 1985). Initial validation studies were promising, but subsequent evaluations (Hankins et al. 1993; Smith et al. 1993) found an uncomfortably high false-positive rate in forensic populations. The accuracy can be improved with the use of Rule-In and Rule-Out scales as proposed by Smith and colleagues (1993). Despite these difficulties, the M test continues to be used as a screening instrument for malingered psychotic disorders because it is brief and easy to administer. For NGRI evaluations, the M test adds little compared with more proven tests such as the MMPI-2 and SIRS.

Projective Techniques

The Rorschach Test, the Thematic Apperception Test, the Sentence Completion Test, and the Group Personality Projective Test are psychometric tests that evaluate a person's personality based on the premise that the evaluee "projects" his or her personality onto the intrinsically neutral test. Although proponents claim that projective tests cannot be faked, substantial research has indicated that these tests are vulnerable to successful malingering (Schretlen 1997). Use of projective techniques to evaluate malingering in an insanity defense case is unwise.

Malingered Hallucinations

Defendants reporting hallucinations with any atypical features should be questioned in great detail about the nature of their symptoms. Both patients with psychotic disorder (Goodwin et al. 1971) and patients with acute schizophrenia (Mott et al. 1965; Small et al. 1966) show a 76% rate of hallucinations in at least one sensory modality. The reported incidence of auditory hallucinations in schizophrenic patients is 66% (Mott et al. 1965; Small et al. 1966); 64% of the hallucinating patients described hallucinations in more than one modality (Small et al. 1966). The incidence of visual hallucinations in psychotic patients is estimated at 24% (Mott et al. 1965) to 30% (Small et al. 1966). Hallucinations usually (88%) are associated with delusions (Lewinsohn 1970). Hallucinations are also generally intermittent rather than continuous (Goodwin et al. 1971).

Auditory Hallucinations

Goodwin et al. (1971) described the following characteristics of auditory hallucinations. Of the patients in their study, 75% heard both male and female voices. Two-thirds of the hallucinating subjects could identify the person speaking (Goodwin et al. 1971; Kent and Wahass 1996; Leudar et al. 1997). The message usually was clear; it was vague in only 7% of the patients. The content of the hallucinations was accusatory in about one-third of the patients. Small et al. (1966) reported that the major themes in auditory hallucinations of schizophrenic patients were persecution and instructions.

Auditory hallucinations usually consist of single words or phrases, especially early in the disease process (Leudar et al. 1997; Nayani and David 1996). Hallucinated voices tend to become more complex over time—from single words to entire sentences. The number of voices heard also increases (Leudar et al. 1997). The syntax of long-standing auditory hallucinations usually is in complete sentences and mirrors the syntax typically used by the patient (Nayani and David 1996). In mood disorders, the content of the hallucination usually is mood congruent and related to delusional beliefs (Asaad 1990).

Schizophrenic hallucinations tend to consist of ego-dystonic, derogatory comments about the patient or the activities of others (Goodwin et al. 1971; Leudar et al. 1997; Oulis et al. 1995). Nayani and David (1996) found that the most common hallucinations were simple terms of abuse. Female subjects described terms of abuse conventionally directed at women (e.g., *slut*). Men described male insults such as those imputing homosexuality.

About one-third of the persons with auditory hallucinations reported that voices asked them questions. Voices never sought information such as "What time is it?" or "What is the weather like?" Instead they asked questions such as "Why are you smoking?" or "Why didn't you do your essay?" (Leudar et al. 1997).

Command hallucinations are auditory hallucinations that instruct a person to act in a certain manner. Command hallucinations are easy to fabricate to support an insanity defense (*People v. Schmidt* 1915). They usually will not serve as a basis for an insanity defense in a jurisdiction limited to a McNaughten wrongfulness test unless the defendant had a concurrent delusion that it was right to obey the command. However, in states that have an insanity test with a volitional arm, a command hallucination to commit a crime may qualify for NGRI if the defendant can show that he or she could not refrain from carrying out the act. Most commands to commit dangerous acts are not obeyed. Thus the examiner must be alert to the possibility that a defendant will fake an exculpatory command hallucination or lie about an inability to refrain from a genuine or faked hallucination. Knowledge of the frequency of command hallucinations and the factors associated with obeying commands will be helpful in examining the authenticity of such claims.

Hellerstein et al. (1987) found in a retrospective chart review that 38% of all patients with auditory hallucinations reported commands. Studies of schizophrenic auditory hallucinations found that 30%–64% included commands or instructions (Goodwin et al. 1971; Hellerstein et al. 1987; Mott et al. 1965; Small et al. 1966). Command hallucinations occurred in 30% (Goodwin et al. 1971) to 40% (Mott et al. 1965) of alcoholic withdrawal hallucinations. Patients with affective disorders reported that 46% of their hallucinations were commands (Goodwin et al. 1971).

Hellerstein et al. (1987) found that the content of command hallucinations was as follows: 52% suicide, 5% homicide, 12% nonlethal injury of self or others, 14% nonviolent acts, and 17% unspecified. The research method of reviewing charts, rather than making direct inquiries, probably increased the relative proportion of violent commands because these are more likely to be charted.

Earlier research suggested that patients generally ignore hallucinatory commands (Goodwin et al. 1971; Hellerstein et al. 1987). However, Junginger (1990) reported that 39% of the patients with command hallucinations obeyed them. Those patients with hallucination-related delusions and hallucinatory voices that they could identify were more likely to comply with the commands. Kasper et al. (1996) reported that 84% of the psychiatric inpatients with command hallucinations had obeyed them within the last 30 days. Rogers et al. (1990) found that 44% of a forensic population with command hallucinations reported that they frequently responded with unquestioning obedience. Among those reporting command hallucinations in a second forensic population, 74% indicated that they acted in response to some of their commands during the episode of illness (Thompson et al. 1992).

Junginger (1995) studied the relation between command hallucinations and dangerousness. He found that 43% of the subjects reported full compliance with their most recent command hallucination. Compliance with commands is much less likely if the commands are dangerous (Junginger 1995; Kasper et al. 1996). A defendant alleging an isolated command hallucination in the absence of other psychotic symptoms should be viewed with great suspicion. Noncommand auditory hallucinations (85%) and delusions (75%) usually are present with command hallucinations (Thompson et al. 1992).

Leudar et al. (1997) found that most patients in their study engaged in an internal dialogue with their hallucinations. Many were able to cope with chronic hallucinations by incorporating them into their daily life as a kind of internal adviser. They considered their advice in the context of the moment. Interestingly, sometimes the hallucinated voices would insist on certain actions after the patient refused to carry them out. The voices would rephrase their requests, speak louder, or curse the patient for being noncompliant. In contrast, malingerers are more likely to claim that they were compelled to obey commands without further consideration. Some malingerers describe voices in a stilted manner, such as "Go commit a sex offense." Other malingerers describe far-fetched commands, such as a robber who alleged that (malingered) voices kept screaming, "Stick up, stick up, stick up!"

Defendants suspected of feigning auditory hallucinations should be asked what they do to make the voices go away or diminish in intensity. Genuine patients often are able to stop auditory hallucinations when their schizophrenia is in remission but not during the acute phase of their illness (Larkin 1979). Frequent coping strategies among actual schizophrenic patients are 1) engaging in specific activities (working or watching television), 2) changing posture (e.g., lying down or walking), 3) seeking out interpersonal contact, and 4) taking medication (Falloon and Talbot 1981; Kanas and Barr 1984). Schizophrenic hallucinations tend to diminish when patients are involved in activities (Goodwin et al. 1971).

The suspected malingerer also may be asked what makes the voices worse. Eighty percent of the persons with genuine hallucinations reported that being alone worsened their hallucinations (Nayani and David 1996). Voices also were worsened by listening to the radio and watching television (Leudar et al. 1997). Television news programs were particularly hallucinogenic.

Visual Hallucinations

Visual hallucinations are volunteered much more often (46% vs. 4%) by malingerers than by genuinely psychotic individuals (Cornell and Hawk 1989). Dramatic, atypical visual hallucinations should definitely arouse suspicions of malingering (Powell 1991).

Visual hallucinations usually are of normal-sized people and are seen in color (Goodwin et al. 1971). Alcohol-induced hallucinations are more likely to contain animals (Goodwin et al. 1971). Visual hallucinations in psychotic disorders appear suddenly and typically without prodromata (Asaad and Shapiro 1986). Psychotic hallucinations usually do not change if the eyes are closed or open. In contrast, drug-induced hallucinations are more readily seen with the eyes closed or in darkened surroundings (Asaad and Shapiro 1986).

Occasionally, small (lilliputian) people are seen in alcoholic, organic (Cohen et al. 1994), or toxic psychosis (D.J. Lewis 1961), especially anticholinergic drug toxicity (Asaad 1990). The little people are sometimes 1 or 2 inches tall and at other times are up to 4 feet in height. Lilliputian hallucinations are rarely seen in schizophrenia (Leroy 1922). Only 5% of the visual hallucinations in the Goodwin et al. (1971) study consisted of miniature or giant figures.

Malingered Delusions

Delusions are not merely false beliefs that cannot be changed by logic. A delusion is a false statement made in an inappropriate context and, most important, with inappropriate justification. Nondelusional people can give reasons, can engage in a dialogue, and can consider the possibilities of doubt. Persons with true delusions cannot provide adequate reasons for their statements.

Delusions vary in content, theme, degree of certainty, degree of systemization, and degree of relevance to the person's life in general. The more intelligent the person, the more elaborate his or her delusional system usually will be. According to Spitzer (1992), most delusions involve the following general themes: disease (somatic delusions), grandiosity, jealousy, love (erotomania), persecution, religion, being poisoned, and being possessed. Delusions of nihilism, poverty, sin, and guilt are commonly seen in depression. Technical delusions refer to the influence of items such as telephones, telepathy, and hypnosis. By technical means, signals and voices can be transmitted to patients. Delusions of technical content occur seven times more often in men than in women (Kraus 1994).

Persecutory delusions are more likely to be acted on than are any other type of delusion (Wessely et al. 1993). Persons who report delusional symptoms involving perceived threat or control override are more likely to act aggressively. These delusions (Link and Stueve 1994; Swanson et al. 1997) include the belief that 1) one's mind is dominated by forces beyond one's control, 2) thoughts are being put into one's head, 3) there are people who wish one harm, and 4) one is being followed. Examples of delusions that are not associated with increased aggression are 1) feeling dead, dissolved, or not existing; 2) feeling that one's thoughts are broadcast; and 3) feeling that thoughts are being removed by an external force. The MacArthur Violence Risk Assessment Study, however, did not find that threat control override delusions were associated with more violence; in fact the authors found that no delusions were associated with an increase in violence in the first year after patients were released from psychiatric hospitals (Appelbaum et al. 2000).

A malingering defendant may claim the sudden onset of a delusion. In reality, systematized delusions usually take several weeks to develop. As true delusions diminish, they first become somewhat less relevant to the everyday life of the patient, but the patient still adheres to the delusional belief. A decrease in preoccupation with delusions may be the first change seen with adequate treatment. In a later stage, the patient might admit to the possibility of error but only as a possibility. Only much later will the patient concede that the ideas were, in fact, delusions (Sachs et al. 1974). Thus, malingering should be suspected if a defendant claims that a delusion suddenly appeared or disappeared.

In assessing the genuineness of delusions, their content and associated behavior should be considered. The content of feigned delusions is generally persecutory, occasionally grandiose, but seldom self-deprecating (Davidson 1952; East 1927). Malingerers' behavior usually does not conform to their alleged delusions, whereas acute schizophrenic behavior usually does. However, "burned out" schizophrenic patients may no longer behave in a manner consistent with their delusions after a year. Table 5–1 summarizes suspect hallucinations and suspect delusions.

Table 5–1.   Suspect hallucinations and delusions

Malingering should be suspected if any of the following are observed:

Auditory hallucinations

Continuous rather than intermittent hallucinations

Vague or inaudible hallucinations

Hallucinations not associated with delusions

Stilted language reported in hallucinations

Inability to state strategies to diminish voices

Hallucinated questions seeking information

Self-report that all command hallucinations were obeyed

Visual hallucinations

Black and white rather than color

Dramatic, atypical visions

Schizophrenic hallucinations that change when the eyes are closed

Only visual hallucinations in schizophrenia

Miniature or giant figures

Visions unrelated to delusions or auditory hallucinations

Delusions

Abrupt onset or termination

Eagerness to call attention to delusions

Conduct not consistent with delusions

Bizarre content without disordered thinking

Malingered Psychosis

All malingerers are actors who portray psychoses as they understand them (Ossipov 1944). Malingerers often overact their part (Wachspress et al. 1953). Malingerers sometimes mistakenly believe that the more bizarrely they behave, the more psychotic they will appear. As observed by Jones and Llewellyn (1917, p. 80), the malingerer

> sees less than the blind, he hears less than the deaf, and he is more lame than the paralyzed. Determined that his insanity shall not lack multiple and obvious signs, he, so to speak, crowds the canvas, piles symptom upon symptom and so outstrips madness itself, attaining to a but clumsy caricature of his assumed role.

Malingerers are eager to call attention to their illnesses, in contrast to schizophrenic patients, who are often reluctant to discuss their symptoms (Ritson and Forest 1970). Some malingerers limit their symptoms to repeatedly volunteering one or two blatant "delusions" (MacDonald 1976). One malingerer stated that he was an "insane lunatic" when he killed his parents at the behest of hallucinations that "told me to kill in my demented state." Malingering defendants may try to take control of the interview and behave in an intimidating, bizarre manner. The clinician should avoid the temptation to terminate such an interview prematurely. Malingerers sometimes accuse clinicians of regarding them as faking. Such behavior is extremely rare in genuinely psychotic persons.

It is more difficult for malingerers to successfully imitate the form than the content of schizophrenic thinking (Sherman et al. 1975). Derailment, neologisms, and incoherent word salads are rarely simulated. Positive symptoms of schizophrenia are faked more often than negative symptoms.

Malingerers give more approximate answers to questions than do schizophrenic patients, such as "There are 53 weeks in the year" (Bash and Alpert 1980; Powell 1991). Defendants malingering psychosis often choose to fake intellectual deficits also (Bash and Alpert 1980; Powell 1991; Schretlen 1988). For example, a man who completed 1 year of college alleged that he did not know the colors of the American flag. Malingerers are more likely to answer "I don't know" to detailed questions about psychotic symptoms, such as hallucinations and delusions. This response may simply mean that they do not know what to say when questioned about the details of their alleged delusions and hallucinations. When asked whether an alleged voice was male or female, one malingerer replied, "It was *probably* a man's voice."

A crime without apparent motive, such as killing a stranger, lends credence to the presence of true mental disease. Genuine psychotic explanations for rape, robbery, or check forging are unusual. Malingerers are more likely to have contradictions in their accounts of their illness. The contradictions may be evident within the story itself or between the malingerer's version and other evidence. When malingerers are caught in contradictions, they may either sulk or laugh with embarrassment (MacDonald 1976).

Defendants who have true schizophrenia may malinger additional symptoms to escape criminal responsibility. These are the most difficult cases to accurately assess. Clinicians have a lower index of suspicion for malingering in these patients because of the history of psychiatric hospitalizations and the presence of residual schizophrenic symptoms. These defendants are able to draw on their prior experience with hallucinations and their observations of other psychotic people. They know what questions to expect from clinicians. If they spend time in a forensic psychiatric hospital, they are likely to learn how to modify their story to fit the exact criteria for an insanity defense. Clinicians should not think of malingering and psychosis from an either-or perspective (Rogers et al. 1994). Defendants with genuine psychosis must be scrutinized for superimposed malingered symptoms.

Malingered Insanity

In assessing defendants for criminal responsibility, clinicians must determine whether defendants report malingered symptoms at the time of the act and/or malinger symptoms at the time of the examination (Hall 1982) (see Table 5–2). Some malingerers mistakenly believe that they must show ongoing symptoms of psychosis to succeed with an insanity defense. When defendants report psychiatric symptoms at the time of their examination, the clinician has the opportunity to determine whether the alleged symptoms are consistent with genuine illness and current psychological testing results.

Table 5–2. Conceptualization of malingered insanity

Faking psychosis while actually committing the crime (rare)
In the evaluation, faking having had psychosis during the crime and either
   Claiming to be well now or
   Still faking psychosis
Actually being psychotic during the crime but superimposing faked exculpatory
  symptoms at the evaluation; either
   Still psychotic at the evaluation or
   No longer psychotic at the evaluation

Faking mental illness during the crime itself is a rare occurrence. Persons who plan to commit a crime ordinarily do not plan to use an insanity defense. In fact persons found NGRI spend slightly more time in a psychiatric hospital than they would have spent in prison if they had been convicted (Perlin 1989–1990). More often, a defendant will discover after he or she is arrested that the prosecutor has sufficient evidence to convict him or her. Because a plea of not guilty will not succeed, the defendant then may decide to fake insanity. However, by that point the defendant already may have done several things that indicate that he or she knew the wrongfulness of his or her act when he or she committed it. For example, a defendant may have wiped off fingerprints, hid the murder weapon, or lied to the police. Thus, even if a defendant is skillful in faking mental illness, he or she still may be adjudicated legally sane because of evidence that he or she knew that his or her act was wrong.

Faking insanity after a crime can be facilitated by jailhouse discussions of "beating the rap," television reports, or research in public or prison libraries (Jaffe and Sharma 1998; Resnick 1997). Case histories and anecdotal reports that portray skilled malingering abound in both the clinical and the forensic literature (Abrahamson 1983; Coons 1991; Faust et al.

1988). In cases in which the stakes are high enough to pursue a malingered insanity defense, the forensic evaluator must assume that the malingerer has planned his or her "strategy" in detail and may even have been coached.

Several clues can assist clinicians in the detection of fraudulent NGRI defenses (see Table 5–3). A psychotic explanation for a crime should be questioned if the new offense matches the same pattern as the defendant's previous convictions. Malingering should be suspected in defendants pleading insanity if a partner was involved in the crime. Most accomplices of normal intelligence will not participate in psychotically motivated crimes. The clinician may explore the validity of such a claim by questioning the codefendant. In a study at the Michigan Center for Forensic Psychiatry, 98% of the successful NGRI acquittees acted alone (Thompson et al. 1992). A malingerer may tell a far-fetched story to fit the facts of a crime into a mental disease model. One malingerer with prior armed robbery convictions claimed that he robbed only on the commands of auditory hallucinations and gave away all the stolen money to "bums" in the street.

Table 5–3.   Clues to malingered insanity defenses

Malingering should be suspected if any of the following are present:
   A nonpsychotic, alternative, rational motive for the crime
   Suspicious hallucinations or delusions (see Table 5–1)
   Current crime fitting an established pattern of prior criminal conduct
   Absence of any active or subtle signs of psychosis during the evaluation
   Report of a sudden irresistible impulse
   Presence of a partner in the crime
   Double denial of responsibility (e.g., disavowal of the crime plus attributing the
      crime to psychosis)
   Far-fetched story of psychosis to explain the crime
   Alleged intellectual deficit coupled with alleged psychosis
   Alleged illness inconsistent with documented level of functioning

---

Malingering defendants are more likely to present themselves as blameless within their feigned illness (Resnick 1984). This tendency was illustrated by a man who pled insanity to a charge of stabbing an 11-year-old boy 60 times with an ice pick. He reported that for 1 week before the homicide, he was constantly pursued by an "indistinct, human-like, black blob." He stated that he was sexually excited and intended to force homosexual acts on the victim but abandoned his plan when the boy began to cry. When he started to leave, 10 faces in the bushes began chanting, "Kill him, kill him, kill him." He yelled, "No," and struck out at the faces with an ice pick. The next thing he knew, "the victim was covered with blood." The autopsy showed a cluster of stab wounds in the victim's head and neck—which was inconsistent with the defendant's claim that he struck out randomly at multiple faces in the bushes. His visual hallucination was atypical. His version showed a double avoidance of responsibility: 1) the faces told him to kill, and 2) he claimed to have attacked the hallucinated faces, not the victim. After his conviction, he confessed to six unsolved sadistic homosexual killings.

Malingered Amnesia

Complaints of memory difficulties are common in criminal cases. Defendants may report that they are unable to remember events from their past (retrograde amnesia), that they are unable to retain new information (anterograde amnesia), or that they have circumscribed amnesia for the crime itself (dissociative amnesia). Although legal decisions (*Wilson v. United States* 1968) have dictated that permanent amnesia for a crime may not render the defendant incompetent to stand trial, amnesia may be faked by a defendant in an attempt to evade criminal responsibility.

Dissociative amnesia is an episodic disorder characterized by the sudden onset of memory loss involving important personal information, usually in response to severe emotional trauma. Sometimes undisturbed "islands" of memory occur within the amnesic period. The disorder may persist for more than a year without resolution. When evaluating claims of dissociative amnesia, the clinician should seek confirmation of previous episodes of amnesia because the disorder tends to recur over the person's life span. Histrionic personality traits with the defense mechanism of denial are likely to be associated with dissociative amnesia, whereas antisocial personality traits militate toward faked amnesia. Patients with genuine amnesia tend to be disturbed by their memory loss and will be agreeable to attempts to regain it, whereas malingerers are more likely to insist that no amount of hints will improve their recall (Schacter 1986).

Defendants who malinger insanity for the commission of a crime or fake psychosis commonly also pretend to have ongoing cognitive deficits (anterograde amnesia) (Brandt et al. 1985). They may claim the loss of procedural memory (e.g., how to ride a bicycle or drive a car), but this type of memory is not actually affected by psychosis or dissociative amnesia. Such malingerers sometimes perform more poorly on portions of an interview labeled "memory testing" than they do in recalling other memories.

Psychometric techniques used to detect faked memory problems use one of two basic designs: *floor effect* and *forced choice*. In the floor-effect strategy, the test is designed to be simple but appear difficult on the presumption that malingerers will overplay their deficit (Rogers et al. 1993). An example of this is the Rey 15-item test.

To administer the Rey test, a test card is presented to the defendant; it contains five rows of three related items each (e.g., numerals, Roman numerals, letters). The difficulty of the test is emphasized in the verbal instructions. In reality, only severely impaired individuals will fail to recall most of the test items. Lezak (1983) recommended that anyone unable to remember at least 9 items should be suspected of malingering amnesia. However, later studies of the Rey 15-item test have shown low specificity and sensitivity with a variety of cutting scores (Guilmette et al. 1994; Schretlen et al. 1991). Griffin et al. (1997) suggested use of a redesigned version of the test with a more formalized scoring procedure, but further studies of this redesigned test are not available. The Rey test may be used in screening for malingered amnesia, but it is not reliable as a solitary test to diagnose malingering with acceptable accuracy. Concerns about low specificity and sensitivity of this and other floor-effect tests have spurred the development of newer tests based on forced-choice testing strategies such as symptom-validity testing.

In symptom-validity testing, the evaluee is presented with a series of stimuli, followed by a forced-choice test of item recognition. Persons who perform statistically significantly worse than chance are presumed to be malingering because a 50% accuracy rate would be expected simply by guessing with no recall at all. The Test of Memory Malingering (TOMM) was developed by Tombaugh (1996) as a specific test for malingered memory problems. The test exposes the evaluee to pictures of 50 common objects. In two further trials, the evaluee is asked to choose the object seen in the first trial rather than a novel object. Development of the TOMM was prompted by difficulties with traditional forced-choice approaches, such as reliance on below-chance performance without more precise cutoff criteria, high false-negative rates, and questionable face validity. In a series of experiments reported by Rees et al. (1998), the TOMM was able to detect malingering of memory deficits with high sensitivity and specificity in a variety of populations. Its use in forensic evaluations has not yet been validated, but it should be considered as an adjunct to traditional memory testing techniques when malingering is suspected.

Forced-choice recognition also can be used to assess the validity of circumscribed dissociative amnesia for a crime. Thirty pieces of information about the crime are taken from police reports that would only be known to the perpetrator of the crime. Thirty incorrect distractor items are added randomly. If a defendant gets a large percentage of the forced-choice questions wrong (well beyond the 50% one would expect with no knowledge), it provides evidence that the defendant actually remembers the crime (Frederick et al. 1995).

Malingered Posttraumatic Stress Disorder

PTSD is extremely easy to fake because it is defined almost completely by subjective criteria. Lists of symptoms associated with PTSD can be found easily in books, in magazine articles, on the Internet, and even as part of popular rap songs. Although the usual motive to malinger PTSD is financial gain, criminal defendants also may claim PTSD to exculpate themselves from criminal responsibility. To evaluate the genuineness of alleged PTSD, the clinician must examine the reasonableness of the relation between the reported symptoms and the stressor, the time elapsed between the stressor and the development of symptoms, and the relation between current symptoms and psychiatric problems before the stressor.

Detection of malingered PTSD requires a meticulous history of current symptoms, treatment efforts, and careful corroboration of information. In addition, the clinician must obtain a detailed history of the defendant's living patterns and psychiatric symptoms preceding the stressor. Collateral information is essential in establishing the presence of symptoms—for example, co-workers and friends can describe the defendant's typical daily patterns, and sleeping partners can comment on the presence of recurrent nightmares, body movement, or sleeplessness.

The examiner should insist on detailed descriptions of symptoms. Malingering defendants may know which symptoms to report but may be unable to give convincing descriptions or examples from their personal life. Behavioral observations during the examination may assist in evaluating symptoms of irritability, exaggerated startle response, and difficulty concentrating. Malingering defendants also may exaggerate the severity of the stressor. Combat stressors should be authenticated by military unit logs. Malingerers may give a neat recitation of symptoms seemingly taken straight from the diagnostic manual. In addition, malingerers are likely to concentrate on reliving the trauma, whereas genuine PTSD patients focus more on the phenomenon of psychic numbing (Melton 1984).

In true posttraumatic dreams, the typical pattern is a few dreams that reenact the traumatic event, followed by nightmares that are "variations" on the traumatic theme in which other elements of the defendant's daily life are incorporated into the dreams (Garfield 1987). Malingerers may claim repetitive dreams that exactly re-create the trauma night after night without variation. Posttraumatic dreams are frequently accompanied by body movements and thrashing in bed, in contrast to nontraumatic dreams (van der Kolk et al. 1984). The person may awake suddenly in a state of panic. Middle insomnia is specifically associated with PTSD, as opposed to initial insomnia or early awakening (Mellman et al. 1995).

The themes of intrusive recollections and dreams are different in true and malingered PTSD. Military veterans with combat PTSD often report themes of helplessness, guilt, or rage. Dreams in true PTSD generally convey a theme of helplessness with regard to the particular traumatic events that occurred during combat. In malingered PTSD, the themes of intrusive recollections are more often anger toward generalized authority; dreams emphasize themes of grandiosity and power (Melton 1984). The reexperienced "trauma" in malingerers often is not consistent with their self-reports of the original trauma (D. Smith, personal communication, May 1987).

Differences have been observed between veterans with true and malingered PTSD in their expression and acknowledgment of feelings. In true PTSD, the veteran often denies or has numbed the emotional effect of combat. In malingered PTSD, the veteran often will make efforts to convince the clinician how emotionally traumatizing combat was for him or her by "acting out" the alleged feelings. The true PTSD veteran generally *downplays* symptoms, whereas the malingerer *overplays* them. For instance, the veteran with true PTSD tries not to bring attention to his or her hyper-alertness and suspicious eye movements. In contrast, the PTSD malingerer presents his or her suspiciousness with a dramatic quality, as if he or she were trying to draw attention to it. Another example is that the PTSD malingerer may volunteer that he or she thinks of nothing but combat and "relishes" telling his or her combat memories (Melton 1984).

An important characteristic of PTSD is the avoidance of environmental conditions associated with the trauma. For example, the PTSD veteran may stay home on hot rainy days because of the resemblance to Vietnam weather. Camping may be avoided because the veteran finds himself or herself looking for trip wires in the bush. In addition, crowds may be avoided because combat usually occurred "in a crowd." In malingered PTSD, the veteran is unlikely to report having such postcombat reactions to environmental stimuli (Melton 1984).

Psychological testing is generally unhelpful in detecting malingered PTSD. Studies show that the disorder can be feigned convincingly on most tests (Resnick 1997). Psychophysiological testing, which includes measurements of heart rates, blood pressure, skin conductance, and muscle tension in response to script-driven imagery of the reported trauma, has proven more useful in studies but cannot be used alone to classify malingering of PTSD hyperarousal symptoms (Orr et al. 1993; Pitman et al. 1994; Shalev et al. 1993).

Malingered Dissociative Identity Disorder

Controversy Surrounding the Diagnosis of Dissociative Identity Disorder

In DSM-IV-TR, dissociative identity disorder is defined by "the presence of two or more distinct identities or personality states (each with its own relatively enduring pattern of perceiving, relating to, and thinking about the environment and self)" that "recurrently take control of the person's behavior" (American Psychiatric Association 2000, p. 529). An additional criterion is an "inability to recall important personal information that is too extensive to be explained by ordinary forgetfulness" (p. 529). Dissociative identity disorder has been successfully used to justify an insanity defense on numerous occasions (Steinberg et al. 1993).

Critics of dissociative identity disorder assert that the disorder is easy to malinger and may be largely iatrogenic in susceptible patients (Coons 1991; Orne et al. 1984). Others point out that even in the presence of dissociative identity disorder, there is no reason to assume that it would affect a person's ability to understand wrongfulness or refrain from wrongful behaviors (Dinwiddie et al. 1993). Authors who argue persuasively for the existence of dissociative identity disorder as a separate diagnostic entity (Saks 1994) admit that objective measures such as psychological testing, memory testing, and physiological tests cannot, by themselves, conclusively differentiate dissociative identity disorder from other forms of psychopathology. These factors make dissociative identity disorder a difficult diagnostic entity even in the presence of an ongoing clinical relationship (Putnam 1989) and even more so in the highly charged atmosphere of an insanity evaluation.

Evaluation of Defendants Claiming Dissociative Identity Disorder

Clinicians who work frequently with patients who have dissociative identity disorder claim that malingerers would have difficulty replicating the complex spectrum of symptoms seen in these patients (Kluft 1987; D.O. Lewis and Bard 1991). Evaluators who lack substantial clinical experience with patients who have dissociative identity disorder may be ill prepared to distinguish malingerers from those with genuine dissociative identity disorder in a forensic context. Examiners may be easily misled by a convincing performance, especially without collateral confirmation (Coons 1991). Therefore, forensic evaluators must be prepared to conduct an extensive evaluation of any defendant claiming dissociative identity disorder. When dissociative identity disorder serves as a basis for an insanity defense, prosecutors will carefully scrutinize psychiatric testimony (D.O. Lewis and Bard 1991). Reliance on personal intuition can be disastrous for the forensic examiner (Coons 1991; Kluft 1987).

When dissociative identity disorder is claimed or suspected, the evaluator should seek access to all sources of independent information. This should include interviews with family members, friends, and co-workers of the defendant. The evaluator must be careful to avoid "fishing" for confirmatory data by asking leading questions. Documentation of dissociation should be sought: for example, changes in preoffense handwriting samples from checks, journals, and so forth; provision of different personal information (e.g., age, name) on applications or medical information forms without an obvious motivation (such as using an alias); periods of amnesia or bizarre behaviors noted by others in the absence of substance abuse; and prominent changes in voice and demeanor on multiple occasions. Because many of these changes occur in individuals without dissociative identity disorder on occasion, the evaluator must seek detailed information to verify a persistent pattern of dissociation.

Clinical Interview of Defendants Claiming Dissociative Identity Disorder

During the interview, defendants malingering dissociative identity disorder are apt to claim stereotyped "good/bad" divisions between personalities; few will claim more than three personalities (Coons 1991; Kluft 1987). Malingerers will be eager to blame their crimes on their "evil alters" and will emphasize their symptoms, in contrast to legitimate patients' tendencies to downplay their illness and accept blame when confronted with evidence of guilt. Unsophisticated malingerers usually will not report symptoms common to patients with dissociative identity disorder such as not being able to account for the presence of objects in their possession, severe headaches, refractory somatic symptoms, frequently being called a liar as a child, and abrupt changes in school or work performance (Kluft 1987).

Malingerers may playact one or more alternate personalities during a brief interview, whereas genuine unforced dissociation typically occurs between 2.5 and 4 hours after the start of an extended interview (Kluft 1987). Malingered presentations of alternate personalities are more likely to be inconsistent and stereotyped; differences in thoughts and memories usually are cognitive. In contrast, differences between true alternate personalities are fairly consistent and have affective as well as cognitive components. Inpatient evaluation may determine that "switching" and other dissociative symptoms do not occur spontaneously and appear limited to periods when the defendant is aware of being observed.

Attention to nonverbal cues in the evaluation of defendants claiming dissociative identity disorder can be problematic. Lying to please a therapist or to protect a perceived self-interest is common in patients with dissociative identity disorder. Catching the defendant in a lie, therefore, does not by itself confirm malingering. A sense of bewilderment and confusion about experiences is frequently part of dissociative identity disorder, and patients' explanations of their behavior may appear logically inconsistent or preposterous (Kluft 1987; D.O. Lewis et al. 1997).

Other Malingered Disorders

Malingered Mental Retardation

Defendants may attempt to portray themselves as mentally retarded, but this is infrequently successful. A review of school records will identify adequate past intellectual functioning. Military and work records can be used to document a level of psychosocial functioning inconsistent with significant intellectual impairment. During IQ testing, malingerers will frequently miss "easy" questions but answer more difficult questions correctly. Their test results often show wide "scatter" and inconsistent responding.

Malingered Mood Disorders

Depression may be malingered by defendants pursuing an insanity defense. The Beck Depression Inventory and the Hamilton Rating Scale for Depression rely solely on self-report and thus are quite easy to malinger. Although malingerers will claim depressed mood, they are less likely to report subtle symptoms such as poor concentration, early-morning awakening, diurnal variations in mood, psychomotor retardation, or loss of interest in sex. Malingerers may report difficulty falling asleep, but sleep disturbances in depression more typically involve multiple awakenings, especially in the early morning hours. Malingerers rarely present the furrowed brow and restricted range of affect seen in severe depression.

Malingering of mania is unusual. It is likely to be helpful only in those states that have an insanity test with a volitional arm. Defendants may claim a history of manic symptoms, but it is difficult to sustain the flight of ideas, pressured speech, grandiose mood, increased psychomotor activity, and decreased need for sleep seen in true mania. Inpatient evaluation of suspected malingerers usually indicates that these symptoms are absent or present only during periods of face-to-face evaluation. The person most likely to succeed with malingered mania is the genuinely bipolar defendant who falsely claims that he or she was manic at the time of the act. Close scrutiny of witness and police accounts is critical in these cases.

Malingered Mutism

Malingered mutism is difficult to maintain for extended periods, but some defendants will attempt to avoid evaluation by pretending to be unable to talk. Genuine mutism is seen primarily in mood disorders, schizophrenia, and medical disorders (e.g., head injuries, Wernicke's encephalopathy, and diabetic ketosis) (Altshuler et al. 1986). It may occur with or without catatonia. Malingered catatonia is extremely difficult to sustain and usually can be unmasked by close observation in an inpatient setting. It may result from extreme paranoia or extended isolation and has been produced by corticosteroids and antihypertensive agents (Altshuler et al. 1986). It also can be produced by drugs, most notably phencyclidine. Persons with true mutism usually try to communicate with gestures and noises, but malingerers rarely do so. Faked mutism sometimes can be detected by awakening the defendant suddenly from a deep sleep and asking a simple question; the malingerer may reply before remembering to be mute.

Sometimes it is difficult to distinguish malingered mutism from a conversion disorder. The key distinction between the two is whether the mutism is under the defendant's voluntary control. The exact details of the onset of mutism are important because a crime that involved "unspeakable horror" may have been traumatic enough to induce a conversion disorder. Persons with true conversion mutism usually can write and may be able to speak in whispers (Cummings 1994). They are likely to have a history of past conversion symptoms, show evidence of repression and dissociation, and be suggestible. In contrast, a malingerer is more likely to have a history of antisocial conduct, lying, and past malingering (Daniel and Resnick 1987).

Malingered Ganser Syndrome

Ganser syndrome is seen most often in convicted prisoners, so it infrequently comes up in the evaluation of defendants pleading insanity (Davidson 1952). In Ganser syndrome, an examinee provides absurd answers and approximate answers to questions (such as $2+2=5$), a phenomenon known as *vorbeireden* (German, "talk around " or "evade" [a point, a question]). Ganser syndrome is now classified among the dissociative disorders in DSM-IV-TR. Some authors (Anderson et al. 1959) concluded that Ganser syndrome is a form of malingering. Others pointed out that Ganser's original description of the syndrome included other symptoms, such as clouding of consciousness and amnesia (Whitlock 1967) and that Ganser himself was convinced that his patients were not malingering. Nonetheless, some research showed that giving approximate answers is common in malingering and is not unique to Ganser syndrome (Anderson et al. 1959; Powell 1991). Evaluators still should suspect malingering in any NGRI defendant who gives approximate answers.

Conclusion

The insanity defense was created to maintain the dignity and fundamental fairness of the criminal process while meeting society's need for justice and protection. The goal of this chapter is to assist clinicians in assessing the veracity of alleged symptoms to ensure that the insanity defense is not misused by clever criminals. Indeed, clinicians who do insanity evaluations bear considerable responsibility to assist society in differentiating the truly insane from those with manufactured madness.

References

Abrahamson D: The Mind of the Accused: A Psychiatrist in the Courtroom. New York, Simon & Schuster, 1983

Adelman RM, Howard A: Expert testimony on malingering: the admissibility of clinical procedures for the detection of deception. Behav Sci Law 2:5–20, 1984

Altshuler LL, Cummings JL, Mills MJ: Mutism: review, differential diagnosis and report of 22 cases. Am J Psychiatry 143:1409–1414, 1986

American Law Institute: Model Penal Code, Proposed Official Draft. Philadelphia, PA, American Law Institute, 1962

American Psychiatric Association: Diagnostic and Statistical Manual of Mental Disorders, 4th Edition, Text Revision. Washington, DC, American Psychiatric Association, 2000

Anderson EW, Trethowan WH, Kenna JC: An experimental investigation of simulation and pseudo-dementia. Acta Psychiatrica et Neurologica Scandinavia 34:1–132, 1959

Appelbaum PS, Robbins PC, Monahan J: Violence and delusions: data from the MacArthur Violence Risk Assessment Study. Am J Psychiatry 157:566–572, 2000

Arbisi PA, Ben-Porath YS: An MMPI-2 infrequent response scale for use with psychopathological populations: the Infrequency-Psychopathology Scale, F(p). Psychological Assessment 7:424–431, 1995

Asaad G: Hallucinations in Clinical Psychiatry: A Guide for Mental Health Professionals. New York, Brunner/Mazel, 1990

Asaad G, Shapiro B: Hallucinations: theoretical and clinical overview. Am J Psychiatry 143:1088–1097, 1986

Bagby RM, Rogers R, Nicholson R, et al: Does clinical training facilitate feigning schizophrenia on the MMPI-2? Psychological Assessment 9:108–112, 1997

Bash I, Alpert M: The determination of malingering. Ann N Y Acad Sci 347:86–99, 1980

Beaber RJ, Marston A, Michelli J, et al: A brief test for measuring malingering in schizophrenic individuals. Am J Psychiatry 142:1478–1481, 1985

Brandt J, Rubinsky E, Lassen G: Uncovering malingered amnesia. Ann N Y Acad Sci 444:502–503, 1985

Brittain RP: The history of legal medicine: the assizes of Jerusalem. Medicolegal Journal 34:72–73, 1966

Cohen MA, Alfonso CA, Haque MM: Lilliputian hallucinations and medical illness. Gen Hosp Psychiatry 16:141–143, 1994

Collinson GD: A Treatise on the Law Concerning Idiots, Lunatics, and Other Persons Non Compo Mentis. London, W Reed, 1812

Coons P: Iatrogenesis and malingering of multiple personality disorder in the forensic evaluation of homicide defendants. Psychiatr Clin North Am 14:757–768, 1991

Cornell DG, Hawk GL: Clinical presentation of malingerers diagnosed by experienced forensic psychologists. Law Hum Behav 13:375–383, 1989

Cummings JL: Mutism: evaluation and differential diagnosis. Psychiatric Times, November 1994, pp 24–25

Daniel AE, Resnick PJ: Mutism, malingering, and competency to stand trial. Bulletin of the American Academy of Psychiatry and the Law 15:301–308, 1987

Davidson HA: Forensic Psychiatry. New York, Ronald Press, 1952

Dinwiddie MD, North CS, Yutzy SH: Multiple personality disorder: scientific and medicolegal issues. Bulletin of the American Academy of Psychiatry and the Law 21:69–79, 1993

East NW: An Introduction to Forensic Psychiatry in the Criminal Courts. London, J & A Churchill, 1927

Ekman P: Telling Lies: Clues to Deceit in the Marketplace, Politics, and Marriage. New York, WW Norton, 1985

Falloon I, Talbot R: Persistent auditory hallucinations: coping mechanisms and implications for management. Psychol Med 2:329–339, 1981

Faust D, Hart K, Guilmette TJ, et al: Neuropsychologists' capacity to detect adolescent malingerers. Professional Psychology: Research and Practice 19:508–515, 1988

Frederick RI, Carter M, Powel J: Adapting symptom validity testing to evaluate suspicious complaints of amnesia in medicolegal evaluations. Bulletin of the American Academy of Psychiatry and the Law 23:231–237, 1995

Garfield P: Nightmares in the sexually abused female teenager. Psychiatric Journal of the University of Ottowa 12:93–97, 1987

Goodwin DW, Alderson P, Rosenthal R: Clinical significance of hallucinations in psychiatric disorders: a study of 116 hallucinatory patients. Arch Gen Psychiatry 24:76–80, 1971

Gough HG: The *F* minus *K* dissimulation index for the MMPI. Journal of Consulting Psychology 14:408–413, 1950

Graham JR: MMPI-2: Assessing Personality and Psychopathology. New York, Oxford University Press, 2000

Graham JR, Watts D, Timbrook TE: Detecting fake-good and fake-bad MMPI-2 profiles. J Pers Assess 57:264–277, 1991

Greene R: Assessment of malingering and defensiveness by multiscale personality inventories, in Clinical Assessment of Malingering and Deception. Edited by Rogers R. New York, Guilford, 1997, pp 169–207

Griffin GAE, Glassmire DM, Henderson EA, et al: Redesigning the Rey Screening Test of Malingering. J Clin Psychol 53:757–766, 1997

Guilmette TJ, Hart KJ, Guilianao AJO, et al: Detecting simulated memory impairment: comparison of the Rey 15-Item Test and the Hiscock Forced-Choice Procedure. Clinical Neuropsychologist 8:283–294, 1994

Hall HV: Dangerousness predictions and the maligned forensic professional. Criminal Justice and Behavior 9:3–12, 1982

Hankins GC, Barnard GW, Robbins L: The validity of the M test in a residential forensic facility. Bulletin of the American Academy of Psychiatry and the Law 21:111–121, 1993

Hathaway SR, McKinley JC: Minnesota Multiphasic Personality Inventory—2 (MMPI-2). Minneapolis, MN, University of Minnesota Press, 1989

Hellerstein D, Frosch W, Koenigsberg HW: The clinical significance of command hallucinations. Am J Psychiatry 144:219–225, 1987

Iacono WG, Lykken DT: The scientific status of research on polygraph tests: the case against polygraph tests, in Modern Scientific Evidence. Edited by Faigman DL, Kaye D, Saks MJ, et al. St. Paul, MN, West Publishing, 1997, 592–618

Jaffe ME, Sharma K: Malingering uncommon psychiatric symptoms among defendants charged under California's "three strikes and you're out" law. J Forensic Sci 43:549–555, 1998

Jones AB, Llewellyn J: Malingering. London, Heinmann, 1917

Junginger J: Predicting compliance with command hallucinations. Am J Psychiatry 147:245–247, 1990

Junginger J: Command hallucinations and the prediction of dangerousness. Psychiatr Serv 46:911–914, 1995

Kanas N, Barr MA: Self-control of psychotic productions in schizophrenics (letter). Arch Gen Psychiatry 41:919–920, 1984

Kasper ME, Rogers R, Adams PA: Dangerousness and command hallucinations: an investigation of psychotic inpatients. Bulletin of the American Academy of Psychiatry and the Law 24:219–224, 1996

Kent G, Wahass S: The content and characteristics of auditory hallucinations in Saudi Arabia and the UK: a cross-cultural comparison. Acta Psychiatr Scand 94:433–437, 1996

Kluft RP: The simulation and dissimulation of multiple personality disorder. Am J Clin Hypn 30:104–118, 1987

Kraus A: Phenomenology of the technical delusion in schizophrenia. Journal of Phenomenological Psychology 25:51–69, 1994

Kucharski LT, Ryan W, Vogt J, et al: Clinical symptom presentation in suspected malingerers: an empirical investigation. Bulletin of the American Academy of Psychiatry and the Law 26:579–585, 1998

Larkin AR: The form and content of schizophrenic hallucinations. Am J Psychiatry 136:940–943, 1979

Lees-Haley PR, Dunn JT: The ability of naïve subjects to report symptoms of mild brain injury, post traumatic stress disorder, major depression, and generalized anxiety disorder. J Clin Psychol 50:252–256, 1994

Lees-Haley PR, English LT, Glenn WJ: A fake bad scale on the MMPI-2 for personal-injury claimants. Psychol Rep 68:203–210, 1991

Leroy R: The syndrome of lilliputian hallucinations. J Nerv Ment Dis 56:325–333, 1922

Leudar I, Thomas P, McNally D, et al: What voices can do with words: pragmatics of verbal hallucinations. Psychol Med 27:885–898, 1997

Lewinsohn PM: An empirical test of several popular notions about hallucinations in schizophrenic patients, in Origin and Mechanisms of Hallucinations. Edited by Keup W. New York, Plenum, 1970, pp 401–403

Lewis DJ: Lilliputian hallucinations in the functional psychoses. Canadian Psychiatric Association Journal 6:177–201, 1961

Lewis DO, Bard JS: Multiple personality and forensic issues. Psychiatr Clin North Am 14:741–756, 1991

Lewis DO, Yeager CA, Swica Y, et al: Objective documentation of child abuse and dissociation in 12 murderers with dissociative identity disorder. Am J Psychiatry 154:1703–1710, 1997

Lezak MD: Neuropsychological Assessment, 2nd Edition. New York, Oxford University Press, 1983

Link BG, Stueve CA: Psychotic symptoms and the violent/illegal behavior of mental patients compared to community controls, in Violence and Mental Disorder: Developments in Risk Assessment. Edited by Monahan J, Steadman H. Chicago, IL, University of Chicago Press, 1994, 137–160

Lovinger RJ: Theoretical affiliations in psychotherapy. Psychotherapy 29:586–590, 1992

MacDonald J: The simulation of mental disease, in Psychiatry and the Criminal. Edited by MacDonald J. Springfield, IL, Charles C Thomas, 1976, pp 425–441

Masling J: Role related behavior of the subject and psychologist and its effect upon psychological data. Nebr Symp Motiv 14:67–104, 1966

Mellman TA, Kulick-Bell R, Ashlock LE, et al: Sleep events among veterans with combat-related posttraumatic stress disorder. Am J Psychiatry 152:110–115, 1995

Melton R: Differential diagnosis: a common sense guide to psychological assessment. Vet Center Voice Newsletter V:1–12, 1984

M'Naghten, 8 Eng Rep 718 (1843)

Miller H, Cartlidge N: Simulation and malingering after injuries to the brain and spinal cord. Lancet 1:580–585, 1972

Mott RH, Small IF, Andersen JM: Comparative study of hallucinations. Arch Gen Psychiatry 12:595–601, 1965

Nayani TH, David AS: The auditory hallucination: a phenomenological survey. Psychol Med 26:177–189, 1996

Orne MT: The use and misuse of hypnosis in court. Int J Clin Exp Hypn 27:311–341, 1979

Orne MT, Dinges DF, Orne EC: On the differential diagnosis of multiple personality in the forensic context. Int J Clin Exp Hypn 32:118–169, 1984

Orr SP, Pitman RK, Lasko NB, et al: Psychophysiological assessment of post-traumatic stress disorder imagery in World War II and the Korean combat veterans. J Abnorm Psychol 102:620–624, 1993

Ossipov VP: Malingering: the simulation of psychosis. Bull Menninger Clin 8:31–42, 1944

Oulis PG, Mavreas VG, Mamounas JM, et al: Clinical characteristics of auditory hallucinations. Acta Psychiatr Scand 92:97–102, 1995

People v Schmidt, 216 NY 324 (1915)

People v Shirley, 181 Cal Rptr 243 (1982)

Perlin ML: Unpacking the myths: the symbolism mythology of insanity defense jurisprudence. Case Western Reserve University Law Review 40:599–725, 1989–1990

Pitman RK, Saunders LS, Orr SP: Psychophysiologic testing for post-traumatic stress disorder. Trial, April 1994, pp 22–26

Powell KE: The Malingering of Schizophrenia. Ph.D. thesis, University of South Carolina, 1991

Putnam FW: Diagnosis and Treatment of Multiple Personality Disorder. New York, Guilford, 1989

Redlich RC, Ravitz LJ, Dession GH: Nacroanalysis and the truth. Am J Psychiatry 107:586–593, 1951

Rees LM, Tombaugh TN, Gansler DA, et al: Five validation experiments of the Test of Memory Malingering (TOMM). Psychological Assessment 10:10–20, 1998

Resnick PJ: The detection of malingered mental illness. Behav Sci Law 2:21–38, 1984

Resnick PJ: Malingered psychosis, in Clinical Assessment of Malingering and Deception. Edited by Rogers R. New York, Guilford, 1997, pp 47–67

Ritson B, Forest A: The simulation of psychosis: a contemporary presentation. British Journal of Medical Psychology 43:31, 1970

Robins LN: Epidemiology: reflections on testing the validity of psychiatric interviews. Arch Gen Psychiatry 42:918–924, 1985

Rogers R: Assessment of malingering within a forensic context, in Law and Psychiatry: International Perspectives. Edited by Weisstub DW. New York, Plenum, 1987, 209–237

Rogers R: Structured interviews and dissimulation, in Clinical Assessment of Malingering and Deception. Edited by Rogers R. New York, Guilford, 1997, pp 301–327

Rogers R, Shuman D: Conducting Insanity Evaluations, 2nd Edition. New York, Guilford, 2000

Rogers R, Wettstein RM: Drug-assisted interviews to detect malingering and deception, in Clinical Assessment of Malingering and Deception. Edited by Rogers R. New York, Guilford, 1997, pp 239–251

Rogers R, Gillis JR, Turner RE, et al: The clinical presentation of command hallucinations. Am J Psychiatry 147:1304–1307, 1990

Rogers R, Bagby RM, Dickens SE: Structured Interview of Reported Symptoms (SIRS) and Professional Manual. Odessa, FL, Psychological Assessment Resources, 1992

Rogers R, Harrell EH, Liff CD: Feigning neuropsychological impairment: a critical review of methodological and clinical considerations. Clin Psychol Rev 13:255–274, 1993

Rogers R, Sewell KW, Goldstein AM: Explanatory models of malingering: a prototypical analysis. Law Hum Behav 18:543–552, 1994

Rogers R, Sewell KW, Ustad KL: Feigning among chronic outpatients on the MMPI-2: a systematic examination of fake-bad indicators. Assessment 2:81–89, 1995

Rosenberg CE: The Trial of the Assassin Guiteau. Chicago, IL, University of Chicago Press, 1968

Rosenhan DL: On being sane in insane places. Science 179:250–258, 1973

Rowan C: Cleveland Plain Dealer, June 21, 1982, p 10B (editorial column)

Sachs MH, Carpenter WT, Strauss JS: Recovery from delusions. Arch Gen Psychiatry 30:117–120, 1974

Saks ER: Does multiple personality disorder exist? the beliefs, the data, and the law. Int J Law Psychiatry 17:43–78, 1994

Schacter DL: Feeling-of-knowing ratings distinguish between genuine and simulated forgetting. J Exp Psychol Learn Mem Cogn 12:30–41, 1986

Schretlen D: The use of psychological tests to identify malingered symptoms of mental disorders. Clin Psychol Rev 8:451–476, 1988

Schretlen D: Dissimulation on the Rorschach and other projective measures, in Clinical Assessment of Malingering and Deception. Edited by Rogers R. New York, Guilford, 1997, pp 208–222

Schretlen D, Brandt J, Krafft RV, et al: Some caveats in using the Rey 15-item memory test to detect malingered amnesia. Psychological Assessment: A Journal of Clinical and Consulting Psychology 3:667–672, 1991

Sewell KW, Rogers R: Response consistency and the MMPI-2: development of a simplified screening scale. Assessment 1:293–299, 1994

Shalev AY, Orr SP, Pitman RK: Psychophysiologic assessment of traumatic imagery in Israeli civilian post-traumatic disorder patients. Am J Psychiatry 150:152–159, 1993

Sherman M, Trief P, Sprafkin QR: Impression management in the psychiatric interview: quality, style and individual differences. J Consult Clin Psychol 43:867–871, 1975

Small IF, Small JG, Andersen JM: Clinical characteristics of hallucinations of schizophrenia. Diseases of the Nervous System 27:349–353, 1966

Smith GP, Borum R, Schinks JA: Rule-out and rule-in scales for the M test for malingering. Bulletin of the American Academy of Psychiatry and the Law 21:107–110, 1993

Spitzer M: The phenomenology of delusions. Psychiatric Annals 22:252–259, 1992

State v Hurd, 173 NJ Super 333, 414 A2d 291 (1980)

Steinberg M, Bancroft J, Buchanan J: Multiple personality disorder in criminal law. Bulletin of the American Academy of Psychiatry and the Law 21:345–356, 1993

Swanson J, Borum R, Swartz M, et al: Violence and severe mental disorder in clinical and community populations: the effects of psychotic symptoms, comorbidity, and lack of treatment. Psychiatry 60:1–22, 1997

Thompson JS, Stuart GL, Holden CE: Command hallucinations and legal insanity. Forensic Reports 5:29–42, 1992

Tombaugh TN: The Test of Memory Malingering (TOMM): normative data from cognitively intact and cognitively impaired individuals. Psychological Assessment 9:260–268, 1996

van der Kolk B, Blitz R, Burr W, et al: Nightmares and trauma: a comparison of nightmares after combat with lifelong nightmares in veterans. Am J Psychiatry 141:187–190, 1984

Wachspress M, Berenberg AN, Jacobson A: Simulation of psychosis. Psychiatr Q 27:463–473, 1953

Wessely S, Buchanan A, Reed A, et al: Acting on delusions, I: prevalence. Br J Psychiatry 163:69–76, 1993

Whitlock FA: The Ganser syndrome. Br J Psychiatry 113:19–29, 1967

Wilson v United States, 391 F.2d 460 (D.C. Cir. 1968)

Yates BD, Nordquist CR, Schultz-Ross RA: Feigned psychiatric symptoms in the emergency room. Psychiatr Serv 47:998–1000, 1996

Ziskin J: Challenging the assessment of malingering or credibility, in Coping With Psychiatric and Psychological Testimony, 5th Edition, Vol II: Special Topics. Los Angeles, CA, Law & Psychology Press, 1995, pp 135–187

6

Murder, Suicide, Accident, or Natural Death?

Assessment of Suicide Risk Factors at the Time of Death

Robert I. Simon, M.D.

Y̶ou only die once—but did you intend it? Or did somebody else intend it? Or was it accidental or natural? Forensic clinicians are frequently asked to assist in answering these questions, especially to help determine for insurance purposes whether an individual's death was a suicide or was accidental (Nolan 1988; Simon 1990, 1996).

In criminal investigations, forensic psychiatric and psychological expertise may be useful in distinguishing suicide from homicide as the cause of death. As I described in Chapter 1 in this volume, on August 5, 1962, Marilyn Monroe was found dead in her bed. She was lying nude, face down, with a sheet pulled over her body. No suicide note was found. Her neigh-

---

Portions of this chapter are adapted from Simon 1998b.

bors heard no disturbance. An autopsy was conducted by Deputy Coroner Thomas Noguchi, M.D., on the morning after her death. The Los Angeles coroner rendered a preliminary judgment 5 days later—Marilyn Monroe died of possible acute barbiturate poisoning from an overdose. The judgment was amended to probable suicide on August 17. The coroner issued his final judgment 10 days later, determining that Marilyn Monroe died of acute barbiturate poisoning following an overdose. Decades later controversy remains over the cause of her death. Was it suicide? Was it accidental overdose? Or was it, as some have hinted darkly, murder staged as a suicide?

Robert Maxwell, the billionaire publishing magnate, suddenly and without explanation ordered the captain of his yacht to sail for Madeira and Tenerife Island, off the northwestern coast of Africa. The captain reached Grand Canary Island and sailed around it. Maxwell had decreed no particular course. At approximately 5:00 A.M. on November 4, 1991, Maxwell called the bridge to complain that his room was too cold. Then, without being seen by anyone, he made his way up to the deck and either fell, jumped, or was pushed to his death. His naked body was later found floating in the calm waters off Grand Canary Island. Was it an accident, a suicide, or a murder? The answer was extremely important. A huge scandal concerning the disappearance of corporate assets and monies from pension funds awaited his return to England. Personal disgrace and the possibility of imprisonment were a distinct reality. The family also was in a position to collect $36 million from his life insurance policy.

Theories about the cause of his death proliferated; they included that he had a multiple personality and was killed by a murderous alter that emerged under the extreme stress of events. Maxwell also had many enemies who would have wanted him dead. Another real possibility was that the personal humiliation and the destruction of his self-invented, larger-than-life image could have led to suicide. On the other hand, the explanation of his death could be much simpler: a Spanish pathologist observed that Maxwell's stomach contained a barely digested banana and theorized that he could have slipped on a banana peel and fallen to his death (Simon 1996).

If Maxwell's death was accidental, the cause of the accident was unusual. The most frequent situations in which the question of suicide versus accident arises occur in injection drug overdose and in motor vehicle deaths. A common cause of confusion between suicide and accidental death in young men is autoerotic asphyxiation errors.

Around noon on Tuesday, July 20, 1993, White House Counsel Vincent W. Foster Jr. walked out of his office in the West Wing of the White House. He told his secretary to have some M&M's candy left on his lunch tray. Foster drove his car to Virginia, taking the George Washington Parkway to a scenic and secluded spot in Fort Marcy Park. There he shot and killed himself. Or did he? Conspiratorial theories of murder continue to surround Foster's death. Doubts that Foster committed suicide still linger despite the fact that a special prosecutor ruled his death a suicide (Schmidt 1997).

Psychiatrists and psychologists are increasingly called on to consult in cases suspected of being "suicide by cop" or unwitting police-assisted suicides. Some persons intentionally create and escalate life-threatening situations for the police or for the general public or both, provoking and forcing the police to assist unwittingly in their suicide (Hutson et al. 1998; Wilson et al. 1998). The deaths usually are certified as homicides, even when "suicide by cop" is suspected. The retrospective suicide risk assessment method proposed in this chapter also can by used in investigating allegations of unwitting police-assisted suicides.

Murder Masquerading as Suicide

Murder masquerading as suicide is rare. It is less likely to occur with a public figure or celebrity because close scrutiny may uncover the deception. Murder masquerading as a suicide is more likely to go undetected or remain unsolved when the individual murdered has a history of mental illness (Simon 1998b).

Case Example 1: Murder or Suicide?[1]

Angela, a 36-year-old married but separated woman, was found hanging naked in her bedroom closet by her landlord. Her knees were approximately 4 inches above the floor. Neighbors complained of a foul odor coming from Angela's apartment. The police were called. They found no signs of a struggle in the apartment. No suicide note was found. Angela told friends and co-workers that she was taking a few days off to put the finishing touches on a novel she was writing. A manuscript was found on her desk. Angela did not have significant financial problems.

The body was cut down so as to preserve the knot made for the noose. Fingerprints were obtained but were inconclusive. The forensic pathologist retained by the prosecution opined in her report that the death was suspicious. She noted that suicide by hanging is not a preferred method for women. The slipknot that was used contained clumps of the deceased's hair tangled within the knot. The forensic pathologist stated

---

[1]For heuristic purposes a number of facts of the original case have been changed (*People v. Darrell Younger,* Sonoma County Superior Court Case Number SCR-24618; Sonoma County District Attorney Case Number DAR-330986).

that persons who hang themselves usually do so with a simple slipknot that is not intertwined with their hair. The slipknot is tied first and then the noose is placed over the head without entangling the hair in the knot. The rope around Angela's neck was in a horizontal plane, as if it were tightened first before any strain was applied. The forensic pathologist explained that a diagonal misplacement is more pronounced in suicides. The rope's impression on Angela's neck was not as pronounced as seen in hanging deaths. Moreover, the forensic pathologist observed that women who kill themselves do not ordinarily do so in a naked state. Furthermore, it could not be determined whether Angela sustained any trauma to her body because of advanced bodily decay. Evidence of a sexual assault was not apparent. Blood analysis did not indicate any evidence of drugs or alcohol. The pathologist concluded that Angela was murdered.

The defense forensic pathologist's report stated that it is not uncommon for hair to become entangled in a noose. He further stated that no conclusions should be drawn from the knots used. Moreover, his experience was that women hang themselves in various states of undress. Also, the angle of the ligature was an equivocal piece of evidence. The pathologist concluded that Angela's death was a "garden variety" suicide.

After further investigation, the police learned that Angela's husband, age 49, had a police record for spousal abuse. Angela was planning a divorce after 10 years of marriage. Angela had obtained a protective order against her husband for stalking 1 year before her death. Neighbors and co-workers reported that Angela worried about being stalked again by her husband whom she greatly feared. Witnesses testified that Angela's husband had once threatened to kill her while in a rage. She had begun a romantic relationship at work. Angela told friends that her husband said that he would kill her rather than "give her up" to another man.

Hair samples found in Angela's apartment matched those of her husband. Her fingernail clippings were unrevealing. The husband was questioned about his wife's death but denied any knowledge of the death. He claimed that he had not spoken to his wife in more than a year. Angela's husband stated that she had an extensive psychiatric history, attempting suicide on several occasions. His alibi was that he was out of town attending a regatta during the time his wife died, but the alibi could not be substantiated. (The husband is a retired military officer whose hobby is sailing.)

Neighbors provided sworn statements that they heard loud, angry voices and the sound of furniture falling over at about the time of Angela's death. One witness saw the husband's car in the parking lot and observed him entering the apartment building where Angela lived around the time of her death.

Because of the suspicious circumstances, the district attorney requested a postmortem psychiatric assessment to determine the presence or absence of suicide risk factors at the time of Angela's death. Witness statements (friends, co-workers, family, neighbors) were reviewed. Angela's medical and psychiatric records were obtained. The psychiatric records indicated that she had developed bulimia nervosa at age 17. The breakup of a romantic relationship had resulted in depression, superficial wrist cutting, and a brief hospitalization at age 19. A maternal grand-mother had attempted suicide following postpartum depression. The in-patient psychiatrist made a diagnosis of adjustment disorder with depression.

Angela had married at age 26, after graduating from college with a master's degree in business administration. She sought outpatient treat-ment because of the physical and psychological abuse by her husband. The decision to seek psychiatric treatment was made after a particularly violent beating by her husband. Her injuries included six fractured ribs and a facial fracture of the right zygomatic process. Her husband was ar-rested, briefly jailed, and ordered to attend a treatment program for wife abusers. The psychiatrist diagnosed dysthymic disorder (chronic depres-sion) in Angela. He noted that Angela had experienced brief flurries of un-bidden suicidal thoughts after being assaulted by her husband but had no suicidal intent or plan. As a way of medicating her marital stress symp-toms, she occasionally drank wine excessively. Angela received 3 years of psychiatric treatment, which ended 1 year before she obtained the protec-tive order against her husband. Treatment frequency varied from once a week at the beginning of therapy to once a month during the last year of treatment. The psychiatrist noted that a solid therapeutic alliance existed with the patient.

Angela's parents revealed that she was about to receive a $500,000 in-heritance from an aunt who had recently died. Angela and her husband knew of this bequest. Angela's husband was a secondary beneficiary of the inheritance as long as the couple remained officially married.

Case Example 2: Guilty of Murder[2]

On November 4, 1996, Ms. Elizabeth Stolpinski died from a gunshot wound to her head. The autopsy report determined that the manner of death was "homicide (shot by another person)." When the rescue squad responded to her husband's 911 call, Mr. Raymond Stolpinski told a fire-man, "I think my wife shot herself." The grand jury returned an indict-ment for murder in the second degree (intentional murder). The forensic psychiatrist was asked by the prosecution to conduct a postmortem psy-chiatric assessment for the presence or absence of suicide risk factors.

At the time of her death, Ms. Stolpinski was 27 years old. She had been married to Mr. Stolpinski for approximately 4 years. On September 24, 1996, she had given birth to a daughter by cesarean delivery because of the infant's breech presentation. Ms. Stolpinski was thrilled with the birth of their daughter, especially after attempting to become pregnant on numerous occasions. No evidence of postpartum depression was observed either by her obstetrician or by the other interviewees (family members, co-workers, and friends). Ms. Stolpinski had no history of psychiatric ill-ness or treatment.

---

[2] *People of the State of New York v. Raymond Stolpinski*, Rich Co Ind No 290/97.

Ms. Stolpinski kept a diary of her infant's feeding schedule, indicating that she was conscientious and taking good care of her child. This was confirmed by all the interviewees who observed her with the infant. The infant had to wear a hip harness because of a "hip problem." Ms. Stolpinski was realistically concerned but was reassured by her family physician that the infant's hip would heal normally with conservative treatment.

Many of the interviewees saw the marital relationship as troubled. Several interviewees observed verbal abuse. No evidence of physical abuse was found.

At the time of her death, Ms. Stolpinski had been enthusiastically making plans to return to part-time work 3 days a week. Her employer (dentist) and his staff were "happy to have her back." The dentist and her co-workers described Ms. Stolpinski as a reliable, hardworking individual who was "very kind and good with patients." Ms. Stolpinski had worked for the dentist as a dental assistant for approximately 5 years. The dentist and her co-workers never observed any mental or emotional problems.

Several interviewees said that Ms. Stolpinski had been looking forward to upcoming events in her life. For example, on the evening before she died, Ms. Stolpinski had written invitations for the infant's christening that was scheduled for December 1, 1996. Ms. Stolpinski had been enthusiastically making plans for this event. According to the dentist's wife (former co-worker), Ms. Stolpinski also was planning to come to her wedding shower. The dentist remarked that Ms. Stolpinski was excited about attending his wedding on December 8, 1996. She was one of the first to RSVP.

Based on the interview of the family members and individuals who knew Ms. Stolpinski and the review of the records provided by the district attorney,[3] the forensic psychiatrist found no evidence in the postmortem psychiatric assessment that Ms. Stolpinski manifested any suicide risk factors (see Table 6–1). The district attorney informed the forensic psychiatrist that he would be asked to testify as a rebuttal witness if the defense presented testimony that Ms. Stolpinski had committed suicide. The day before the scheduled trial date, faced with the evidence against him, which included gunshot residue analysis, ballistics, and computer reconstructions of the crime scene, the defendant entered an *Alford* plea of guilty to manslaughter 1. An *Alford* plea permits a competent defendant to plead guilty when denying guilt.

Postmortem Suicidal Risk Assessment

Suicide risk factors can be classified as individual, clinical, interpersonal, situational, and statistical (see Table 6–1). An example of a unique, highly individual suicide risk factor occurred in a patient with severe depression whose stuttering would clear prior to the onset of suicidal ideation. As his

---

[3]Prosecuting attorneys Eric Nelson and David Frey.

Table 6–1. Assessment of suicide risk

Risk factors	Facilitating suicide	Inhibiting suicide	Acute	Chronic
Individual (unique patient factors)	0			
Clinical				
Current attempt (lethality)	0			
Suicidal ideation: syntonic or dystonic—current[a]	0			
Suicide intent[a]	0			
Suicide plan	0			
Panic attacks[b]	0			
Psychic anxiety[b]	0			
Loss of pleasure and interest[b]	0			
Alcohol abuse[b]	L			X
Depressive turmoil[b]	0			
Diminished concentration[b]	0			
Global insomnia[b]	0			
Recent discharge from psychiatric hospital (within 3 months)[b]	0			
Hopelessness[a]		M		
Shame	0			
Psychiatric diagnoses (Axes I and II)—current	0			
Symptom severity	0			
Prior attempts (lethality)[a]	L			X
Family history of suicide	L			X
Impulsivity (violence, driving, money)	L			X
Preparations for death (e.g., wills)	0			
Drug abuse	0			
Physical illness	0			
Mental competency		H		
Interpersonal				
Therapeutic alliance with patient	0			
Other relationships (work, partner or spousal, family)	0	H		
Situational				
Specific situational factors	M		X	
Living circumstances		M		
Employment status		H		
Financial status	0			
Availability of guns		M		

Table 6–1.   Assessment of suicide risk *(continued)*

Risk factors	Facilitating suicide	Inhibiting suicide	Acute	Chronic
Statistical (age, sex, marital status, race)	L		X	X

Note.   Clinically judge overall suicide risk as high, moderate, or low. Rating system: L=low factor; M=moderate factor; H=high factor; 0=nonfactor.
[a]Long-term indicators associated with suicide 2–10 years following assessment.
[b]Short-term indicators are risk factors found to be statistically significant within 1 year of assessment.

depression improved, the stuttering would return. Another patient never hummed and whistled except when he was sinking into a suicidal depression. Short-term risk factors are statistically significant within 1 year of assessment (derived from prospective studies of completed suicides of patients with major affective disorders). Long-term traditional suicide risk factors are significantly associated with suicides completed 2–10 years after assessment (derived from community-based psychological autopsies and the retrospective studies of completed suicide by psychiatric patients) (Fawcett et al. 1998; Roy 1992). A major mental illness was a primary factor in suicide in 93% of the adult cases. The most common diagnoses from retrospective studies have been major depression (40%–60%), chronic alcoholism (20%), and schizophrenia (10%). Thus, groups of persons with the greatest vulnerability to suicide can be identified (Fawcett et al. 1993).

In clinical practice, however, no standard of care exists for predicting which patients will attempt or commit suicide (Simon 1992a). The standard of care does require that the clinician gather relevant information and assess the patient's level of suicide risk, which informs clinical interventions (Simon 1998a). The assessment of a patient's suicide risk bears an analogy to weather forecasting (Monahan and Steadman 1996; Simon 1992a). Although eclipses can be predicted with 100% accuracy, the weather can be forecasted only within certain probabilities. Moreover, like weather forecasts, time attenuates suicide risk assessments, which are only "here-and-now" gauges. Frequent updates are required. Suicide risk assessment is not an event, like an eclipse, but a process, like weather forecasting, requiring ongoing assessment and revision.

When performing a postmortem assessment of suicide risk, the forensic clinician gathers information from death scene evidence, witnesses' statements, pathologist's findings, medical-psychiatric records, and any other relevant sources to determine the presence or absence of suicide risk factors at the time of death. For example, the careful analysis by experts of knots in hangings can yield important information about whether a death was a suicide, homicide, or accident (Spitz 1993). Paradoxically, the forensic examiner may obtain more data when assessing suicide risk factors of the deceased than in the clinical setting with a live uncooperative, disorganized, or dissembling suicidal patient. Table 6–1 describes one method of suicide risk assessment adapted from clinical practice (Simon 1992b). Other methods of suicide risk assessment also are available (Blumenthal 1990; Chiles and Strohsall 1995; Maris et al. 1992). The assessment of suicide risk factors can be applied to both the living and the dead (Tanay 1989). Regardless of the method used, the quality of suicide risk assessments significantly depends on the training, knowledge, experience, and clinical judgment of the evaluator.

An important caveat is that no suicide risk assessment model has been empirically tested for reliability and validity (Simon 1998c). Busch et al. (1993) observed that no standardized suicide prediction scale can identify which patients will commit suicide. At best, patients from certain diagnostic groups—such as those with major depression, chronic alcoholism, schizophrenia, and borderline personality disorder—are at increased risk of suicide, but it is not possible to identify precisely which patients will commit suicide (Fawcett et al. 1993).

The inability to predict suicide was shown in a classic study by Pokorny (1983). This prospective study of 4,800 consecutive patients attempted to identify which psychiatric patients would commit suicide. Twenty-one items were used to identify a subsample of 803 patients who were considered suicidal risks. Of the 67 patients who committed suicide during the 5-year follow-up period, only 30 were in the 803-patient subsample; 37 suicides (>50%) were not among those identified as at risk. Furthermore, 766 of the 803 at-risk patients did not commit suicide. This overprediction of suicide risk and the high number of missed or undetected suicides (error rate) are consistent with other research in future behavior prediction (Melton et al. 1997; Pokorny 1993). Pokorny (1993) reanalyzed his data with logistic regression. The results were the same as in his previous study.

As in clinical practice, postmortem psychological analysis requires the identification and assessment of suicide risk factors present at the time of death. Various suicide risk assessment models are available to clinicians (Chiles and Strohsall 1995; Clark and Fawcett 1992; Maris et al. 1992). Table 6–1 is schematically designed for heuristic purposes to encourage a systematic approach to suicide risk assessment. Suicide risk factors may be assigned different weights according to the clinician's professional judgment and the patient's clinical presentation. Table 6–1 allows the clinician to consider factors that both facilitate and inhibit suicide risk. A symptom, condition, or situation that clearly is the diametric opposite of a suicide risk factor (e.g., hopefulness vs. hopelessness), when present clinically, should be rated as a factor inhibiting suicide risk. Some suicide risk factors (facilitating) can be further divided into acute and chronic duration (Simon 1998c). Chronic suicide risk factors are present for a year or longer before evaluation. For example, statistical (demographic) factors are considered to be relatively static, chronic measures of suicide risk. Acute risk factors are the focus of current, ongoing clinical assessment. Patients with comorbid Axis I and Axis II disorders often have both acute and chronic risk factors. A suicide risk factor also may be rated as both acute and chronic. For example, a recurrent depression can be an acute and a chronic suicide risk factor.

Assessment of Suicide Risk Factors

Assessment of Angela's (Case Example 1) suicide risk factors at the time of her death, using the material in Table 6–1, indicated that no uniquely individual risk factors or risk factors associated with short-term anxiety could be identified (Fawcett et al. 1990). No indication of anxiety symptoms was found. She maintained a loving interest in her three young nephews. At the time of her death she had also been pursuing numerous interests, such as oil painting, stained glass work, and had had a passion for reading. Her friends did not notice any change in her interests and usual high level of functioning. Angela saw her parents and sister frequently. They heard no complaints of sleep or appetite problems and did not observe any evidence of depression. Angela's family was out of town at the time of her death.

Angela's relationships with her friends, family, and new boyfriend were important and supportive. No evidence of depression or hopelessness existed. Angela was pursuing personal plans and life goals. For example, at the time of her death, Angela was planning a 30-day trip through Europe with friends for the next year. She also intended to use her inheritance to make a major career change. She was applying to graduate school to pursue her literary interests. Angela was looking forward to publishing her first novel. The fact that Angela was hopeful, future-oriented, and avidly pursuing life goals was rated as moderately inhibiting of suicide in Table 6–1 opposite the risk factor "hopelessness."

As an adolescent, Angela had been hospitalized after making an impulsive suicide gesture by superficially cutting her wrists. In her therapy as an adult, the psychiatrist noted that she entertained suicidal thoughts following abusive episodes with her husband. She never acted on her thoughts. The therapist observed that Angela's "impulsive streak" moderated as she matured, being channeled more into making sound intuition-based business decisions. The psychiatrist recorded that Angela had thoughts of overdosing with pain medications that she would take occasionally for a chronic ankle injury. Her recent psychiatrist was contacted and indicated that Angela was never at risk for suicide during her treatment. No witness reported any evidence of suicidal ideation or behaviors at any time. In fact, friends and relatives described Angela as quite happy, particularly after she obtained the protective order against her husband.

At the time of Angela's death, no evidence indicated that she had symptoms of psychiatric distress or communicated suicidal intent to anyone. Clark and Fawcett (1992) reported that direct communication of suicidal intent to significant others occurred in two-thirds of the completed suicides in the weeks before death. Clark and Horton-Deutsch (1992), in their study of suicide completers, observed that twice as many males as females committed suicide, that the decedents almost always qualified for a psychiatric diagnosis, and, more often than not, that the persons had communicated their suicide intent. They also found that 93%–95% of all cases of completed suicide met the diagnostic criteria for one or more DSM-III-R (American Psychiatric Association 1987) diagnoses.

Angela's living circumstances were comfortable. She earned a substantial salary as a very competent public relations consultant. Angela was respected by both her co-workers and her boss. These items were rated as highly inhibiting of suicide on Table 6–1 under "employment status." Angela was separated and pursuing a divorce, placing her in a class that was at an increased but low acute and chronic risk for suicide under the risk category "statistical." However, she considered divorce as a liberation from her abusive husband. Nonetheless, Angela kept a gun under her mattress for protection. She had the means to obtain and accumulate a lethal supply of pain medications (acetaminophen) prescribed by her physician for a chronic ankle injury. The fact that Angela did not take a lethal overdose, a preferred method in female suicides, makes it unlikely that she would commit suicide by hanging. Thus a violent death by hanging appeared to be a less likely choice than suicide by overdose. A moderate rating for inhibiting suicide under the "availability of guns" category was made.

The therapist's notes clearly stated that Angela's suicidal thoughts were dystonic; that is, she felt that they were unbidden and unwanted. At the time of her death, no evidence existed of any current suicidal ideation, intent, plan, or behavior. No conclusion could be drawn from the absence of a suicide note. Only 10%–35% of the persons who commit suicide leave notes (Evans and Faberow 1988).

The presence of a family history of depression with suicide attempt was rated on Table 6–1 as a low chronic facilitating factor. Even though Angela had impulsively made a suicide gesture as an adolescent, at the time of her death, all who knew her considered her to be a reasonably prudent and careful person. Nonetheless, a history of adolescent impulsivity was rated as a low chronic facilitating factor. No current evidence of drug or sustained alcohol abuse was detected. Angela's occasional self-medication with alcohol during stressful marital situations in the past was rated as a low chronic factor, even though toxicology was negative for drugs and alcohol. She was in excellent physical health except for a chronic ankle injury. Angela was a high-functioning, competent person. If she were depressed and suicidal, it is highly likely that she would have obtained professional help based on her seeking of psychiatric treatment in the past under similar circumstances and the existence of a solid therapeutic alliance with her psychiatrist. Thus, "mental competency" on Table 6–1 was rated as highly inhibiting suicide.

Angela had told her parents and friends that she was apprehensive that her husband would start stalking again. She feared that her husband would harm her after he had threatened to kill her if she had a relationship with another man. Being terrorized by a stalker can cause despair and depression. No evidence, however, indicated that Angela was in despair or was depressed at the time of her death. The fear of being stalked was rated as a moderate acute facilitating suicide risk factor under "specific situational factors."

A postmortem overall assessment of Angela's suicide risk factors indicated a low or minimal suicide risk at the time of death. The few risk factors facilitating suicide were far outweighed by the presence of factors that tend to exclude suicidal risk. Heavy weight was given to the absence of any overt symptoms of psychiatric disorder, no evidence of suicidal ideation, no alcohol or drug abuse, future orientation, and factors indicating good interpersonal and occupational functioning. This suicide risk assessment method is qualitative and, as with the living patient, relies heavily on the clinical judgment and experience of the evaluating clinician or expert in determining the weight given to the various risk factors.

The forensic psychiatrist retained by the prosecution was unable to testify with reasonable medical certainty that Angela did not commit suicide by hanging or that she was murdered by her husband or, for that matter, by someone else. However, it was possible to testify with reasonable medical certainty that the postmortem suicide risk assessment indicated that Angela was at low risk for suicide at the time of her death. The defense psychiatrist testified that suicide could not be ruled out because of Angela's psychiatric history of a prior impulsive suicide attempt, psychiatric hospitalization, chronic depression, and recurrent suicidal thoughts triggered by spousal abuse. She could not definitively rule out murder either. Did Angela commit suicide, or was she murdered? And, if so, by whom? These were the ultimate questions placed before the jury. Courts are skeptical of prejudicial psychiatric or psychological testimony that claims to resolve how an individual died (Biffl 1996).

The prosecution argued that Angela's husband strangled her because of intense jealousy and to obtain her sizable inheritance, staging the murder as a suicide. The defense argued that Angela had a long psychiatric history with a prior suicide attempt and subsequent psychiatric hospitalization. She continued to experience suicidal thoughts following the emotional and physical abuse by her husband. The defense further argued that Angela's fear that her husband would harm her because of a romantic relationship she had begun led to depression and suicide.

Angela's husband was charged with first-degree murder and found guilty by the jury. He was given a sentence of 25 years to life. No eyewitnesses had been present to the alleged crime. No single piece of evidence or testimony was conclusive by itself in determining how Angela died. After hearing more than 100 witnesses, the jury determined that the prosecution had constructed a compelling mosaic of facts that implicated the husband, supporting a verdict of guilty of first-degree murder beyond a reasonable doubt. The postmortem suicide risk assessment was an important piece in the mosaic of facts put together by the prosecution.

On appeal, the case was remanded to the Trial Court for retrial on technical legal issues.

Postmortem Suicidal Risk Assessment and *Daubert*

The competent assessment of suicide risk factors is an essential part of the standard of care in the clinical management of potentially suicidal patients (Simon 1992a). Practice parameters for the assessment of suicide risk have been promulgated by professional organizations such as the American Academy of Child and Adolescent Psychiatry (Shaffer et al. 1997). The academy's recommendations in official practice guidelines usually indicate the degree of importance or certainty of each recommendation (Shaffer et al. 1997). For example, *minimal standards* are recommendations based on substantial empirical evidence (such as well-controlled double-blind studies), overwhelming clinical consensus, legal and regulatory requirements, or all of the above. Minimal standards are expected to pertain more than 95% of the time—for instance, in almost all cases. If the clinician does not follow this standard in a particular case, the reason should be documented in the medical record.

Clinical guidelines are recommendations that are based on empirical evidence such as open trials and clinical studies or on strong clinical consensus or on both. Clinical guidelines apply approximately 75% of the time. The clinician always should consider these recommendations, but exceptions to their application exist.

Options are practical recommendations that are acceptable but not required. Insufficient empirical evidence is available to support recommending these practices as minimal standards or clinical guidelines. In some instances the practice may be entirely appropriate, whereas in other situations it should be avoided.

The category of *not endorsed* refers to practices that are known to be useless or contraindicated.

By these definitions, the recommendation to perform formal (systematic) suicide risk assessments on patients at risk for suicide is endorsed by overwhelming clinical consensus, thus meeting the criteria for minimal standards of practice. Postmortem assessment of clinically based suicide risk factors in questionable suicide cases also should meet the evidentiary criteria for probative testimony (Biffl 1996).

In *Daubert v. Merrell Dow Pharmaceuticals, Inc.* (1993), the United States Supreme Court held that the "general acceptance" test established under *Frye v. United States* (1923) had been superseded by the "reasonableness" standard of the Federal Rules of Evidence. Thus *Daubert* shifted the focus from the general acceptance of the conclusion of expert testimony to the underlying soundness of the methodology (Slovenko 1995). *Daubert* applies to federal courts but also has been adopted by some states. *Daubert* criteria include testability of scientific knowledge, its peer review and publication, factors affecting potential error rate, and general acceptability by the relevant scientific community. Clinically based standard suicide risk assessments should meet process-driven *Daubert* criteria. Even if a court were to find that postmortem suicide risk assessment was not scientific in a strict sense, it should meet the relevant criteria of general acceptance among mental health professionals.

In *Kumho Tire Co. v. Carmichael* (1999), the United States Supreme Court addressed the testimony of a tire failure analyst. The Court held that the *Daubert* gatekeeping obligation applies to all expert testimony, not only to "scientific" testimony. Federal Rule of Evidence 702 (helpfulness of expert testimony) does not distinguish between scientific knowledge and "technical" or "other specialized" knowledge. Postmortem suicide risk assessment is specialized knowledge. *Daubert* referred only to scientific knowledge because of the nature of the expertise at issue in that case. Federal Rules of Evidence 702 and 703 grant all expert witnesses—not just scientific experts—testimonial latitude that is not available to other witnesses, on the assumption that the expert's opinion will be based reliably on the knowledge and experience of his or her discipline. A trial judge may consider one or more of the specific *Daubert* factors. The *Daubert* factors do not constitute a definitive checklist because they may or may not be pertinent in assessing reliability, which depends on the nature of the issue, the expert's particular expertise, and the subject of the testimony. In determining the reliability of expert testimony, the trial court should consider the specific *Daubert* factors that are reasonable measures of reliability.

The admissibility of psychiatric and psychological testimony likely will be determined on a case-by-case basis. *Daubert* hearings, in which motions *in limine* are introduced to exclude psychiatric or psychological testimony on the retrospective assessment of an individual's mental state, will be a likely venue for such determinations. As courts struggle with this issue, it remains to be seen what accommodations will be worked out under *Daubert* for testimony based on clinical medicine and the social sciences. Meanwhile, the traditional means of challenging expert testimony will continue to be rigorous cross-examination, the presentation of contrary evidence, and careful instruction on the burden of proof.

The issue is not so much deciding how and exactly when *Daubert* applies. Instead, the legal system is telling experts to "prove it." Judges can no longer accept the testimony of experts on faith, merely based on their academic degrees. For altruistic reasons and because it harms the profession, ethical codes and task force reports provide guidelines for fact-based psychiatric and psychological testimony (American Academy of Psychiatry and the Law 1995; "American Psychiatric Association Resource Document on Peer Review of Expert Testimony," 1997).

Generally, appellate courts have been receptive to the use of psychological autopsy methodology as providing helpful testimony. In *United States v. St. Jean* (1995), the court admitted suicide profiles and psychological autopsy testimony in a murder trial. The defendant was charged with the premeditated murder of his wife. The defense claimed that reasonable doubt existed about his guilt because the evidence was just as consistent with suicide. The prosecution's expert testified that the wife manifested none of the suicide risk factors associated with persons who commit suicide. The defense asserted that testimony based on psychological autopsies is inherently unreliable under Federal Rules of Evidence 702 and 403 (prejudicial vs. probative value of evidence) (28 USCA §§ 2071–2074). The court ruled that the expert's testimony was helpful regarding the issue of the wife's suicidal risk. The expert testified that the suicide assessment method was reliable and accepted by the psychiatric and psychological professions.

Psychological autopsy evidence also has been accepted by courts in child abuse cases when the child committed suicide (*Jackson v. State* 1989; *State v. Huber* 1992). Standard suicide risk assessment methods are the stock-in-trade of psychiatrists and other mental health professionals, having been used beneficially in clinical settings for many years. The *Kumho* court admonished the expert witness to approach her or his opinion with "the same intellectual rigor that characterizes the practice of an expert in the relevant field" (*Kumho Tire Co. v. Carmichael* 1999). Testimony concerning a deceased's mental state or the presence or absence of suicide risk factors should satisfy this *Kumho* requirement.

The psychological autopsy was proposed by Shniedman (1973) as a clinical tool. It has proved useful and found general acceptance among forensic psychiatrists and psychologists for its use in litigation (Jacobs and Klein-Benheim 1995). Shneidman (1973, p. 132) stated, "the psychological autopsy is no less than a reconstruction of the motivations, philosophy, psychodynamics, and existential crises of the decedent." Biffl (1996) noted that before psychological autopsy testimony is admissible, the court will require that the evidence is relevant under Federal Rule of Evidence 401, that the expert is qualified in this area under Federal Rule of Evidence 702, and that the testimonial evidence will be helpful to the jury and is reliable under Federal Rules of Evidence 702 and 703, using either *Frye* or *Daubert*. The court also must consider whether prejudicial factors outweigh the probative value of the evidence under Federal Rule of Evidence 403.

The Centers for Disease Control and Prevention developed the 16-item Empirical Criteria for the Determination of Suicide to address criticism that the psychological autopsy lacks psychometric properties such as reliability and validity (Jobes et al. 1991). It has been shown to be 92% accurate in differentiating between suicide and accident. The Empirical Criteria for the Determination of Suicide is useful as an adjunctive tool to professional clinical judgment.

Attempting to reconstruct the mental state or intention of the deceased is more difficult than retrospectively assessing the presence or absence of suicide risk factors alone. As stated in Chapter 1, Oliver Wendell Holmes observed that "even a dog knows the difference between being tripped over and being kicked" (Keeton et al. 1984, p. 34). Nonetheless, the legal concept of intent as applied to suspicious suicide cases is complicated. Retrospectively assessing the presence or absence of suicide risk factors may help clarify the question of suicide intent. However, attempting to discern the motives for suicide can be a daunting task (Simon 1998b). A person's intentions or subjective mental states may be opaque, even after direct psychiatric examination.

Conclusion

Forensic psychiatrists and psychologists are increasingly retained in suspicious suicide cases in both civil and criminal litigation. They can be of considerable assistance in these cases if their expert opinions are based on careful postmortem suicide risk assessment that includes the review of relevant collateral sources of information, death scene analysis, and autopsy findings. In patients with complex medical-psychiatric-life histories, the suicide risk assessment may prove inconclusive. A history of mental illness may obscure the cause of death, even though it may not have been a factor. In cases of murder masquerading as suicide, the crime is more likely to be undetected if a mental illness history is present.

Expert opinions should avoid conclusive statements that invade the province of the fact-finder in determining criminal responsibility. After *Daubert* and *Kumho*, the appropriate question is not invasion of the province of the trier of fact but the availability of reliable and valid methods and procedures to support the conclusions reached. After careful evaluation of the data, probabilistic assessments of suicide risk such as low, moderate, or high at the time of death will be the most helpful to the trier of fact.

The deaths of Marilyn Monroe and Robert Maxwell remain shrouded in mystery despite numerous attempts to determine their causes. The death of Vincent W. Foster Jr., officially ruled a suicide, has quieted political controversy but not the conspiracy theories. Forensic psychiatrists and psychologists who are retained in high-profile cases of celebrity deaths must maintain their usual ethical stance of striving for objectivity and honesty amid media distractions and intense pressure for certainty (American Academy of Psychiatry and the Law 1995). The same professionalism is required of the assessment in the suspicious deaths of ordinary citizens.

References

28 USCA §§ 2071–2074

American Academy of Psychiatry and the Law: American Academy of Psychiatry and the Law Ethical Guidelines for the Practice of Forensic Psychiatry. Bloomfield, CT, American Academy of Psychiatry and the Law, 1995

American Psychiatric Association: Diagnostic and Statistical Manual of Mental Disorders, 3rd Edition, Revised. Washington, DC, American Psychiatric Association, 1987

American Psychiatric Association resource document on peer review of expert testimony. J Am Acad Psychiatry Law 25:359–373, 1997

Biffl E: Psychological autopsies: do they belong in the courtroom? American Journal of Criminal Law 24:123–145, 1996

Blumenthal SJ: An overview and synopsis of risk factors, assessment, and treatment of suicidal patients over the life cycle, in Suicide Over the Life Cycle. Edited by Blumenthal SJ, Kupfer DJ. Washington, DC, American Psychiatric Press, 1990, pp 685–733

Busch KA, Clark DC, Fawcett J, et al: Clinical features of inpatient suicide. Psychiatric Annals 23:256–262, 1993

Chiles JH, Strohsall K: The Suicidal Patient: Principles of Assessment, Treatment and Case Management. Washington, DC, American Psychiatric Press, 1995

Clark DC, Fawcett J: An empirically based model of suicide risk assessment of patients with affective disorders, in Suicide and Clinical Practice. Edited by Jacobs DJ. Washington, DC, American Psychiatric Press, 1992, pp 55–74

Clark DC, Horton-Deutsch S: Assessment in absentia: the value of the psychological autopsy method for studying antecedents of suicide and predicting future suicides, in Assessment and Prediction of Suicide. Edited by Maris R, Berman A, Maltsberger J, et al. New York, Guilford, 1992, pp 144–182

Daubert v Merrell Dow Pharmaceuticals, Inc., 509 US 579 (1993)

Evans G, Faberow NL: The Encyclopedia of Suicide. New York, Facts on File, 1988, pp 212–213

Fawcett J, Scheptner WA, Fogg L, et al: Time-related predictors of suicide in major affective disorder. Am J Psychiatry 147:1189–1194, 1990

Fawcett J, Clark DC, Busch KA: Assessing and treating the patient at risk for suicide. Psychiatric Annals 23:244–255, 1993

Frye v United States, 293 F 1013 (DC Cir 1923)

Hutson HR, Anglin D, Yarbrough J, et al: Suicide by cop. Ann Emerg Med 32:665–669, 1998

Jackson v State, 553 So2d 719 (Fla Dist Ct App 1989)

Jacobs DJ, Klein-Benheim ME: The psychological autopsy: a useful tool for determining proximate causation in suicide cases. Bulletin of the American Academy of Psychiatry and the Law 23:165–182, 1995

Jobes DA, Caseys JO, Berman AL, et al: Empirical criteria for the determination of suicide manner of death. J Forensic Sci 36:244–256, 1991

Keeton W, Dobbs D, Keeton R, et al: Intentional interference with the person, in Prosser and Keeton on Torts, 5th Edition. St. Paul, MN, West Publishing, 1984, p 34

Kumho Tire Co. v Carmichael, 526 US 137 (1999)

Maris RW, Berman AL, Maltsberger JT, et al: Assessment and Prediction of Suicide. New York, Guilford, 1992

Melton GB, Petrila J, Poythress NG, et al: Psychological Evaluations for the Courts, 2nd Edition. New York, Guilford, 1997

Monahan J, Steadman HJ: Violent storms and violent people: how meteorology can inform risk communication in mental health law. Am Psychol 51:931–938, 1996

Nolan J (ed): Suicide: The Suicide Case: Investigation and Trial of Insurance Claims. Chicago, IL, American Bar Association, 1988

People of the State of New York v. Raymond Stolpinski, Rich Co Ind No 290/97

People v. Darrell Younger, Sonoma County Superior Court Case Number SCR-24618; Sonoma County District Attorney Case Number DAR-330986

Pokorny AD: Prediction of suicide in psychiatric patients: report of a prospective study. Arch Gen Psychiatry 40:249–257, 1983

Pokorny AD: Suicide prediction revisited. Suicide Life Threat Behav 23:1–10, 1993

Roy A: Risk factors for psychiatric patients. Arch Gen Psychiatry 39:1084–1095, 1992

Schmidt S: Starr's probe concludes Foster committed suicide. Washington Post, July 16, 1997, pp A1, A7

Shaffer DA, Pfeffer CR, Bernet W, et al: Practice parameters for the assessment and treatment of children and adolescents with suicidal behavior. J Am Acad Child Adolesc Psychiatry 40(7, suppl):245–515, 1997

Shniedman ES: Deaths of Man. New York, Quadrangle New York Times Book, 1973

Simon RI: You only die once—but did you intend it? Psychiatric assessment of suicide intent in insurance litigation. Tort and Insurance Law Journal 25:650–662, 1990

Simon RI: Clinical risk management of the suicidal patient, in Clinical Psychiatry and the Law, 2nd Edition. Washington, DC, American Psychiatric Press, 1992a, pp 277–281

Simon RI: Clinical risk management of suicidal patients: assessing the unpredictable, in American Psychiatric Press Review of Clinical Psychiatry and the Law, Vol 3. Edited by Simon RI. Washington, DC, American Psychiatric Press, 1992b, pp 3–63

Simon RI: Bad Men Do What Good Men Dream: A Forensic Psychiatrist Illuminates the Darker Side of Human Behavior. Washington, DC, American Psychiatric Press, 1996

Simon RI: Concise Guide to Psychiatry and Law for Clinicians, 2nd Edition. Washington, DC, American Psychiatric Press, 1998a, pp 143–144

Simon RI: Murder masquerading as suicide: post-mortem assessment of suicide-risk factors at the time of death. J Forensic Sci 43:1129–1133, 1998b

Simon RI: Psychiatrists awake! Suicide risk assessments are all about a good night's sleep. Psychiatric Annals 28:479–485, 1998c

Slovenko R: Psychiatry and Criminal Culpability. New York, Wiley, 1995, pp 375–376

Spitz WV: Asphyxia, in Medicolegal Investigation of Death: Guidelines for the Application of Pathology to Crime Investigations, 3rd Edition. Edited by Spitz WV. Springfield, IL, Charles C Thomas, 1993, p 465

State v Huber, 597 NE2d 570 (Ohio CP 1992)

Tanay E: The psychological autopsy, in Medicolegal Death Investigation:ttreatises in the Forensic Sciences. Edited by Caplan YH. Colorado Springs, CO, Forensic Sciences Foundation Press, 1997, pp 237–247

United States v St. Jean, WL 106960 (AF Ct Crim App 1995)

Wilson EF, Davis JH, Bloom JD, et al: Homicide or suicide: the killing of suicidal persons by law enforcement officers. J Forensic Sci 43:46–52, 1998

7

Retrospective Assessment of Children's Mental States

Nancy E. Walker, Ph.D., M.L.S.

Consider the case of young Brian Dailey, age 5 years 9 months, defendant in an action for battery brought by the plaintiff, Ms. Garratt, an elderly and arthritic woman (*Garratt v. Dailey* 1955). Ms. Garratt sued Brian in tort for damages resulting from a hip fracture that occurred when she fell to the ground after laboriously attempting to sit in a chair that was, as it turns out, not beneath her. Young Brian contended that he had tried to help Ms. Garratt by placing a chair under her as she was about to fall but that he was too small to move it into place. A conflicting account of the incident was offered by the plaintiff's sister, also present at the occasion, who claimed that the arthritic Ms. Garratt had begun the slow process of seating herself when the defendant quickly removed the chair from beneath her and seated himself on it. Furthermore, she asserted that Brian *knew* that Ms. Garrett would attempt to sit in the place where the chair had been.

The trial court found for the defendant. However, unlike the trial court, the appellate court focused its attention on the "substantial certainty test." According to the appellate court, the crucial issue in this case was not whether the chair was outside Ms. Garrett's backward aim but rather *whether Brian knew with substantial certainty* that the plaintiff would attempt to sit down in the spot where the chair had been. On appeal from the trial court's judgment in favor of young Brian, the Washington Supreme Court noted that "a battery would be established if, in addition to plaintiff's fall, it was proved that, when Brian moved the chair, *he knew with substantial certainty* that the plaintiff would attempt to sit down where the chair had been" (p. 1094, emphasis added).

In other words, the court had to make a retrospective assessment of Brian's state of mind at the time of the incident. When the trial judge reconsidered the evidence under this standard, he awarded a judgment of $11,000 to Ms. Garratt, which was upheld on appeal.

Attorneys, physicians, psychiatrists, psychologists, social workers, teachers, and other professionals all may be required to conduct retrospective assessments of children's mental states at some point during their careers. In many cases these assessments occur in nonlegal contexts. For example, teachers and principals who conduct disciplinary hearings must assess the state of a child's mind at some prior point in time, such as when interpersonal conflict occurred at school. Similarly, in mental health treatment settings, psychiatrists or psychologists may be called on to assess what a child's mental state was during a significant incident that occurred earlier in the child's life. In such cases, neither criminal nor civil litigation typically is on the horizon.

Although it is important to conduct an accurate retrospective assessment of a child's mental state even when litigation is not involved, it is especially important to do so in legal contexts because fundamental rights such as life or liberty may be implicated. In this regard, one commentator noted that

> if the initial interview is improperly conducted, like Humpty-Dumpty, the child's account can never be put together again. Without exaggeration, the investigative interview is the single most important component of any trial involving a child witness. The skill of the interviewer is more important than the sophistication of the judge or jury assigned to decide the case, more important than any of the other players—the lawyers and their experts. A skilled interviewer can empower the child to capture his or her experiences while memory of them is most fresh and vibrant. When the child's memories are carefully and neutrally extracted, both the needs of the legal system and the child are well served. In contrast, when the interview is inartfully conducted, the "Humpty-Dumpty Effect" is set in motion. (McGough 1996, p. 189)

Legal Contexts in Which Retrospective Assessment of a Child's Mental State May Be Required

In the legal arena, retrospective assessments of children's mental states generally occur in one of three contexts: criminal, civil, and juvenile court. The child whose mental state is under review may be a plaintiff, a defendant, a victim, or a witness.

Criminal Litigation Contexts

A child's prior mental state may need to be assessed during the course of criminal litigation. For example, the statutes of several states provide that the juvenile court's jurisdiction over a child who has been charged with committing a serious crime may be waived in favor of criminal court adjudication (Cauffman et al. 1999). For the child who, by this means, becomes a defendant in adult criminal proceedings, a retrospective assessment of mental state may be necessary to assist in the determination of mens rea, or legal culpability for the act allegedly committed. Children also may be asked to testify as witnesses in criminal litigation; for example, a child may be the sole living witness to homicide or arson. More commonly, children may be asked to describe domestic assaults they witnessed at some point in the past. Alternatively, children may be required to give testimony as victim-witnesses in cases of alleged sexual or physical assault or neglect. In each of these cases, the interviewer must assess not only the accuracy of the basic facts reported but also any potential motivations to exaggerate or diminish the importance of reported events. In other words, mental states must be assessed to determine how those states might influence the veracity of the report communicated.

Civil Litigation Contexts

A child also may be a party to or may testify in civil litigation. For example, in the case of divorce, a child may be asked to provide an opinion about not only the current situation but also events that occurred during prior points in time. Less commonly, a child may be asked to provide testimony regarding an alleged tort that occurred at some point in the past, particularly if that child is a party to the lawsuit (see, e.g., *Garratt v. Dailey* 1955, described in the introductory text of this chapter). In these civil contexts, as in the criminal arena, retrospective assessments of a child's mental state may provide information that can assist the trier of fact to determine whether the child was motivated to exaggerate, diminish, or otherwise alter the account reported.

Juvenile Court Contexts

Juvenile courts, first established in 1899, were designed to "free children from the harsh and punitive effects of the adult criminal justice system" (Nguyen 1995, p. 403). The system recognized the unique needs of children and emphasized treatment and rehabilitation rather than incarceration and punishment (Gardner 1997). The system even developed its own professional jargon: juveniles were to be "detained" (not arrested) and "treated" (not punished) (Gardner 1997).

In the juvenile court's rehabilitative context, therefore, the reason for conducting a retrospective assessment may diverge, at least to some degree, from that in the criminal and civil contexts mentioned above. In this case, the retrospective assessment may focus on whether the child's mental state at the time of an action suggests that the child is amenable to rehabilitation. If so, the child then may be adjudicated in the juvenile system; if not, the juvenile court's jurisdiction over the child may be waived (Gardner 1997). Even with the recent trend toward a more punitive (rather than rehabilitative) focus in juvenile court proceedings, the issue of assessing the child's potential for rehabilitation remains.

Juvenile courts also have authority to deal with children who commit status offenses. *Status offenses* are offenses that would not be a crime if committed by an adult—that is, acts that are offenses solely because of the perpetrator's status as a juvenile (Gardner 1997). Status offenses include truancy, running away from home, incorrigibility, and unruly behavior. For the latter categories, in particular, retrospective assessment of a child's mental state may prove useful to the court. For example, the court may well react differently if a child's status offenses result from the need to escape abuse as opposed to the need for attention or even infamy.

Finally, juvenile or family courts may handle dependency hearings, foster care placements, cases involving termination of parental rights, and adoptions. In these cases, assessments of a child's current state of mind may be more relevant than retrospective assessments, but the latter may come into play as well. For example, assessments of a child's prior mental states and patterns of behavior may provide helpful information about that child's likely future demeanor in various placements.

Thus, in each of these legal contexts (criminal, civil, and juvenile), professionals may need to conduct retrospective assessments of a child's state of mind. The professionals involved must conduct forensic interviews that are most likely to produce complete and accurate reports and least likely to induce suggestibility in the child. To do so, the professionals involved should have some understanding of children's developing abilities in memory, language, and communication as well as common pitfalls to avoid when engaging in retrospective assessment of children's mental states.

Development of Children's Abilities in Memory, Language, and Communication

The critical task in conducting retrospective assessments of children's mental states is to determine which factors, if any, impinge on their ability to comprehend, accurately recall, and report past events. For example, did the child have some ulterior motive for falsification, withholding, or fabrication of information? At the time in question, did the child have the capacity to understand the events that transpired? Did the child, at that point in time, understand the difference between right and wrong? Did the child have the ability to comprehend and act on *Miranda* warnings or other legal procedures? Whether we approach such questions from a psychological or a legal perspective, the essential question is, "How do internal mental states affect historical accuracy in remembering and reporting events?"

To answer this fundamental question, professionals who conduct retrospective assessments of children's mental states should be well grounded in child development as well as in the scientific literature on memory and suggestibility. It is, however, outside the scope of this chapter to provide a comprehensive review; for the purposes of this chapter, a succinct overview of child development will suffice. Interested readers may consult other sources for more information (see, e.g., Perry 1987; Perry and Wrightsman 1991; Poole and Lamb 1998).

Memory

The first steps in remembering an event are to perceive it and to pay attention to it. Interestingly, young children are not less aware of their surroundings than are older children and adults. In general, alertness changes little after the first few months of life (Gibson and Radner 1979). However, as children mature, they develop the ability to focus their attention in task-specific ways, so their capacity for reporting what they perceive improves (Poole and Lamb 1998).

A child interviewed retrospectively must have sufficient ability not only to perceive and attend to an event but also to remember the event. The child's memory of the event may be tested through different means, including recognition, reconstruction, and recall.

Recognition is the simplest form of remembering because it requires only that the child perceive an object as something that was perceived previously. Recognition is within the capacity of very young infants and even of animals (see Piaget and Inhelder 1973). Recognition memory improves rapidly as children mature (see, e.g., Myers and Perlmutter 1978) and functions particularly well during the elementary-school years (Perry and Wrightsman 1991). It is tempting, therefore, to incorporate recognition tasks in interviews of children. One risk of this approach, however, is that it may foster suggestive interviewing, thereby leading to incorrect or tainted reports of memory.

Reconstruction is a specialized method of retrieving material from memory that involves reproducing the form of information that was seen in the past. Reconstructing the scene of a crime is an example. Some forensic interview protocols, such as the Cognitive Interview (Fisher and Geiselman 1992), recommend using a reconstruction technique called context reinstatement. In this technique, interviewees are encouraged to re-create the scene of an event mentally and to report everything they can remember by focusing on the surroundings, the smells and sounds, the temperature, the location of the furniture, or anything else about the event that may elicit memories they could not otherwise recall. Use of reconstruction techniques generally leads to recall of more correct details than does a standard interview, although some confabulated details may increase as well (Memon et al. 1997).

Recall is the most complex form of memory test because it requires that previously observed events be retrieved from storage with few or no prompts. Unlike the simpler forms of memory assessment, recall ability is strongly age-related (see, e.g., Marin et al. 1979). It is important to note, however, that although younger children may be able to recall less information, if they are interviewed nonsuggestively, the details they do report often have lower error rates than do those of older children and adults (Marin et al. 1979). Perry and Teply (1984–1985) drew the following conclusions about research on children's memory:

> In the context of a legal interview or examination, this research suggests that when children are simply asked to tell what they can remember about an event, the quality of the narrative of older children will be better than that of younger ones, but neither will give as full a narrative as an adult. It also suggests, however, that even young children (kindergarten-first grade) have sufficiently developed ability to remember past events and that simple, direct (nonleading) questions or recognition recall [i.e., cued recall] appear to be viable means of finding out factual information from them. Using those methods, their answers apparently are no less credible than those of an adult, absent other influences. (p. 1389)

Another aspect of memory relevant to interviewers conducting retrospective assessments is the issue of *source monitoring*, or the process of identifying the origin of one's knowledge of event memories. For example, source monitoring is involved when a person struggles to decide whether an event was personally experienced, was experienced by a friend who reported it, was viewed on television, or was described in a book.

Young children generally are more likely than their older counterparts to have difficulty in determining whether the information they "know" came from their own experiences or from other sources. One explanation for this problem is that young children have immature frontal lobe development (Schacter et al. 1995). As their brains develop, so too does their ability to monitor the sources of their knowledge, although even adults may have considerable difficulty with this task.

Research on interview techniques to combat the problem of source monitoring is scant. Poole and Lindsay (1995, 1996) found that children were more likely to include information from the wrong source when interviewers asked closed questions that limited response options (e.g., "Did he...") rather than providing open-ended prompts (e.g., "Tell me what happened"). In addition, children who attribute information to the wrong source sometimes can reconstruct what they actually experienced when interviewers explicitly ask them to do so, although this ability is limited at ages 3 and 4 years (Lindsay et al. 1995; Poole and Lindsay 1996). Finally, Poole and Lamb (1998) noted that

> For children, evidently, information obtained from parents and other sources is "real," and therefore references to "what really happened" do not always prompt the distinction between information obtained by personal experience and information that was only heard. It is difficult to rephrase such questions, however, because many young children have not yet mastered the distinctions among mental verbs such as *remember, know,* and *guess.* (p. 45)

Language and Communication

Children who are retrospectively interviewed also must have the ability to report information about an experienced event. Poole and Lamb (1998) noted that research on the relation between language comprehension and attention suggests that, regardless of age, children may attend to interviews more successfully when they have a better understanding of the interview purpose and processes. However, important differences between the autobiographical reports of preschool children and those of older children also must be taken into consideration.

Younger children, for example, have more difficulty recognizing which event is under discussion during an interview (see, e.g., Poole and Lindsay 1995, 1996; Steward and Steward 1996). Also, even when children begin talking about target events, as questioning continues they tend to stray from the original topic (Poole and Lindsay 1996). In this regard, Poole and Lamb (1998) noted that

> Topic drifts...can have serious implications in forensic contexts, leading to bizarre interpretations of the child's experiences or even false accusations of other adults who happen to be mentioned. Topic drift might also lead adults to consider the child an unreliable witness. Interviewers therefore must be especially careful to ensure that children start, and stay, on topic. A simple strategy is to reword ambiguous prompts (e.g., "Can you tell me more?") into topic-focus prompts (e.g., "Can you tell me more about that time at the cottage?"). (p. 40)

Another source of potential communication errors occurs when children are interviewed more than once about the same event or events. Because younger children are particularly likely to focus on different topics during the various interviews, their repeated accounts of the events involved appear to be less consistent than those provided by older children (Poole and Lamb 1998). In reviewing the research in this area, Poole and Lamb (1998) concluded that

> Content analyses of the children's narratives surprisingly revealed no decrease across sessions in either the total amount of information or the amount of descriptive information recalled, even after a 1-year delay. The children reported different pieces of information across sessions, however, recalling less than 10% of their information during each of two consecutive sessions. This pattern of session-to-session inconsistency is a well-documented pattern. (pp. 40–41)

Moreover, although information reported for the first time during a second interview is less accurate on average than information also reported during the first interview, information is not necessarily unreliable simply because it was not mentioned earlier.

In addition, interviewers should be familiar with common errors in children's communications (see, e.g., Perry and Wrightsman 1991). For example, young children often engage in *overextension*, which is extending the meaning of a word to encompass actions or objects for which a child has no word. For example, young children may consider elbows and knees to be "private parts" because they often are covered by clothing. Children also tend to *underextend* the meanings of words; that is, they attribute to a word only part of the meaning the term has for adults. For example, a child may deny that abuse occurred at "home" if the actions occurred in an apartment as opposed to a house.

Another potential source of error in communication with children is *syntax*, or the ordering of words to convey meaning. This problem is particularly apparent when adults use the passive voice as opposed to the active voice. For example, when a child hears, "You said your mom *was hit by* your dad," the child may visualize the scene as Mom hitting Dad, an error that may be avoided by using the active voice statement, "You said your dad *hit* your mom."

Finally, although children may use "big" words, their understanding often is more limited than their vocabularies. Researchers have found that sophisticated vocabulary—as well as complex syntax, use of negatives and double negatives, and multipart and forced-choice questions—reduces by nearly one-half the ability of interviewees to comprehend questions and to answer correctly, whether the respondents are children or adults (Perry et al. 1995; N.E. Walker et al. 1996). Therefore it is especially important that interviewers use simple words and define and explain jargon.

The Problem of Distinguishing Truths, Lies, and False Beliefs

It is difficult to determine the point at which children understand the difference between a "lie" and a "truth," for these concepts are multifaceted. Perry (1995) explains:

> A truthful statement is characterized by five elements: (1) the statement is true; (2) the speaker believes the statement to be true; (3) in uttering the statement, the speaker intends the statement to be truthful; (4) the speaker wants to convey truthfulness; and (5) the speaker expects the listener to believe the statement because, of course, it is truthful. (p. 75)

Some research evidence suggests that young children's definitions of truthfulness may differ from those of older children and adults. For instance, 4-year-old children may label any verbal indiscretion (such as swearing) a lie (see, e.g., Haugaard 1992), and even most 6-year-olds do not consider the speaker's intention (i.e., "good" or "bad") when assessing whether an inaccurate statement is a mistake or a lie (Wimmer et al. 1984). Some time between ages 6 and 10 years, children begin to place more emphasis on the belief system of the speaker than on the factuality of the statement (Strichartz and Burton 1990). In other words, with increasing age, they begin to focus more on whether the speaker *believes* the statement to be true than on the objective truth of the utterance. (See Ceci et al. 1992 and Perry 1995 for reviews of the development of truth-lie understanding.)

In general, the ability to distinguish between lies and truth varies as a function of two factors: 1) the form of the questions posed and 2) the topic of discussion (Poole and Lamb 1998). Poole and Lamb (1998) identified three major limitations to incorporating truth-lie discussions into investigative interviews. First, children who "pass" so-called truth-lie tests are not necessarily more accurate or less suggestible than same-age peers who fail. Thus truth-lie tests do not predict well which children will be accurate reporters. Second, no evidence indicates that standard truth-lie tests encourage children to filter out inaccurate information. Third, young children's inaccuracies in reporting may be more a result of errors in complying with the perceived demands of the interview situation and errors in memory than intentional deception. Thus Poole and Lamb (1998) noted: "Current competency procedures do not address many of the reasons why children sometimes misreport events" (p. 48). Although revised procedures seem warranted, research on this topic is insufficient to make specific recommendations for practice.

The Problem of Suggestibility

Suggestibility refers to the tendency to make errors elicited by exposure to information that is false, to misleading questions or statements, and to social pressures that encourage particular types of answers. During the past quarter century, the literature on interviewing children has been replete with discussions of the perils associated with suggestive questioning and of the interview techniques likely to induce suggestibility (see Ceci and Bruck 1993 for a review of this topic). Although several factors influence eyewitness reports (e.g., time since event and interview procedures), research studies that have manipulated these variables suggest some general conclusions regarding children's suggestibility. Poole and Lamb (1998) described relevant research in this area and offered the following conclusions:

- Younger children tend to be more vulnerable to suggestion than are older children. Preschoolers in particular have difficulty rejecting misleading information even after adults tell them that they were misinformed.
- Children are better able to resist suggestions about significant body-related events than suggestions about other details or events.
- Specific misleading questions are very likely to produce erroneous responses.
- Factors that generally impair memory (e.g., longer time lags before interviewing and questions about less salient events) also increase suggestibility.

- Interviewers who have a bias about what might have happened tend to elicit more false information from children.
- Nonsuggestive, open-ended interviewing cannot ensure that children will provide accurate reports, especially if those children have been exposed to misinformation in prior interviews or by other sources.
- In certain contexts, errors induced by misinformation procedures show disturbing stability over time and in repeated interviews, although such errors tend to drop out of children's reports at a faster rate than do either spontaneous errors or accurate details.

Poole and Lamb (1998) concluded that

> it is not the case that children's event reports are generally distorted and unreliable, nor is it the case that children cannot be prompted to falsely report events that might be considered abusive. Rather, the quality of children's testimony is a joint product of their cognitive and social maturity, their experiences outside formal interviews, and the interviewing context. (p. 69)

Legal Scrutiny of Forensic Interviewing Practices

The problems associated with retrospective assessments of children's mental states came to national attention during the 1980s and 1990s in a series of highly publicized trials of day-care staff. In the McMartin Preschool Trial (*People v. Buckey* 1990), more than 350 children were alleged to have been molested at the preschool and at other public locations, including a market, a car wash, and a church. During interviewing, some children reported that, in addition to being sexually abused, they had been taken on airplane rides and forced to drink blood and to watch animals being mutilated. Prosecutors said that the suggestive techniques used to elicit retrospective reports from such young children were appropriate, whereas the defense claimed that the interviewing and videotaping procedures were inept. When the trial ended in January 1990, several jurors reported that they believed that some of the children had in fact been molested but that the state had failed to prove the identity of the perpetrator(s). This 3-year trial—the longest running criminal trial in the history of the United States—cost taxpayers $13–$15 million, produced no convictions, and destroyed the lives of many individuals connected to the case (Perry and Wrightsman 1991). In the end, it was not possible to determine whether the retrospective reports provided by the children interviewed were accurate.

Research completed since the McMartin trial shows that the skill of the interviewer directly influences whether a child relates a true memory, discusses a false belief, affirms details suggested by others, embellishes fantasies, or provides no information at all (see, e.g., Garven et al. 1998; Gilstrap et al. 1999; Perry et al. 1995; N.E. Walker and Hunt 1998; Warren et al. 1996). For example, Garven and colleagues (1998) reported that the types of techniques used by interviewers in the McMartin case (e.g., telling the child that the interviewer already had received information from another person regarding the topics of the interview, making positive and negative consequences contingent on the child's responses, repeating questions already asked and answered by the child, and inviting speculation about past events) elicited substantially more false allegations from children than did simple suggestive questions. This finding is particularly important given the fact that suggestive questions have long been known to negatively affect the quality of children's reports. (See Ceci and Bruck 1993 and Poole and Lamb 1998 for reviews of the suggestive questioning literature.) When exposed to the "McMartin techniques" for less than 5 minutes, children in the Garven et al. study showed error rates of nearly 60%. Moreover, children subjected to social influence techniques became more acquiescent as the interview proceeded.

Other researchers have investigated different aspects of the ways in which interviewer skill affects children's reports. For example, Warren et al. (1996) analyzed the questions posed in 42 Child Protective Service interviews of children who alleged that they had been sexually abused. Among other findings, they reported that interviewers only infrequently asked open-ended questions that invited narrative responses from children. When invitational utterances were used, however, they prompted longer and more detailed responses from the children.

N.E. Walker and Hunt (1998) conducted further analyses of Warren et al.'s 42 Child Protective Service interviews. These researchers identified several types of questions that compromised interview integrity. Faulty techniques included instances in which the interviewer modified the child's statement, used forced-choice questions that limited the responses the child could give, and used multipart questions. These faulty techniques increased the likelihood that children became inappropriately compliant (e.g., when children failed to correct the interviewer's modifications), that children chose one of the options offered by the interviewer regardless of whether it was correct (in the case of forced-choice questions), or that children became confused (e.g., when confronted with multipart questions).

In a laboratory study of children's and adults' comprehension of various question forms, Perry and colleagues (1995) found that even kindergarten-age children could correctly answer most (75%) simply phrased, straightforward questions about a recently viewed event and that older children and adults correctly answered approximately 90% of the simply phrased questions. In contrast, children, adolescents, and young adults alike were befuddled by convoluted question forms requesting the same information; participants correctly answered only about 55% of those complex questions.

These studies found that the specific techniques used by an interviewer have a direct effect on the quality of the retrospective report obtained; this conclusion has been heeded in appellate court opinions. For example, in *State v. Michaels* (1993), the New Jersey Supreme Court considered whether the state's interview techniques in the case had been "so coercive or suggestive that they had a capacity to distort substantially the children's recollections of actual events and thus compromise the reliability of the children's statements and testimony based on their recollections" (p. 1377). An amicus curiae brief signed by more than 40 scientists provided the appellate court with a summary of research relevant to issues associated with the forensic interviewing of children and showed the causative link between the use of highly suggestive interviewing techniques and children's flawed memories (Bruck and Ceci 1995). The information presented in the brief contributed to the appellate court's decision to reverse the defendant's conviction.

As the McMartin Preschool and *State v. Michaels* cases illustrate, truth finding that involves retrospective assessments of children's mental states may be seriously compromised, if not completely obscured, by faulty interviewing techniques. In the remainder of this chapter, therefore, I focus on the legal standards for assessing the admissibility of interview evidence and on empirically based procedures for conducting sound forensic interviews of children.

Legal Standards for Assessing the Admissibility of Interview Evidence

In a case that involves retrospective assessment of a child's mental state, the assessment must be relevant to the issues at bar and material to the case. In addition, the assessment should facilitate truth finding without being either unfairly prejudicial or confusing to the jurors or judge. Some jurisdictions require additional criteria—for example, that the assessment methods have been "generally accepted" by the relevant scientific community (the *Frye* test) or that they have been subjected to rigorous scientific scrutiny (the *Daubert* standard). A retrospective assessment may be supported or attacked on any of these grounds.

The practitioner who conducts retrospective assessments of children's

mental states, therefore, must be familiar not only with the scientific literature on memory and suggestibility but also with the legal rules in the relevant jurisdiction. An interviewer who completes a retrospective
assessment with faulty or problematic techniques, such as those described
in the previous section, risks having the evidence thrown out of court—and
appropriately so. No interview is perfect, of course, so interview evidence
should not be ruled inadmissible simply because a few minor errors were
committed. However, as the number of faulty techniques increases, and as
the egregiousness of the errors escalates, it becomes increasingly appropriate to invoke either the *Frye* test of general acceptance or the *Daubert* criteria of scientific rigor in 1) ruling on the admissibility of the interview
evidence or 2) determining the weight to be accorded that evidence.

Under the Federal Rules of Evidence

More than 50% of the states follow the Federal Rules of Evidence (Lilly
1996). Under Federal Rule of Evidence 702, the court has discretion to admit expert testimony if it will assist the jury:

> If scientific, technical, or other specialized knowledge will assist the trier
> of fact to understand the evidence or to determine a fact in issue, a witness
> qualified as an expert by knowledge, skill, experience, training, or educa-
> tion, may testify thereto in the form of an opinion or otherwise. (Lilly
> 1996, p. 642)

Admission or exclusion of expert testimony must not be capricious,
however; rather, the court must use standards of admissibility. In jurisdictions that follow the Federal Rules of Evidence, the admissibility of a retrospective assessment of a child's mental state offered by an expert witness
will be evaluated on the criteria of relevance; materiality; probative value;
and lack of unfair prejudice, confusion, or potential to mislead the fact-
finders. Federal Rules of Evidence 401, 402, and 403 speak to these issues.
Federal Rule 401 defines *relevant evidence* as "evidence having any tendency to make the existence of any fact that is of consequence to the determination of the [legal] action more probable or less probable than it would
be without the evidence" (Lilly 1996, p. 629) Federal Rule 402 states that
"[a]ll relevant evidence is admissible....Evidence which is not relevant is
not admissible" (Lilly 1996, p. 629)
Two tests of relevance must be met: materiality and probative value. If the
evidence is offered to prove a proposition that is not at issue, the evidence is
immaterial and therefore irrelevant. For example, if evidence regarding retrospective assessment of a child's mental state has no bearing on the facts of a
case, the evidence is immaterial and therefore will not be admitted. Even if the

evidence directly addresses a fact of central concern to the substantive law (and therefore is material to the case), it will not be admitted unless the evidence "provides insight into the likelihood that the fact at issue exists" (Monahan and Walker 1998, p. 122). This criterion is the test of probative value. In a case involving alleged sexual abuse of a child, for example, evidence regarding retrospective assessment of the child's mental state at the time of the alleged abuse may provide considerable insight into whether the alleged abuse in fact occurred. Did the child have some motivation for fabrication (such as revenge), for recantation (e.g., threats or promises of reward), or for truthfulness? Finally, even if both material and probative, relevant evidence may be excluded if "its probative value is substantially outweighed by the danger of unfair prejudice, confusion of the issues, or misleading the jury" (Federal Rule 403, in Lilly 1996, p. 629).

Courts have used a variety of criteria for assessing probative value when a purportedly scientific technique or method (such as retrospective assessment of a child's mental state) is introduced into legal proceedings. Two of the widely used criteria are known as the *Frye* test (*Frye v. United States* 1923) and the *Daubert* standard (*Daubert v. Merrell Dow Pharmaceuticals, Inc.* 1993). Depending on the jurisdiction, either standard may be invoked in evaluating the probative value of a retrospective assessment technique.

Under the *Frye* Standard

In *Frye v. United States* (1923), the United States Court of Appeals for the D.C. Circuit ruled that the trial judge's exclusion of a purportedly scientific procedure was appropriate. Frye, the defendant in a murder case, had sought to prove his innocence by introducing into evidence favorable results of a "systolic blood pressure deception test" he had taken. In upholding the trial judge's exclusion of the blood pressure evidence, the appellate court commented:

> Just when a scientific principle or discovery crosses the line between the experimental and demonstrable stages is difficult to define. Somewhere in this twilight zone the evidential force of the principle must be recognized, and while courts will go a long way in admitting expert testimony deduced from a well-recognized scientific principle or discovery, the thing from which the deduction is made must be sufficiently established to have gained *general acceptance* in the particular field in which it belongs. (p. 1014)

Moreover, any technique (including means for conducting retrospective assessment of a child's mental state) may be 1) valid and reliable as well as generally accepted, 2) valid and reliable but not generally accepted, or 3) invalid and/or unreliable but generally accepted. The *Frye* test is met in either the first or the third case, but it is met appropriately only in the first instance; furthermore, the test fails to meet the court's objective in the second case. Because of these problems with the *Frye* test, courts have searched for other means to assess the probative value of purportedly scientific methods.

Under the *Daubert* Standard

Under the *Daubert* standard, courts must ensure that the proposed expert testimony meets the basic test of relevance. In addition, they must determine whether experts' testimony reflects "scientific knowledge," whether their findings are "derived by the scientific method," and whether their work product amounts to "good science." Although *Daubert* did not set out a definitive checklist or test of admissibility, the United States Supreme Court articulated four factors that would be helpful for judges to consider:

1. Whether the technique can be (and has been) tested
2. Whether the theory or technique has been subjected to peer review and publication
3. The known or potential error rate and the existence and maintenance of standards controlling the operation of a particular scientific technique
4. "General acceptance" within a relevant scientific community

Some methods for conducting retrospective assessment of a child's mental state generally meet all four factors; other methods meet only some, or even none, of the factors. The next section provides recommendations for best practice in forensic interviewing of children. These recommendations are based on empirical findings that have been subjected to peer review and publication and that appear to meet the test of "general acceptance" within the community of researchers of forensic interviewing techniques. These recommendations for best practice, therefore, should satisfy judicial scrutiny under *Frye*, *Daubert*, or the Federal Rules of Evidence.

Recommendations for Best Practice in Forensic Interviewing of Children

Although professional disagreements have been aired with respect to specific aspects of interviewing practice (e.g., assessment of truth-lie distinctions, individual questioning techniques), experts' recommendations for proper interviewing of children are remarkably consistent (Home Office 1992; Orbach et al. 2000; Poole and Lamb 1998; N.E. Walker and Hunt 1998; N.E. Walker and Nguyen 1996).

Developmentally Appropriate Language

Adults who interview children need to understand some basic principles of child development. Interviewers need to understand that significant differences exist in language comprehension and usage between children and adults (see the "Language and Communication" section above). Without that foundation, interviewers risk obtaining either contaminated information or poor-quality retrospective reports from children. The comprehensive guidelines for interviewing child witnesses in criminal proceedings developed by the United Kingdom's Home Office in 1992, known as the *Memorandum of Good Practice*, caution that "all interviews should be undertaken only by those with training, experience and an aptitude for talking to children" (p. 3).

Despite this caution, some researchers have documented the deleterious effects of adults' use of confusing language when questioning children (Brennan and Brennan 1990; Kranat and Westcott 1994; Perry et al. 1995; A.G. Walker 1993; N.E. Walker and Hunt 1998; Warren et al. 1996). For example, Perry and colleagues (1995) questioned kindergartners, fourth-graders, ninth-graders, and college students about a videotaped scenario. Some questions were phrased in "lawyerese" (i.e., including negatives, double negatives, multiple parts, difficult vocabulary, or complex syntax). Other questions, matched for content with the "lawyerese" forms, were phrased simply. Across age groups, participants correctly answered almost twice as many simply phrased questions as "lawyerese" questions. Moreover, participants of all ages accurately judged how well they understood and could answer the simply phrased questions 90% of the time, but the "lawyerese" questions only 55% of the time. Thus adults risk miscarriage of justice when they use complex language and question forms in interviewing children.

Based on research findings, N.E. Walker and Nguyen (1996) suggested several specific strategies for increasing the likelihood that an interview of a child will be developmentally appropriate:

- Use active rather than passive voice.
- Avoid negatives and double negatives.
- Include only one query per question.
- Use simple words.

- Use simple phrases.
- Use the child's terms.
- Be alert to any signals that the child is having difficulty comprehending the questions asked.

Interview Protocol

Many experts (e.g., Home Office 1992; N.E. Walker and Nguyen 1996; Poole and Lamb 1998; N.E. Walker and Memon 2000; Orbach et al. 2000) agree on the elements of a sound basic protocol for interviewing children, elements based on the results of empirical studies. These elements include establishing rapport, explaining the interview purpose, discussing interview "ground rules," emphasizing the use of open-ended questions, limiting the use of demonstrative aids (such as anatomically detailed dolls), and formally closing the interview. Each of these elements is described below, including descriptions of relevant research findings.

Establish Rapport

The goal of the first phase of the interview is to establish rapport between the interviewer and the child so that the child can feel as relaxed and comfortable as possible in the interview situation. This phase serves as more than an ice-breaker, however. If correctly conducted, the rapport-building phase can "supplement the interviewer's knowledge about the child's social, emotional and cognitive development, and particularly about his or her communication skills and degree of understanding" (Home Office 1992, pp. 15–16). Moreover, Lamb and colleagues (1996) found that when child abuse interviewers spent adequate time on rapport-building activities, the first substantive open-ended question about abuse produced four times as much information as when inadequate time was spent on building rapport.

Explain the Interview Purpose

The adult should tell the child, in language the child can understand, why the interview is being conducted. The interviewer should emphasize that the child is the one who has all the information, that the interviewer was not present at the event(s) that took place in the past, and that he or she therefore cannot know what happened unless the child describes the event(s) completely.

Discuss the Interview Ground Rules

Like adults, children have a right to know what will happen to them in legal proceedings, including interviews. They need to know which behaviors are permissible and which are prohibited. N. E. Walker and Memon (2000) recommended the following guidelines for establishing interview ground rules:

- Emphasize the importance of telling the truth.
- Explicitly request detailed information, explaining that the interviewer cannot possibly know the correct details because the interviewer was not there at the time of the incident.
- Teach the child how to appropriately use the "I don't know" response. One research study found, for example, that kindergarten, second-grade, and fifth-grade children who had been trained to use the "I don't know" response generally used it appropriately and used it significantly more often than did children who had not been so trained (N. E. Walker et al. 1996).
- Give the child permission to indicate when he or she does not understand a question. Although children do not always know when they do not comprehend something, even many kindergarten-age children can signal lack of comprehension if given the opportunity to do so in an interview (Perry et al. 1995).
- Explain that asking a question more than once does not mean that the child answered the question incorrectly; the important point is for the child to understand the importance of answering each question truthfully each time it is asked.
- Encourage the child to correct the interviewer if he or she incorrectly paraphrases a response or makes another mistake.
- Emphasize that the *child* is the one who will be doing most of the talking, not the interviewer.

(See Poole and Lamb 1998 for further detail on ground rules.)

Emphasize the Use of Open-Ended Questions

Children's spontaneous, free-recall reports, although typically less detailed than those elicited by specific questioning, tend to be more accurate than reports obtained through direct questioning (Dent 1991). Research suggests, however, that only a small fraction of interviewers typically ask open-ended questions when interviewing children (N. E. Walker and Hunt 1998; Warren et al. 1996). One explanation for this phenomenon is that children often are reluctant to provide free narrative accounts. An adult who creates a comfortable atmosphere for the interview, who takes time to establish rapport, and who is patient and calm is more likely to elicit informative free narrative accounts (see, e.g., Lamb et al. 1996).

It may be appropriate, and even necessary, to ask direct questions following the free narrative portion of the interview, especially when questioning younger children. Here, the interviewer must balance competing interests in resolving an apparent paradox: young children in particular may need help recalling experiences, but the use of direct questions and specific memory prompts may be especially likely to distort memory and increase suggestibility. Therefore, many experts wisely urge interviewers to ask direct questions only if necessary, that is, if the free narrative does not provide sufficient information.

Limit the Use of Demonstrative Aids

Especially when talking with children, interviewers may be tempted to use props (such as anatomically detailed dolls or drawings) or other cues to aid memory and communication. As Poole and Lamb (1998) noted, two primary concerns are associated with using props and cues in investigative interviews:

> First, the presence of relevant cues might lead some children to elaborate from general knowledge or fantasy, thereby increasing the amount of inaccurate information they report. Second, the presence of irrelevant cues could be inherently suggestive, leading the investigators who selected the cues in the first place to confirm their a priori beliefs. (p. 196)

After reviewing relevant research studies, Poole and Lamb (1998) drew four general conclusions about the use of cues and props in investigative interviews of children:

1. Demonstrative aids (such as props and cues) often, but not always, help children report additional information.
2. Some of the additional information elicited through the use of props and cues is erroneous.
3. Real objects facilitate accurate recall more effectively than do toys.
4. The use of cues magnifies age differences in the completeness of recall during the preschool years but decreases age differences during the school years.

The benefits of using cues and props therefore must be weighed against the risk that their presence might result in more inaccuracies in children's reports. As several experts recommend, interviewers should use cues in therapeutic and forensic settings with great caution and typically only as a last resort (see, e.g., Poole and Lamb 1998; N.E. Walker and Nguyen 1996). Such demonstrative aids should be used only to encourage children to expand on information that already has been discussed.

Close the Interview

Just as it is important to open the interview in a positive manner, it is essential to close the interview gracefully. N.E. Walker and Nguyen (1996) noted that good closure has several advantages, including 1) providing an opportunity to thank the child, 2) allowing the interviewer to summarize what the child discussed and to ask once again for verification of the veracity of the interviewer's summary, 3) allowing the interviewer to explain what may happen next in legal proceedings, 4) giving the interviewer an opportunity to provide the child with a contact name and telephone number, 5) permitting the child to ask any remaining questions, and 6) offering a few moments to return to neutral topics.

Published Guidelines for Forensic Interviewing of Children

Today, it is reasonable to conclude that general consensus exists in the scientific community regarding procedures for conducting high-quality forensic interviews of children, including those that involve retrospective assessments of mental state. Not surprisingly, therefore, both governmental and nongovernmental organizations are beginning to publish and distribute recommended guidelines.

The British Home Office has been a leader in this effort. The *Memorandum of Good Practice*, first published by the Home Office in 1992, provides concrete recommendations for good practice in making videotapes of child interviews to be used in criminal proceedings in the United Kingdom. Although intended for this specific purpose, the memorandum provides sound guidelines for interviewing children in a variety of situations.

The United States recently followed the United Kingdom's lead. Although no national guidelines have been adopted in the United States, several groups have published their recommendations for forensic interviewing of children. For example, the National Institute of Child Health and Human Development recently published its protocol for investigative interviews of alleged sex-abuse victims (Orbach et al. 2000). The state of Michigan (1998) published the *Forensic Interviewing Protocol*, whose purpose is "to prepare local investigators to conduct competent child interviews which will reduce trauma to children, make the information gained more credible in the court process, and protect the rights of the accused" (Introduction). The American Professional Society on the Abuse of Children (APSAC) is also in the process of publishing guidelines for investigative interviewing in child abuse cases (A. Kaufman, Managing Editor,

APSAC Adviser, personal communication, February 23, 2000).

Like the *Memorandum of Good Practice,* the protocols developed in the United States generally are intended for use in specific circumstances (e.g., criminal investigations of child sexual abuse), but the principles they recommend have broader application. Professionals who conduct retrospective assessments of children's mental states thus may benefit from becoming familiar with these protocols.

Conclusion

It is important to conduct an accurate retrospective assessment of a child's mental state even when litigation is not involved, but it is especially important to do so in legal contexts, particularly when fundamental rights may be implicated. Whether an interviewer is conducting a retrospective assessment of a child's mental state in a criminal, civil, or juvenile court context, the interviewer must have a basic understanding of the processes of child development, including the development of children's abilities in memory, language, communication, and moral reasoning. The interviewer also must be familiar with means for avoiding suggestibility problems. He or she should be aware of the legal standards for assessing the admissibility of interview evidence in the relevant jurisdiction (e.g., Federal Rules of Evidence, *Frye* test, *Daubert* standard) as well as any interviewing protocols that may guide practice within that jurisdiction. If the interviewer gains this fundamental knowledge and then follows the recommendations for best practice in forensic interviewing of children described in this chapter, the interviewer more likely will be successful in obtaining complete and accurate retrospective assessments of children's mental states. Moreover, because the scientific experts who have published most widely in this area agree on the basic elements of a sound interviewing protocol, following the recommendations for best practice should meet the *Frye* test of general acceptance in the relevant scientific community, as well as the factors articulated in the *Daubert* standard.

References

Brennan M, Brennan R: Strange Language: Child Victims Under Cross Examination, 4th Edition. Wagga Wagga, NSW, Australia, Charles Sturt University–Riverina, 1990

Bruck M, Ceci SJ: Suggestibility of child witnesses: amicus brief for the case of State of New Jersey v. Michaels prsented by Committee of Concerned Social Scientists. Psychology, Public Policy, and Law 1(2):272–322, 1995

Cauffman E, Woolard J, Reppucci ND: Justice for juveniles: new perspectives on adolescents' competence and culpability. Quarterly Law Review 18:403–419, 1999

Ceci SJ, Bruck M: Suggestibility of the child witness: a historical review and synthesis. Psychol Bull 113:403–439, 1993

Ceci SJ, Leichtman MD, Putnick ME: Cognitive and Social Factors in Early Deception. Hillsdale, NJ, Lawrence Erlbaum, 1992

Daubert v Merrell Dow Pharmaceuticals, Inc., 509 US 579 (1993)

Dent HR: Experimental studies of interviewing child witnesses, in The Suggestibility of Children's Recollections: Implications for Eyewitness Testimony. Edited by Doris J. Washington, DC, American Psychological Association, 1991, pp 138–146

Fisher RP, Geiselman RE: Memory-Enhancing Techniques for Investigative Interviewing: The Cognitive Interview. Springfield, IL, Charles C Thomas, 1992

Frye v United States, 293 F 1013 (DC Cir 1923)

Gardner MR: Understanding Juvenile Law. New York, Matthew Bender, 1997

Garratt v Dailey, 279 P2d 1091 (Wash 1955), rev'd and remanded, 304 P2d 681 (Wash 1956)

Garven S, Wood JM, Malpass RS, et al: More than suggestion: the effect of interviewing techniques from the McMartin Preschool case. J Appl Psychol 83:347–359, 1998

Gibson E, Radner N: Attention: the perceiver as performer, in Attention and Cognitive Development. Edited by Hale GA, Lewis M. New York, Plenum, 1979, pp 1–21

Gilstrap LL, Warren HK, Hewitt S: Are all leading questions created equal?: The effects of various types of questions in unstructured interviews. Presented at the combined meeting of the European Association of Psychology and Law and the American Psychology–Law Society, Dublin, Ireland, July 1999

Haugaard J: Young children's classification of the corroboration of a false statement as the truth or a lie. Paper presented at the biennial meeting of the American Psychology–Law Society, San Diego, CA, March 1992

Home Office: Memorandum of Good Practice. London, England, Home Office, 1992

Kranat VK, Westcott HL: Under fire: lawyers questioning children in criminal courts. Expert Evidence 3:16–24, 1994

Lamb ME, Hershkowitz I, Sternberg KJ, et al: Effects of investigative utterance types on Israeli children's responses. International Journal of Behavioral Development 19:627–637, 1996

Lilly GC: An Introduction to the Law of Evidence, 3rd Edition. St. Paul, MN, West Group, 1996

Lindsay DS, Gonzales V, Eso K: Aware and unaware uses of memories of postevent suggestions, in Memory and Testimony in the Child Witness. Edited by Zaragoza MS, Graham JR, Hall GCN, et al. Thousand Oaks, CA, Sage, 1995, pp 86–108

Marin BV, Holmes DL, Guth M, et al: The potential of children as eyewitnesses. Law Hum Behav 3:295–306, 1979

McGough LS: Commentary: achieving real reform—the case for American interviewing protocols. Monogr Soc Res Child Dev 61(4–5, Serial No 248):188–203, 1996

Memon A, Wark L, Holley A, et al: Eyewitness performance in cognitive and structured interviews. Memory 5:639–659, 1997

Monahan J, Walker L: Social Science in Law: Cases and Materials, 4th Edition. Westbury, NY, Foundation Press, 1998

Myers NA, Perlmutter M: Memory in the years from two to five, in Memory Development in Children. Edited by Ornstein PA. Hillsdale, NJ, Lawrence Erlbaum, 1978, pp 191–218

Nguyen KQ: In defense of the child: a jus cogens approach to the capital punishment of juveniles in the United States. George Washington Journal of International Law and Economics 28:401–443, 1995

Orbach Y, Hershkowitz I, Lamb ME, et al: Assessing the value of structured protocols for forensic interviews of alleged child abuse victims. Child Abuse Negl 24(6):733–752, 2000

People v Buckey (not reported) (Cal 1990)

Perry NW[1]: Child and adolescent development: a psycholegal perspective, in Child Witness Law and Practice. Edited by Myers J. New York, Wiley, 1987, pp 459–525

Perry NW: Children's comprehension of truths, lies, and false beliefs, in Allegations in Child Sexual Abuse Cases: Assessment and Management. Edited by Ney T. New York, Brunner/Mazel, 1995, pp 73–98

Perry NW, Teply LL: Interviewing, counseling, and in-court examination of children: practical approaches for attorneys. Creighton Law Review 18:1369–1426, 1984–1985

Perry NW, Wrightsman LS: The Child Witness: Legal Issues and Dilemmas. Thousand Oaks, CA, Sage, 1991

Perry NW, McAuliff BD, Tam P, et al: When lawyers question children: is justice served? Law Hum Behav 19:609–629, 1995

Piaget J, Inhelder B: Memory and Intelligence. New York, Basic Books, 1973

Poole DA, Lamb ME: Investigative Interviews of Children: A Guide for Helping Professionals. Washington, DC, American Psychological Association, 1998

Poole DA, Lindsay DS: Interviewing preschoolers: effects of non-suggestive techniques, parental coaching, and leading questions on reports of nonexperienced events. J Exp Child Psychol 60:129–154, 1995

Poole DA, Lindsay DS: Effects of parental suggestions, interviewing techniques, and age on young children's event reports. Paper presented at the NATO Advanced Study Institute: Recollections of Trauma: Scientific Research and Clinical Practice, Port de Bourgenay, France, June 1996

---

[1]N.W. Perry is now N.E. Walker, author of this chapter.

Schacter DL, Kagan J, Leichtman MD: True and false memories in children and adults: a cognitive neuroscience perspective. Psychology, Public Policy, and Law 1:411–428, 1995

State of Michigan: Forensic Interviewing Protocol. Available through State of Michigan Governor's Task Force on Children's Justice and Family Independence Agency, Lansing, 1998

State v Michaels, 625 A2d 489 (NJ Super Ct App Div 1993), aff'd, 642 A2d 1372 (NJ 1994)

Steward MS, Steward DS (with Farquhar L, Myers JEB, Reinhart M, et al): Interviewing young children about body touch and handling. Monogr Soc Res Child Dev 61(4–5, Serial No 248), 1996, pp 1–186

Strichartz AF, Burton RV: Lies and truth: a study of the development of the concept. Child Dev 61:211–220, 1990

Walker AG: Questioning young children in court: a linguistic case study. Law Hum Behav 17:59–81, 1993

Walker NE, Hunt JS: Interviewing child victim-witnesses: how you ask is what you get, in Eyewitness Memory: Theoretical and Applied Perspectives. Edited by Thompson CP, Herrmann DJ, Read JD, et al. Mahwah, NJ, Lawrence Erlbaum, 1998, pp 55–87

Walker NE, Memon A: Forensic interviews of children: techniques for improving the accuracy and completeness of children's reports. Workshop presented in Reykjavik, Iceland, April 2000

Walker NE, Nguyen M: Interviewing the child witness: the do's and the don't's, the how's and the why's. Creighton Law Review 29:1587–1617, 1996

Walker NE, Lunning S, Eilts J: Do children respond accurately to forced choice questions? yes or no. Paper presented at the NATO Advanced Study Institute: Recollections of Trauma: Scientific Research and Clinical Practice. Port de Bourgenay, France, June 1996

Warren AR, Woodall CE, Hunt JS, et al: "It sounds good in theory, but…": do investigative interviewers follow guidelines based on memory research? Child Maltreatment 1:231–245, 1996

Wimmer H, Gruber A, Perner J: Young children's conception of lying: lexical realism–moral subjectivism. J Exp Child Psychol 37:1–30, 1984

The Past as Prologue

Assessment of Future Violence in Individuals With a History of Past Violence

Kenneth Tardiff, M.D., M.P.H.

The assessment of the potential for violence by patients is often at the core of clinical practice and the law. As is discussed later in this chapter, assessment of past violence is crucial to the risk of future violence. Malpractice suits for wrongful death or injury examine a clinician's decision as to whether a patient posed an imminent risk of violence to others, and, if so, whether proper measures were taken to protect victims of violence. Clinicians predict the potential for violence many times each day, in evaluating a patient in the emergency room, deciding whether an inpatient should be given a pass or discharged, determining the level of observation for a patient in the inpatient unit, making custody recommendations in cases of child abuse or neglect, and routinely evaluating a patient in outpatient treatment. Involuntary commitment proceedings and preventive hospitalization for patients in involuntary outpatient commitment programs are based on an assessment of a patient's danger to others.

Although the law expects clinicians to predict violence by patients, the question of whether they can predict violence has been a thorny one. Earlier

studies found that psychiatrists and psychologists were not accurate in predicting whether a patient will be violent (Monahan 1981). Later studies showed
that mental health professionals have improved to the point that their predictions of violence are better than one would expect by chance alone (Apperson
et al. 1993; Lidz et al. 1993; Monahan and Steadman 1994; Mossman 1994;
Otto 1994; Quinsey 1995; Serin and Amos 1995; Tardiff 1996). Past patterns
of violent behavior are particularly important in making decisions about future
risk of violence. Several chapters by authoritative authors have expressed confidence that mental health professionals do have some expertise in determining
whether a patient will become violent but only in the near future (Simon 1992;
A.A. Stone 1984; Tardiff 1996).

In this chapter, I scrutinize the current practices in predicting violence
with a high standard, the United States Supreme Court's decision in *Daubert v. Merrell Dow Pharmaceuticals, Inc.* (1993). I have chosen a clinical decision-making model rather than the use of rating instruments. The model
is supported by studies of factors associated with increased risk of violence
among psychiatric patients.

It has been suggested that testimony about future dangerousness
should be based ideally on objective instruments, but in the real world testimony usually is based on practice-based expertise (Mark 1999). Several
instruments have been developed to measure violence potential: the Barratt
Impulsiveness Scale; the Buss-Durkee Hostility Scale; the Past Feeling and
Acts of Violence Scale; the Three Ratings of Involuntary Admissibility and
the Violence Scale; the Anger, Irritability and Assault Questionnaire; and
the Overt Aggression Scale—Modified (Barratt 1959; Borum 1996; Buss
and Durkee 1957; Coccaro et al. 1991; Morrison 1993; Plutchik and van
Praag 1990; Segal et al. 1988a, 1988b). These instruments are used to measure violence and aggression and are not intended to have predictive validity. Another problem with quantitative scales is that a score does not reveal
much about an individual patient. The factors described in a clinical model
for the short-term determination of the risk of violence are weighted by the
clinician based on the individual patient. For one patient recurrence of psychosis might be weighed heavily, whereas for another patient recurrence of
drinking or drug use might be weighed more heavily based on the pattern
of past violence by these patients. The American Psychiatric Association
formed a task force in 1996 to evaluate the reliability and validity of approximately 240 measures used in psychiatry. The work of this task force is contained in a lengthy, definitive book (Rush et al. 2000). The book begins
with this cautionary statement:

> The proper interpretation of the results of these measures requires both
> clinical training and consideration of a variety of other factors. A particu-
> lar result, in and of itself, is never sufficient to determine clinical judg-

ments such as diagnosis of a specific mental disorder, *propensity to violence or self-injury*, or legal or other nonmedical standards of disability or competence. (p. xxi, emphasis added)

Some authors have developed clinical models in deciding whether a patient poses a significant risk of violence in the near future (Appelbaum 1989; Brizer and Crowner 1989; Gross et al. 1987; Monahan and Steadman 1994; Mulvey and Lidz 1995; Simon 1992; Tardiff 1996, 1999; Wack 1993). These models are rather consistent in describing what information should be collected and weighed in the evaluation of a patient to determine the potential for violence.

The model includes information the clinician should collect to determine a patient's potential for violence in the near future (i.e., the next few days or a week at most). Beyond a week, intervening factors may change the state of the patient and the environment at the time of the evaluation of violence potential. These intervening factors include noncompliance with medication, resumption of drinking or substance use, threats of divorce by a spouse, and other stressors.

Before presenting the areas that should be covered in determining risk of violence, several principles should be considered. The essential components of this model for the short-term prediction of violence rely on information collected from the interview with the patient, but other sources of information must be sought. These include past treatment records, police records, and other records such as from school, the military, and employment. The clinician must speak or attempt to speak to the family, therapist, police, and others who may have knowledge of the patient. Some patients, such as those with paranoid delusions, may be reluctant to divulge thoughts of violence, so the clinician must listen carefully and follow up on any hints of violence that may surface during the interview. If the patient has thoughts of violence or even threats, the degree of formulation of the ideas or threats of violence must be assessed. The clinician should be concerned about the risk of violence that a patient poses if he or she has a well-formulated or detailed plan. If a patient has thoughts of harming a specific person, it is important to assess his or her intent to harm the person. Thoughts of violence that occur in a patient's mind may not be sufficient to warrant action by the clinician. Last, the patient's access to the potential victim is important.

Studies of Past Violence and Risk of Future Violence

A history of violence or other impulsive behaviors by the patient is a major factor in the assessment of potential for violence. Davis (1991) reviewed studies that reported a definite link between a history of violence and violence in the future. Most of these studies examined violence in hospitals or violence before hospitalization. Convit et al. (1988) found that a self-reported history of violence toward people in the community and arrests for violent crimes were the strongest discriminators between violent patients and matched control subjects in a state hospital inpatient unit. The study was repeated several years later in the same hospital, and the positive correlation between past violence and violence on the unit was found again (Volavka 1995). Past history of violence before admission was related to an increased risk of violence on units in a variety of other types of hospitals, on a university-based inpatient unit (McNiel and Binder 1991; McNiel et al. 1988), and in two Department of Veterans Affairs (VA) hospitals (Sheridan et al. 1990; Werner et al. 1984).

Other types of studies following up patients after discharge from hospitals found that a history of violence either before admission or during hospitalization was associated with an increased presence of violence after discharge (Klassen and O'Connor 1988, 1989). These studies followed up patients from 6 months to 5 years after hospitalization. Whether violence occurs long after discharge is not as clinically relevant as whether violence occurs shortly after discharge from a hospital because it is not linked to the decision to discharge the patient. Violence shortly after discharge can reflect on the decision to discharge a patient and, presumably, the assessment of the risk of violence at that time. Tardiff et al. (1997a) followed up patients from a university psychiatric hospital for 2 weeks after discharge. A research assistant assessed violence before hospitalization and interviewed patients by telephone after discharge. Patients who were violent in the month before admission were nine times more likely than patients who were not violent in the month before admission to be violent 2 weeks after discharge. For 69% of the patients who were violent after discharge, the target of the violence was the same person who had been attacked before hospitalization, and the circumstances surrounding the violence generally were the same before and after hospitalization.

Evaluation of Past Violence

Past violence predicts future violence. To predict future violence, the clinician must dissect episodes of past violence in a detailed, concrete manner. This includes details of the time and place of the violence, who was present, who said what to whom, what the patient saw, what the patient remembers, what family members and staff remember, why the patient was violent (e.g., delusions vs. anger), and what could have been done to avoid the violent confrontation. Often there is a pattern of escalation of violence over a short time, whether it involves the dynamics of a couple interacting in domestic violence or the schizophrenic patient on the inpatient unit whose violence escalates as interactions with other patients become too intense.

The history of violence should be assessed in terms of the date of onset, frequency, target (directed at other persons vs. self or objects), and severity. Severity is measured by degree of injury to the victims—from pushing, to punching, to causing minor injuries (such as bruises), to causing more severe injuries (such as broken bones, lacerations, and internal injuries), even to causing death. Frequency, severity, and targets of violence may be measured by the Overt Aggression Scale (Yudofsky et al. 1986). The history of suicide attempts should be assessed because suicidal behavior may be related to violence.

Studies of Suicide and Violence

A history of suicide, particularly with impulsivity, may indicate a greater risk of violence in the future due to impulsivity and low self-control. Early studies found that violent patients have a greater history of suicide attempts than do nonviolent patients. This association was found among patients evaluated in an outpatient clinic and an emergency department (Climent and Ervin 1972; Skodal and Karasu 1978). Tardiff and Sweillam (1980a) studied 9,365 patients admitted to public hospitals in a 1-year period and found that patients who were violent 2 weeks before admission were more likely than nonviolent patients to have a history of suicidal behavior at some time in their lives. Patients who were both violent and suicidal in the 2 weeks before admission were more likely to have delusions, hallucinations, belligerence, and antisocial behavior than were patients who were suicidal but not violent (Tardiff and Sweillam 1980b).

There may be a biological link between violence and suicidal behavior. Several studies have found that patients who have been violent and those who have attempted suicide have lower levels of the metabolite of the neurotransmitter serotonin in spinal fluid than do nonviolent or nonsuicidal patients (Brown and Goodwin 1986; Coccaro et al. 1989 ; Linnoila and Virkkunen 1992; Marazziti et al. 1993). These researchers suggested that the common factor linking violence and suicide may be impulsivity caused by low levels of serotonin in the brain.

Psychopathology and Violence

Schizophrenia and Psychosis

Schizophrenia has been found to be associated with an increased risk of violence by psychiatric patients. Four different studies in which patients were interviewed during hospitalization in regard to violence just before admission found that patients with schizophrenia were more likely than patients with other disorders to have been violent (Binder and McNiel 1988; Craig 1982; Rossi et al. 1986; Tardiff 1984). Tardiff (1984) differentiated paranoid from nonparanoid schizophrenia and found no difference between rates of violence and type of schizophrenia. However, Krakowski et al. (1986) pointed out in their review of other studies of inpatient violence and violence before admission that four studies reported higher rates of violence among paranoid schizophrenic patients, two studies found more violence among nonparanoid schizophrenic patients, and one study found no difference between type of schizophrenia and violence.

Two studies of patients living in the community found that a diagnosis of schizophrenia was related to an increased risk of violence (Link et al. 1992; Swanson et al. 1990). In both studies, drug abuse further increased the risk of violence among schizophrenic patients.

Studies of patients who were violent in psychiatric hospitals found that schizophrenia is associated with increased violence (Convit et al. 1988; Tardiff and Sweillam 1982). In two studies schizophrenia was the *only* diagnosis related to violence in hospitals (Lee et al. 1989; Tam et al. 1996). Studies of patients in hospitals allow for better observation in regard to the role of psychosis in violence. They found that psychosis in the form of delusions and hallucinations plays a major role in violence by schizophrenic inpatients (Arango et al. 1999; Benjaminsen et al. 1996; M. Lowenstein et al. 1990).

Taylor and Gunn (1999) and McNiel et al. (2000) explored the role of psychosis—namely, delusions and hallucinations, respectively—in violence by psychiatric patients. Delusions, particularly paranoid delusions, do play an important role in violence by schizophrenic patients, but so do nonparanoid delusions (e.g., erotic delusions about the victim). Hallucinations play an important role in violence by patients (Humphreys et al. 1992). The importance of command hallucinations—in which voices in auditory hallucinations tell the patient to attack the victim—in relation to violence is unclear (Hellerstein et al. 1987; Junginger 1995; Rogers et al. 1988). Studies are conflicted in this matter; some find that command hallucinations do result in violence, whereas others find that patients ignore command hallucinations.

Schizophrenia and Other Causes of Violence

It is important to recognize that schizophrenic patients can be violent for reasons other than psychosis per se. Violence by schizophrenic patients may be due to comorbid alcohol or drug abuse (Lindqvist and Allebeck 1990; Swanson et al. 1990). Violence due to alcohol and drug abuse is discussed later in this chapter (see the section "Substance Abuse"). A concurrent neurological disorder may result in a low threshold for violence (Krakowski et al. 1989) (see section "Organic Mental Disorders" later in this chapter). Mentally retarded schizophrenic patients may resort to violence in response to frustration caused by either demands from family or staff or the inability to verbalize their needs and conflicts.

Comorbid antisocial or borderline personality disorders increase the potential for violence among patients with major mental disorders (Geller 1980; Swanson et al. 1990). Violence can be manipulative, used to control or to express anger by these patients, and not be related to the schizophrenic disorder itself. For example, a paranoid schizophrenic patient with antisocial personality disorder who was no longer psychotic deliberately punched a nurse in the face when the nurse told him that his weekend pass was rescinded.

Delusional Disorder

Delusional disorder, especially with paranoid or jealous themes, can be associated with violent behavior. Patients with a paranoid delusional disorder harbor grudges against those whom they believe have wronged them, such as employers or co-workers (Tardiff 1998b). Patients with delusional disorders of the jealous type retaliate violently against their spouse or the suspected third person in the illicit affair.

Mania

Patients in a manic episode have been found to be more violent than some other types of patients (Binder and McNiel 1988; Janofsky et al. 1988; Tardiff 1984). Violence usually occurs during the acute phase of the manic state and is often associated with psychosis and/or gross disorganization of thoughts and/or behavior (Miller et al. 1993; Yesavage 1983). Targets of violence are often random in these cases. Manic patients who are more intact are violent when they feel restricted or when staff set limits. For example, a middle-aged woman who was manic attacked a female psychiatric resident in the emergency department because the resident told the patient that she would be admitted involuntarily to the hospital. Later when the patient was stabilized and interviewed, she apologized for the attack but commented that she had felt trapped.

Personality Disorders

Patients with personality disorders have an increased risk of violence. Tardiff et al. (1997a, 1997b) found increased violence among patients with personality disorders 2 weeks before admission to a hospital and 2 weeks after discharge. They also found that violence was increased among patients with personality disorders who presented to outpatient clinics for evaluations (Tardiff and Koenigsberg 1985). Miller et al. (1993) found that patients with personality disorders have increased rates of violence in hospitals as well. The two types of personality disorders most likely to be associated with violence are the antisocial and borderline personality disorders (Eronen et al. 1996; Raine 1996).

Antisocial Personality Disorder

Individuals with antisocial personality disorder have disregard for and violate the rights of others, including using violence, which is a criterion for the DSM-IV-TR diagnosis of antisocial personality disorder (American Psychiatric Association 2000). These patients tend to be irritable and repeatedly get into physical fights or otherwise attack others, including spouses and children (Bland and Orn 1986). They destroy property, steal, harass others, and are involved in other criminal activities. They are impulsive and tend not to plan ahead (Hare 1991). Violence and other behaviors that violate the rights of others are not accompanied by remorse or fear of consequences of violence. Instead the violence is rationalized; for example, these individuals think that the victim deserves the violence. Decisions are made quickly without thinking of the consequences to self or others.

Some evidence indicates that the violence and other impulsive behavior in antisocial personality disorder are related to low levels of the serotonin metabolite 5-hydroxyindoleacetic acid (5-HIAA) in spinal fluid and brain (Coccaro et al. 1989, 1992; Roy and Linnoila 1990). Studies have found that inheritance plays a part in antisocial personality disorder (Carey and Goldman 1997). The individual with antisocial personality disorder is at risk for alcohol abuse, perhaps reflecting another genetic association (Miczek et al. 1994). A magnetic resonance imaging study by Raine et al. (2000) found that men with antisocial personality have reductions in prefrontal gray matter. This reduction may result in poor development of the conscience through defective learning.

Borderline Personality Disorder

Individuals with borderline personality disorder have a pervasive pattern of instability in interpersonal relationships, self-image, and emotional states and marked impulsivity (American Psychiatric Association 2000). They make efforts to avoid real or imagined rejection. Abandonment or rejection as seen by these individuals may appear slight to external observers (e.g., someone is a few minutes late for an appointment). They form intense relationships with caregivers or lovers and expect these persons to protect and rescue them (Benjamin 1993). When the caregiver or lover fails to live up to these unrealistic expectations, the individual with borderline personality disorder reacts with rage, verbal and/or physical violence, and suicidal behavior or other self-destructive behaviors. Anger has been traditionally recognized as the main emotion and a core component of borderline personality disorder (Grinker et al. 1968). Impulsivity is severe in borderline personality disorder and causes violence, suicide attempts, and other self-destructive behaviors (M.H. Stone 1990).

Impulsivity may be related to low levels of serotonin; for example, individuals with borderline personality disorder have diminished responsiveness to fenfluramine challenge (Coccaro et al. 1989). Individuals with borderline personality disorder have an increased likelihood of having been physically or sexually abused as children (Perry and Herman 1993). Being physically abused as a child increases the risk of violence as an adult (Widom 1989). Physical abuse, along with impulsivity and substance abuse, contributes to the violent nature of those with borderline personality disorder.

Antisocial personality disorder and borderline personality disorder are both characterized by manipulation and dangerous behaviors. Individuals with antisocial personality disorder manipulate impulsivity to gain profit, power, or some other materialistic goal, whereas individuals with borderline personality disorder manipulate to gain the concern of caregivers or lovers and to express rage at perceived rejection. Individuals with both personality disorders have little remorse or concern for the damage caused by their violence and other dangerous behaviors in other persons around them.

Intermittent Explosive Disorder

Intermittent explosive disorder is characterized by discrete episodes of loss of control resulting in serious violence toward persons or destruction of property (American Psychiatric Association 2000). The violent episode is not due to the physiological effects of a substance or a general medical condition. This syndrome of episodic explosive disorder was described decades ago (Bach-y-Rita et al. 1971; Monroe 1970). The degree of violence is grossly out of proportion to any provocation or environmental stressor. The patient with intermittent explosive disorder may describe the episodes as "spells" or "attacks" in which the violence is preceded by a sense of tension and followed by a sense of relief. As with antisocial and borderline personality disorders, the impulsivity in intermittent explosive disorder may be related to low levels of serotonin in the brain (Linnoila et al. 1983). Unlike patients with antisocial personality and borderline personality, the patient with intermittent explosive disorder feels remorseful and/or embarrassed about the violence after the episode. Between episodes of violence, the individual with intermittent explosive disorder may appear stable and a model employee, spouse, or citizen of the community.

Posttraumatic Stress Disorder

Posttraumatic stress disorder (PTSD) can have violence as one of many symptoms, along with depression, other anxiety disorders, and substance abuse (American Psychiatric Association 2000). Most studies have compared veterans with and without PTSD (Jordan et al. 1992; Lasko et al. 1994). Controlling for substance abuse and personality disorders, veterans with PTSD had higher levels of hostility, anger, and physical violence than did veterans without PTSD. The violence may be diffuse as part of increased arousal with irritability and anger. Conversely, violence may be part of intense psychological distress in response to exposure to external cues that symbolize or resemble an aspect of the traumatic event. An illustration of the latter case is that of a 34-year-old man who was raped just before his release from prison. He developed severe PTSD with depression and alcohol abuse. He made numerous attacks and fought with men who resembled the rapist; he also used violence in situations in which people appeared to be abused—for example, when a foreman of a work crew on the street yelled at a man in the crew.

Substance Abuse

The presence of alcohol or drug abuse increases the risk of violence (Volavka and Tardiff 1999). Among persons residing in the community, substance abuse is the disorder most frequently associated with violence, and the presence of substance and major mental disorders increases the risk of violence beyond that found for the major mental disorders alone (Swanson et al. 1990). Patients in a psychiatric hospital reported violence just before admission twice as often for males and three times more often for females if they had a substance abuse disorder (Tardiff et al. 1997b). Patients are more likely to be violent in hospitals if they have a substance abuse disorder (Davis 1991). Last, after discharge from hospitals, substance abuse was a major factor, alone and co-occurring with a major mental disorder, in determining whether a patient would be violent in the community (Steadman et al. 1998). Alcohol and each drug associated with violence are discussed separately.

Alcohol Use

An extensive literature shows that the use of alcohol is associated with violence and violent crime (Collins and Schlenger 1988; Eronen et al. 1996; Murdoch et al. 1990). Sometimes violence is caused by the overlay of alcohol use and antisocial personality (Abram and Teplin 1990). The mechanism through which alcohol causes violence is complex. Alcohol releases the drinker from personally and socially acceptable inhibitions, so that one acts, in this case violently, on angry urges and thoughts (Taylor and Leonard 1983). Laboratory studies show that alcohol impairs the brain in thinking; thus the person under the influence of alcohol cannot fully use verbal and intellectual skills to deal with conflict or threatening situations (Peterson et al. 1990). Cognitive impairment from alcohol leads to violence because the intoxicated person must rely on physical rather than verbal means of dealing with conflict. Cognitive impairment also may lead to misinterpretation of events or words, such as perceiving an insult from someone. Alcohol lowers levels of serotonin, which itself is associated with impulsive behaviors (Virkkunen and Linnoila 1990).

The surrounding social environment interacts with the intoxicated individual to produce violence (Ito et al. 1996). There are provocations from family and friends, isolation resulting from chronic alcohol use, failure at work, and lower self-esteem, all of which interact with the disinhibited, cognitively impaired brain to produce violence.

Cocaine and Amphetamine Use

Cocaine users have been found to have anger and violent behavior during acute intoxication (Giannini et al. 1993; McCormick and Smith 1995). Smoking crack or intravenous use of cocaine produces a more rapid, intense intoxication than does intranasal use. Smoking or intravenous use produces a more intense "crash," during which a severe craving for cocaine occurs. A cycle of crash, smoking or intravenous injection to avoid a crash, followed by another crash, and so on is set into motion. This produces severe intoxication and irritability and even a delirious state, which can result in severe violence (Brody 1990; D.H. Lowenstein et al. 1987; Mendoza and Miller 1992). Cocaine can produce psychosis with paranoid delusions and hallucinations (Manschreck et al. 1988). In a psychotic state the cocaine user strikes out at persons who the user believes is trying to hurt him or her. Psychosis with delusions may persist for days and result in violence. Cocaine users take alcohol or opiates to counteract the irritability, agitation, and other disturbing side effects of cocaine. These two or more substances combine to produce a degree of violence greater than that with the use of one substance alone (Denison et al. 1997; Salloum et al. 1996). The abuse of amphetamines can produce paranoid delusional thinking similar to that seen with abuse of cocaine, which is associated with violence (Ellinwood 1971).

Phencyclidine Use

Of the hallucinogens, phencyclidine (PCP) is the one most commonly associated with violence as well as self-destructive and other bizarre behaviors. A study of patients presenting to an emergency department found that two-thirds of the patients with PCP intoxication were agitated and/or violent (Bailey 1979). Within an hour of oral use and 5 minutes if smoked or taken intravenously, PCP produces impulsivity, unpredictability, grossly impaired judgment, and violence. Delusional thinking or delirium may occur. Because PCP is an anesthetic, it produces numbness or diminished response to pain, which has resulted in cases in which excessive force by police has been used in arresting persons intoxicated with PCP. As with cocaine, psychopathology such as delusions may persist for days after the use of PCP.

Ecstasy Use

Ecstasy (methylenedioxymethamphetamine) has amphetamine and hallucinogenic properties. It produces confusion, severe anxiety, paranoia, depression, and aggression (National Institute on Drug Abuse 1999). Physical symptoms include muscle tension, involuntary teeth clenching, nausea, blurred vision, rapid eye movement, faintness, chills, sweating, and increased heart rate and blood pressure. It is popular at dance clubs and college scenes.

Anabolic Steroid Use

There have been several reports of violence by athletes using anabolic steroids (Choi et al. 1989; Pope and Katz 1990; Schulte et al. 1993). These athletes were young men with no previous history of aggression or violence. After a month or so of routine use of anabolic steroids, they became irritable and violent. A study of a group of healthy volunteers showed an increase in hostility and impulsivity in the subjects when they were given anabolic steroids (Su et al. 1993).

Organic Mental Disorders

Several large studies of patients found that violence was increased among patients with an *organic mental disorder*, a term no longer in use. Organic mental disorders are cases in which a gross physical or metabolic injury to the brain occurred. Today we use the terms *neurological* and *medical disorders* instead of *organic disorders* (Anderson and Silver 1999).

Among psychiatric inpatients who were interviewed, patients with organic mental disorders, along with schizophrenia and mania, were more likely than patients with other Axis I diagnoses to report violence toward people just before admission (Craig 1982; Tardiff 1984; Tardiff and Sweillam 1982). The risk of violence in hospitals was increased among psychiatric inpatients with organic mental disorders (Convit et al. 1988; Miller et al. 1993; Tardiff and Sweillam 1982).

The more common neurological and medical diseases that are associated with violence are covered in this chapter. Rare diseases associated with violence have been presented in an earlier publication (Tardiff 1998a). These include brain tumors, encephalitis not due to acquired immunodeficiency syndrome (AIDS), Wilson's disease, Huntington's disease, sleep disorders, thyroid diseases, parathyroid diseases, vitamin deficiencies, and toxins.

Dementia

Violence and other behavior problems are common among patients with Alzheimer's disease (Reisberg et al. 1987). Among patients in a long-stay psychogeriatric unit over a 3-day period, 45% of the patients with Alzheimer's disease were aggressive, with 4% rated as severely aggressive and 11% as moderately aggressive (Patel and Hope 1992). In another study of outpatients with dementia, 34% had a history of physical aggression, most often occurring when the patient was told to do something (Hamel et al. 1990). Other studies have found that patients with Alzheimer's disease were most likely violent when they were delusional or when they misidentified the environment as being threatening to them (Deutsch et al. 1991; Reisberg and Ferris 1985).

AIDS Encephalitis

AIDS infection of the brain can cause dementia with irritability, agitation, paranoid delusions, and violence (Nurnberg et al. 1984; Snider et al. 1983). AIDS encephalitis can cause other psychiatric problems such as mania, depression, and confusion. The picture can be very complex because this population of patients is at risk for other disorders related to violence, namely substance abuse and antisocial personality disorder. In addition, some AIDS patients harbor a great amount of anger at having contracted the disease and may vent that anger in the form of physical violence toward others.

Head Trauma

Blunt trauma to the brain often results in irritability and aggressiveness, from 70% to nearly 100% of the time (McKinlay et al. 1981; Rao et al.

1985). Agitation begins in the first few weeks after the brain injury and may persist for several months (Brooke et al. 1992). The patient explodes at the slightest provocation, with violence toward other persons or property. Some patients with traumatic brain injury become delirious with delusions, hallucinations, and confusion, which further lead to violence. Long-term changes in personality and intellect can predispose a patient to violence for years (Fordyce et al. 1993).

Developmental Disorders

Intellectually impaired individuals with mental retardation or autism can be violent, generally in proportion to the severity of the impairment (Bouras and Drummond 1997; Linaker 1994). Much of the violence occurs among inpatients who kick, punch, and push other patients or staff (Ghaziuddin and Ghaziuddin 1992). Intellectually impaired patients who live in the community with family or in supervised housing also have a high rate of violence toward family and roommates (Bouras and Drummond 1997).

Hypoxia and Electrolyte Imbalance

Hypoxia is insufficient oxygen in the blood caused by heart or lung disease, anemia, and vascular problems. Electrolyte imbalance is abnormally low, or there are high levels of elements such as sodium and calcium in the blood caused by kidney disease or intravenous transfusion. Hypoxia and electrolyte imbalance affect the functioning of the brain, which produces delirium with fluctuating levels of consciousness, disorientation, confusion, hallucinations, delusions, and combativeness (Kutzer 1990). Violence can occur because of emotional instability and general agitation or from paranoid delusional thinking or misperception of the environment.

Compliance With Treatment

Therapeutic alliance refers to the quality of the clinician's relationship with the patient and how active a patient is in treatment. It includes compliance with treatment with regular attendance at treatment sessions and taking medication as directed. The strength of the therapeutic alliance has been shown to be related to better outcomes in studies of outpatient psychiatric treatment (Allen et al. 1985; Clarkin et al. 1987). Some have suggested that the strength of the therapeutic alliance could be related to the risk of violence by patients in treatment (Gutheil et al. 1986; Truscott et al. 1995). One study measured the strength of the therapeutic alliance at the time of admission to a hospital and found that it was related to the risk of violence in the hospital (Beauford et al. 1997). Two studies of compliance have examined patients with schizophrenia and medication. In both studies schizophrenic patients who stopped taking antipsychotic medication or who had lower blood levels of antipsychotic medication were more likely to be violent than were those who were compliant (Tiihonen et al. 1996; Yesavage 1983). The Special Hospitals' Research Group (1996) in England recommended the newer antipsychotic medications such as risperidone and clozapine because they produce fewer unpleasant side effects and thus would increase patient compliance and decrease dangerousness.

Summary of Model Practices in Predicting Violence

A clinician should be expected to have the capacity to determine a patient's risk of violence in the near future (i.e., days or a week or so). Information should be sought from the patient and other sources such as the family, police, therapist, and past records. If the patient has ideas about violence, the clinician should assess the degree of formulation, intent to carry out the plan, and access to the potential victim.

The presence of past violent behavior increases the risk of future violence. The pattern surrounding circumstances and the type of victim in past violence often repeat themselves in future violence. If the circumstances appear to be forming again, then the future risk of violence increases. A history of impulsive violence or suicide raises the risk of future violence.

The presence of psychosis with delusions and/or hallucinations increases the risk of violence. An acute psychotic state found in schizophrenia, mania, delusional disorder, or organic mental disorder reflects a high risk of violence if the patient is thinking about violence. Manic patients can be violent when they feel contained or trapped.

Patients with antisocial and borderline personality disorders are often violent as a form of manipulation to get what they want. Violence is not followed by remorse for such behavior. Patients with intermittent explosive disorder are remorseful after being violent. Between violent episodes they are more stable than patients with antisocial or borderline personality disorder. Patients with PTSD often can be violent when confronted with the same or similar cues as in the original traumatic event.

Alcohol disinhibits and impairs cognition, resulting in violence. Cocaine, amphetamine, PCP, and anabolic steroid use produce violence. Polysubstance abuse and alcohol further increase a patient's risk for violence.

Gross impairment of the brain by neurological and medical diseases is associated with an increased risk of violence. The more common diseases linked with violence are dementia, AIDS encephalitis, head trauma, developmental disorders, and hypoxia and electrolyte imbalances.

Noncompliance with treatment, such as a history of missing appointments or not taking medication as prescribed, indicates a risk of future violence.

The presence or absence of these factors is weighed for the specific patient based on a history of violence by that patient and the situation for that patient. The clinician determines whether the patient poses a risk of violence in the near future. If so, the reasoning process is documented, and action is taken to prevent violence. If not, the reasoning process is documented, and no immediate action is necessary. The clinician must document the positive and negative aspects of the information gathered and the decision-making process. For example, a schizophrenic patient with alcohol abuse may have a history of violence resulting from delusional thinking and intoxication but is deemed appropriate for discharge from the hospital because of a rigorous aftercare program with long-term depot haloperidol, Alcoholics Anonymous meetings, and the assignment of a caseworker. In malpractice suits, the medical record is the main source of information in determining whether the clinician met the standard of care, not only in assessing violence potential but also in correctly diagnosing and treating the patient.

Scrutiny of the Model Under *Daubert*

The *Daubert* criteria are described in depth in Chapter 2 of this volume. The method used in expert testimony must be generally accepted by the relevant professional community, be based on scientific research, have a known rate of error, and be subjected to peer review in the scientific literature.

According to the Task Force for the Handbook on Psychiatric Measures of the American Psychiatric Association, it is generally accepted that determination of "propensity for violence" is clinical judgment, and although instruments may be used, they are never sufficient to make that determination (Rush et al. 2000). The elements of a clinical determination of risk of violence include history of violence and psychiatric, neurological, and medical disorders associated with increased risk of violence; the role of substance abuse; and compliance with treatment. The peer-reviewed publications of studies finding increased violence with each of these elements were cited earlier in this chapter.

The clinical "method" of predicting risk of violence has been tested to some extent. Mossman (1994) reviewed the literature on the assessment of risk of violence. He identified 30 publications in which clinical assessment of violence was conducted and patients were followed up to determine whether they were subsequently violent. Only six studies used 1 week or less as the follow-up period. The remaining studies used follow-up periods of months or years. As was explained earlier in this chapter, the short-term prediction of risk of violence is of greater relevance in clinical and legal matters.

The generalizability of the six studies was limited because they used violence by patients in psychiatric hospitals as the outcome measure. Three of the studies used the clinical determination by physicians that the patients were a "danger to others" during commitment proceedings. Yesavage et al. (1982) evaluated and followed up 84 patients for 1 week in the hospital. In their first study McNiel and Binder (1987) evaluated and followed up 101 patients for 3 days in the hospital. McNiel et al. (1988) evaluated and followed up 238 patients for 3 days in the hospital. In all three studies, whether a patient was deemed to be a danger to others was correlated at a statistically significant level to violence in hospital in the follow-up period. Rates of accuracy were calculated. True positive rates were 65%, 67%, and 78%, respectively, and false-negative rates were 35%, 33%, and 22%, respectively (McNiel and Binder 1987; McNiel et al. 1988; Yesavage et al. 1982). In a fourth study by McNiel and Binder (1991), 22 nurses and 41 physicians rated 149 patients at the time of admission as at high, moderate, or low risk for violence and followed up the patients for 1 week to determine whether they were violent in the hospital. Patients who did attack people in the hospital had been rated as a moderate or high risk more than nonviolent patients had. Janofsky et al. (1988) had 2 physicians rate 54 patients at the time of admission and followed up the patients for a week in the hospital. They found no statistically significant correlation between the physicians' ratings and patient violence during the follow-up week. Werner et al. (1984) had 15 psychiatrists rate 40 patients at the time of admission and followed up the patients for 1 week in the hospital. They found no statistically significant correlation between the psychiatrists' ratings and patient violence.

In conclusion, the psychiatric profession believes that prediction of the risk of violence is based on clinical judgment and not instruments alone. The peer-reviewed literature supports elements of a model of prediction. Studies of clinical determination of risk of violence in the near future are divided, but the larger studies by well-known violence researchers do support clinicians' ability to predict violence better than chance alone.

Legal Standards

In 1976, the California Supreme Court recognized that psychiatrists and other therapists have a legal duty to protect potential victims from violence by their patients when a therapeutic relationship exists between the therapist and the patient (*Tarasoff v. Regents of the University of California* 1976). Elements of that duty to protect involve assessment of the threat of dangerousness, identification of the potential object of the threat, and implementation of some affirmative preventive act (Appelbaum 1985). The United States Supreme Court has reinforced the duty to predict violent behavior among patients for the purpose of protection of potential victims and in other legal proceedings despite protests by the profession that it is impossible to predict violence (*Schall v. Martin* 1984).

Beck and Cerundolo (1999) reviewed decisions about duty to protect. They pointed out that approximately 70 published cases have involved allegations that a health care professional breached the duty to protect and that until recently no court has disagreed with the *Tarasoff* decision. Court decisions have found that a duty exists when the violence is foreseeable, when a victim is identifiable, and when a history of violence is present. Court decisions have found that a duty exists to control patients to prevent violence after discharge from the hospital. There have been conflicting decisions in regard to outpatients. In 1991, a Florida court rejected the *Tarasoff* duty (*Boynton v. Burglass* 1991). The family of a victim who was shot by an outpatient sued the patient's doctor. The court affirmed a lower court decision to dismiss the suit. It did not impose liability on the defendant's failure to control the patient because it questioned whether psychiatric predictions of violence are accurate.

Ethical Considerations

Health care professionals have a legal duty to protect potential victims from violence by their patients if a special relationship exists, such as a treatment relationship. This involves gathering information about the potential for violence in the near future, determining the potential for violence, and, if the patient poses a significant risk of violence, intervening to protect the intended victim. If the health care professional does not have a special relationship with someone who intends to harm someone else, he or she has no legal duty; however, I believe that a moral duty exists to do something to prevent injury to a person. For example, if a physician hears about a potentially violent situation from a friend, there is no legal duty to do something, but as a human being the physician would probably take steps or give advice to protect the intended victim.

Breach of confidentiality is discussed frequently in the duty of clinicians to protect potential victims from violence by their patients. Most states allow interventions to protect other than warning an intended victim; thus confidentiality need not be breached in appropriate cases. Confidentiality is breached when the risk of violence is significant and other means of controlling a patient's violence are not appropriate or feasible. Before breaching confidentiality and warning a potential victim, the clinician should discuss the matter with the patient. The therapist should present the warning in a therapeutic sense, not a legal one. For example, the patient should be told something like "I will tell Miss X that you have had thoughts of attacking her since she broke off your relationship. I believe the risk of your doing so is serious. I want to prevent you from doing something that will get you hurt as well as Miss X."

Summary of Prediction of Violence

The assessment of violence potential for the short term (i.e., in days or a week) is analogous to the assessment of suicide potential. The clinician must consider the following:

- Subtle questioning of the patient if violence is not mentioned
- How well planned the threat of violence is
- Available means of inflicting injury
- History of violence and impulsive behavior with attention to frequency, degree of past injuries to others and self, toward whom, and under what circumstances
- Alcohol and drug use
- Presence of other organic mental disorders
- Presence of schizophrenia, mania, or other psychosis
- Presence of certain personality and impulse-control disorders
- Noncompliance with treatment in the past

All of these factors are weighed in the final assessment of whether the patient poses a significant risk to others so that some action is necessary on the part of the evaluator. Action may include hospitalizing the patient or warning the intended victim and/or the police. All of the data on which the decision that the patient is or is not at risk for violence is based must be documented in writing. The thinking process through which the decision was made should be evident in the written documentation. Violence potential should be reassessed at short intervals (e.g., from visit to visit or every few days) if the patient is to continue to be treated outside of the hospital or other institution.

References

Abram KM, Teplin LA: Drug disorder, mental illness and violence. NIDA Res Monogr 103: 222–236, 1990

Allen J, Tranoff G, Coyne I: Therapeutic alliance and long-term hospital treatment outcome. Compr Psychiatry 26:187–194, 1985

American Psychiatric Association: Diagnostic and Statistical Manual of Mental Disorders, 4th Edition, Text Revision. Washington, DC, American Psychiatric Association, 2000

Anderson KE, Silver JM: Neurological and medical diseases and violence, in Medical Management of the Violent Patient: Clinical Assessment and Therapy. Edited by Tardiff K. New York, Marcel Dekker, 1999, pp 87–124

Appelbaum PS: Tarasoff and the clinician: problems in fulfilling the duty to protect. Am J Psychiatry 142:425–429, 1985

Appelbaum PS: Statutory approaches to limiting psychiatrists' liability for their patients' violent acts. Am J Psychiatry 146:821–828, 1989

Apperson LJ, Mulvey EP, Lidz CW: Short-term clinical prediction of assaultive behavior: artifacts of research methods. Am J Psychiatry 150:1374–1379, 1993

Arango C, Barba AC, Gonzalez-Salvador T, et al: Violence in inpatients with schizophrenia: a prospective study. Schizophr Bull 25:493–503, 1999

Bach-y-Rita G, Lion JR, Clement CE, et al: Episodic dyscontrol: a study of 130 violent patients. Am J Psychiatry 127:1473–1479, 1971

Bailey DN: Phencyclidine abuse, clinical findings and concentrations in biological fluids after nonfatal intoxication. Am J Clin Pathol 72:795–799, 1979

Barratt ES: Anxiety and impulsiveness related to psychomotor efficiency. Percept Mot Skills 9:191–198, 1959

Beauford JE, McNiel DE, Binder RL: Utility of the initial therapeutic alliance in evaluating psychiatric patients' risk of violence. Am J Psychiatry 154:1272–1276, 1997

Beck JC, Cerundolo P: The clinician's legal duties when the patient may be violent, in Medical Management of the Violent Patient: Clinical Assessment and Therapy. Edited by Tardiff K. New York, Marcel Dekker, 1999, pp 429–445

Benjamin L: Interpersonal Treatment of Personality Disorders. New York, Guilford, 1993

Benjaminsen S, Botzsche-Larsen K, Norrie L, et al: Patient violence in a psychiatric hospital in Denmark: rate of violence and relation to diagnosis. Nordic Journal of Psychiatry 50:233–242, 1996

Binder RL, McNiel DE: Effects of diagnosis and context on dangerousness. Am J Psychiatry 145:728–732, 1988

Bland R, Orn H: Family violence and psychiatric disorder. Can J Psychiatry 31:129–137, 1986

Borum R: Improving the clinical practice of violence risk assessment: technology, guidelines and training. Am Psychol 51:945–956, 1996

Bouras N, Drummond C: Mental disorders and problematic behaviours in people with intellectual disability. J Intellect Disabil Res 36:440–447, 1997

Boynton v Burglass, 490 So2d 446 (Fla App 1991)

Brizer DA, Crowner ML (eds): Current Approaches to the Prediction of Violence. Washington, DC, American Psychiatric Press, 1989

Brody SL: Violence associated with acute cocaine use in patients admitted to a medical emergency department. NIDA Res Monogr 103:44–55, 1990

Brooke MM, Questad KA, Patterson DR: Agitation and restlessness after closed head injury: a prospective study of 100 consecutive admissions. Arch Phys Med Rehabil 73:320–323, 1992

Brown GL, Goodwin FK: Human aggression and suicide. Suicide Life Threat Behav 16:223–243, 1986

Buss AH, Durkee A: An inventory for assessing different kinds of hostility. Journal of Consulting Psychology 21:343–349, 1957

Carey G, Goldman D: The genetics of antisocial behavior, in Handbook of Antisocial Behavior. Edited by Stoff DM, Breiling J, Moser JD. New York, Wiley, 1997, pp 243–254

Choi PYL, Parrott AC, Cowan D: High dose anabolic steroids in strength athletes: effects upon hostility and aggression. J Psychopharmacol 3:102–112, 1989

Clarkin JF, Hurt SW, Grilly JL: Therapeutic alliance and hospital treatment outcome. Hospital and Community Psychiatry 38:871–875, 1987

Climent C, Ervin F: Historical data in the evaluation of violent subjects. Arch Gen Psychiatry 27:621–624, 1972

Coccaro EF, Siever LJ, Klar HM, et al: Serotonergic studies in patients with affective and personality disorders with correlates of suicidal and impulsive aggressive behavior. Arch Gen Psychiatry 46:587–599, 1989

Coccaro EF, Harvey PD, Kupshaw-Lawrence E, et al: Development of neuropharmacologically based behavioral assessments of impulsive violent behavior. J Neuropsychiatry Clin Neurosci 3:544–551, 1991

Coccaro EF, Kavoussi RJ, Lester JC: Self and other directed human aggression: the role of central serotonergic system. Int J Psychopharmacol 6:70–83, 1992

Collins JJ, Schlenger WE: Acute and chronic effects of alcohol use on violence. J Stud Alcohol 49:516–521, 1988

Convit A, Isay D, Gadioma R: Underreporting of physical assaults in schizophrenic inpatients. J Nerv Ment Dis 176:507–509, 1988

Craig TJ: An epidemiologic study of problems associated with violence among psychiatric inpatients. Am J Psychiatry 139:1262–1266, 1982

Daubert v Merrell Dow Pharmaceuticals, Inc., 509 US 579 (1993)

Davis S: Violence by psychiatric inpatients: a review. Hospital and Community Psychiatry 42:585–590, 1991

Denison ME, Paredes A, Booth JB: Alcohol and cocaine interactions and aggressive behaviors. Recent Dev Alcohol 13:283–303, 1997

Deutsch LH, Bylsma FW, Rovner BW, et al: Psychosis and physical agitation in probable Alzheimer's disease. Am J Psychiatry 148:1159–1163, 1991

Ellinwood EH: Assault and homicide associated with amphetamine abuse. Am J Psychiatry 127:1170–1175, 1971

Eronen M, Hakola P, Tiihonen J: Mental disorders and homicidal behavior in Finland. Arch Gen Psychiatry 53:497–501, 1996

Fordyce DJ, Roueche JR, Prigatano GF: Enhanced emotional reactions in chronic head trauma patients. J Neurol Neurosurg Psychiatry 46:620–624, 1993

Geller MP: Sociopathic adaptation by psychotic patients. Hospital and Community Psychiatry 31:108–112, 1980

Ghaziuddin M, Ghaziuddin N: Violence against staff by mentally retarded inpatients. Hospital and Community Psychiatry 43:503–504, 1992

Giannini AJ, Miller NS, Lioselle RH, et al: Cocaine-associated violence and relationship to route of administration. J Subst Abuse Treat 10:67–75, 1993

Grinker RR, Werble B, Drye RC: The Borderline Syndrome. New York, Basic Books, 1968

Gutheil TG, Bursztajn H, Brodsky J: The multidimensional assessment of dangerousness: confidence assessment in patient care and liability prevention. Bulletin of the American Academy of Psychiatry and the Law 14:123–129, 1986

Hamel M, Gold DP, Andres M, et al: Predictors and consequences of aggressive behavior by community-based dementia patients. Gerontologist 30:206–211, 1990

Hare R: The Hare Psychopathy Checklist—Revised Manual. Toronto, Ontario, Multi-Health Systems, 1991

Hellerstein D, Frosch W, Koenigsberg HW: The clinical significance of command hallucinations. Am J Psychiatry 144:219–221, 1987

Humphreys MS, Johnstone EC, MacMillan JF: Dangerous behavior preceding first admission for schizophrenia. Br J Psychiatry 161:501–505, 1992

Ito TA, Miller N, Pollock VE: Alcohol and aggression: a meta-analysis on the moderating effects of inhibitory cues, triggering events and self-focused attention. Psychol Bull 120:60–82, 1996

Janofsky JS, Spears S, Neubauer DN: Psychiatrists' accuracy in predicting violent behavior on an inpatient unit. Hospital and Community Psychiatry 39:1090–1094, 1988

Jordan BK, Marmar CR, Fairbank JA: Problems in families of male Vietnam veterans with posttraumatic stress disorder. J Consult Clin Psychol 60:916–923, 1992

Junginger J: Command hallucinations and the prediction of dangerousness. Psychiatr Serv 46:911–914, 1995

Klassen D, O'Connor WA: A prospective study of violence in adult male mental health admissions. Law Hum Behav 12:143–158, 1988

Klassen D, O'Connor WA: Assessing the risk of violence in released mental patients: a cross-validation study. Psychological Assessment 1:75–81, 1989

Krakowski M., Volavka J, Brizer D: Psychopathology and violence: a review of literature. Compr Psychiatry 27:131–148, 1986

Krakowski M, Convit A, Jaeger J: Neurological impairment in violent schizophrenic inpatients. Am J Psychiatry 146:849–856, 1989

Kutzer DJ: Psychobiological factors in violent behavior, in Violent Behavior, Vol I: Assessment and Intervention. Edited by Hertzberg LJ, Ostrum GF, Field JR. New York, PMA Publishing, 1990

Lasko NB, Gurvits TV, Kuhne AA: Aggression and its correlates in Vietnam veterans with and without chronic posttraumatic stress disorder. Compr Psychiatry 35:373–381, 1994

Lee HK, Villar O, Juthani N, et al: Characteristics and behavior of patients involved in psychiatric ward incidents. Hospital and Community Psychiatry 40:1295–1297, 1989

Lidz CW, Mulvey EP, Gardner W: The accuracy of predictions of violence to others. JAMA 269:1007–1011, 1993

Linaker OM: Assaultiveness among institutionalised adults with mental retardation. Br J Psychiatry 164:62–68, 1994

Lindqvist P, Allebeck P: Schizophrenia and assaultive behaviour: the role of alcohol and drug abuse. Acta Psychiatr Scand 82:191–195, 1990

Link BG, Andrews H, Cullen FT: The violent and illegal behavior of mental patients reconsidered. American Sociological Review 57:275–292, 1992

Linnoila VM, Virkkunen M: Aggression, suicidality and serotonin. J Clin Psychiatry 53 (suppl):46–51, 1992

Linnoila M, Virkkunen M, Scheinin M, et al: Low cerebrospinal fluid 5-hydroxyindole acetic acid concentration differentiates impulsive from non-impulsive violent behavior. Life Sci 33:2609–2614, 1983

Lowenstein DH, Massa SM, Rowbotham MC, et al: Acute neurologic and psychiatric complications associated with cocaine abuse. Am J Med 83:841–846, 1987

Lowenstein M, Binder RL, McNiel DE: The relationship between admission symptoms and hospital assaults. Hospital and Community Psychiatry 41:311–313, 1990

Manschreck TC, Laughery JA, Weisstein CC, et al: Characteristics of freebase cocaine psychosis. Yale J Biol Med 61:115–122, 1988

Marazziti D, Rotando A, Presta S, et al: Role of serotonin in human aggressive behavior. Aggressive Behavior 19:347–353, 1993

Mark MM: Social science evidence in the courtroom: Daubert and beyond. Psychology, Public Policy and Law 5:175–193, 1999

McCormick RA, Smith M: Aggression and hostility in substance abusers: the relationship to abuse patterns, coping style, and relapse triggers. Addict Behav 20:555–562, 1995

McKinlay WW, Brooks DN, Bond MR, et al: The short-term outcome of severe blunt head trauma as reported by relatives of injured persons. J Neurol Neurosurg Psychiatry 44:527–533, 1981

McNiel DE, Binder RL: Predictive validity of judgments of dangerousness in emergency civil commitment. Am J Psychiatry 144:197–200, 1987

McNiel D, Binder RL: Clinical assessment of the risk of violence among psychiatric inpatients. Am J Psychiatry 148:1317–1321, 1991

McNiel DE, Binder RL, Greenfield TK: Predictors of violence in civilly committed acute psychiatric patients. Am J Psychiatry 145:965–970, 1988

McNiel DE, Eisner JP, Binder RL: The relationship between command hallucinations and violence. Psychiatr Serv 51:1288–1292, 2000

Mendoza R, Miller BL: Neuropsychiatric disorders associated with cocaine use. Hospital and Community Psychiatry 43:677–678, 1992

Miczek KA, Haney M, Tidey JW, et al: Neurochemistry and pharmacotherapeutic management of aggression and violence, in Understanding and Preventing Violence, Vol 2. Edited by Reiss AJ, Miczek KA, Roth JA. Washington, DC, National Academy Press, 1994, pp 245–273

Miller RJ, Zadolinnyj K, Hafner RJ, et al: Profiles and predictors of assaultiveness for different psychiatric ward populations. Am J Psychiatry 150:1368–1373, 1993

Monahan J: The Clinical Prediction of Violent Behavior. Rockville, MD, National Institute of Mental Health, 1981

Monahan J, Steadman H (eds): Violence and Mental Disorder: Developments in Risk Assessment. Chicago, IL, University of Chicago Press, 1994

Monroe RR: Episodic Behavioral Disorders. Cambridge, MA, Harvard University Press, 1970

Morrison EF: The measurement of aggression and violence in hospitalized psychiatric patients. Int J Nurs Stud 30:51–64, 1993

Mossman D: Assessing predictions of violence: being accurate about accuracy. J Consult Clin Psychol 62:783–792, 1994

Mulvey EP, Lidz CW: Conditional prediction: a model for research on dangerousness to others in a new era. Int J Law Psychiatry 18:129–143, 1995

Murdoch D, Pihl RO, Ross D: Alcohol and crimes of violence: present issues. International Journal of the Addictions 25:1065–1081, 1990

National Institute on Drug Abuse: Facts About Ecstasy. NIDA Notes 14(4), 1999

Nurnberg HG, Prudic J, Fiori M, et al: Psychopathology complicating acquired immune deficiency syndrome (AIDS). Am J Psychiatry 141:95–96, 1984

Otto RK: On the ability of mental health professional to predict dangerousness: a commentary on interpretations of the dangerousness literature. Law and Psychology Review 18:43–68, 1994

Patel V, Hope RA: Aggressive behaviour in elderly psychiatric inpatients. Acta Psychiatr Scand 85:131–139, 1992

Perry JC, Herman J: Trauma and defense in the ideology of borderline personality disorder, in Borderline Personality Disorder: Etiology and Treatment. Edited by Paris J. Washington, DC, American Psychiatric Press, 1993, pp 135–139

Peterson JB, Rolhfleisch J, Zelazo PD, et al: Acute intoxication and cognitive functioning. J Stud Alcohol 51:114–122, 1990

Plutchik R, van Praag HM: A self-report measure of violence risk. Compr Psychiatry 31:450–456, 1990

Pope HG Jr, Katz DL: Homicide and near-homicide by anabolic steroid users. J Clin Psychiatry 51:28–31, 1990

Quinsey VL: The prediction and explanation of criminal violence. Int J Psychiatry Law 18:117–127, 1995

Raine A: Autonomic nervous system factors underlying disinhibited antisocial and violent behavior: biosocial perspectives and treatment implications. Ann N Y Acad Sci 794:46–59, 1996

Raine A, Lency T, Bihrle S, et al: Reduced prefrontal gray matter volume and reduced autonomic activity in antisocial personality disorder. Arch Gen Psychiatry 57:119–127, 2000

Rao N, Jellinek HM, Woolston DC: Agitation in closed head injury: haloperidol effects on rehabilitation outcome. Arch Phys Med Rehabil 66:30–34, 1985

Reisberg B, Ferris SH: A clinical rating scale for symptoms of psychosis in Alzheimer's disease. Psychopharmacol Bull 21:101–104, 1985

Reisberg B, Borenstein J, Salbo S, et al: Behavioral symptoms in Alzheimer's disease: phenomenology and treatment. J Clin Psychiatry 48 (suppl 5):9–15, 1987

Rogers R, Nussbaum D, Gillis R: Command hallucinations and criminality: a clinical quandary. Bulletin of the American Academy of Psychiatry and the Law 16:251–258, 1988

Rossi AM, Jacobs M, Monteleone M, et al: Characteristics of psychiatric patients who engage in assaultive or other fear-inducing behaviors. J Nerv Ment Dis 174:154–160, 1986

Roy A, Linnoila M: Monoamines and Suicidal Behavior. New York, Brunner/Mazel, 1990

Rush AJ, Pincus HA, First MB, et al: Handbook of Psychiatric Measures. Washington, DC, American Psychiatric Association, 2000

Salloum IM, Daley DC, Cornelius JR: Disproportionate lethality in psychiatric patients with concurrent alcohol and cocaine abuse. Am J Psychiatry 153:953–955, 1996

Schall v Martin, 467 US 278–279 (1984)

Schulte HM, Hall MJ, Boyer M: Domestic violence associated with anabolic steroid abuse (letter). Am J Psychiatry 150:348, 1993

Segal SP, Watson MA, Goldfinger SM, et al: Civil commitment in the psychiatric emergency room, part I: the assessment of dangerousness by emergency room clinicians. Arch Gen Psychiatry 45:748–752, 1988a

Segal SP, Watson MA, Goldfinger SM, et al: Civil commitment in the psychiatric emergency room, part II: mental disorders indicators and three dangerousness criteria. Arch Gen Psychiatry 45:753–758, 1988b

Serin RC, Amos NL: The role of psychopathology in the assessment of dangerousness. Int J Psychiatry Law 18:231–238, 1995

Sheridan M, Henrion R, Robinson L, et al: Precipitants of violence in a psychiatric inpatient setting. Hospital and Community Psychiatry 41:776–780, 1990

Simon RI: Clinical approaches to the duty to warn and protect, in Clinical Psychiatry and the Law, 2nd Edition. Washington, DC, American Psychiatric Press, 1992, pp 297–343

Skodal A, Karasu T: Emergency psychiatry and the assaultive patient. Am J Psychiatry 135:202–204, 1978

Snider WD, Simpson DM, Nielson S, et al: Neurological complications of acquired immune deficiency syndrome: analysis of 50 patients. Ann Neurol 14:40–418, 1983

Special Hospitals' Research Group: Schizophrenia, violence, clozapine and risperidone: a review. Br J Psychiatry 169 (suppl 31):21–30, 1996

Steadman HJ, Mulvey EP, Monahan J, et al: Violence by people discharged from acute psychiatric inpatient facilities and by others in the same neighborhoods. Arch Gen Psychiatry 55:393–401, 1998

Stone AA: Law, Psychiatry, and Morality. Washington, DC, American Psychiatric Press, 1984, pp 161–190

Stone MH: The Fate of the Borderline Patient: Successful Outcome in Psychiatric Practice. New York, Guilford, 1990, p 173

Su T, Pagliaro M, Schmidt PJ: Neuropsychiatric effects of anabolic steroids in male normal volunteers. JAMA 269:2760–2764, 1993

Swanson JW, Holzer CE, Ganju VK, et al: Violence and psychiatric disorder in the community: evidence from the Epidemiologic Catchment Area surveys. Hospital and Community Psychiatry 41:761–770, 1990

Tam E, Engelsmann F, Fugere R: Patterns of violent incidents by patients in a general hospital psychiatric facility. Psychiatr Serv 47:86–88, 1996

Tarasoff v Regents of the University of California, 118 Cal Rptr 129, 529 P2d 553 (1974)

Tardiff K: Characteristics of assaultive patients in private hospitals. Am J Psychiatry 141:1232–1235, 1984

Tardiff K: Assessment and Management of Violent Patients, 2nd Edition. Washington, DC, American Psychiatric Press, 1996

Tardiff K: Unusual diagnoses among violent patients. Psychiatr Clin North Am 21:567–579, 1998a

Tardiff K: The potential for violence among employees with psychiatric disorders, in Violence in the Workplace. Edited by Wilkinson C. Rockville, MD, Government Institutes, 1998b

Tardiff K (ed): Medical Management of the Violent Patient: Clinical Assessment and Therapy. New York, Marcel Dekker, 1999

Tardiff K, Koenigsberg H: A study of assaultive behavior among psychiatric outpatients. Am J Psychiatry 142:960–963, 1985

Tardiff K, Sweillam A: Assault, suicide, and mental illness. Arch Gen Psychiatry 37:164–169, 1980a

Tardiff K, Sweillam A: Factors related to increased risk of assaultive behavior in suicidal patients. Acta Psychiatr Scand 62:63–68, 1980b

Tardiff K, Sweillam A: Assaultive behavior among chronic inpatients. Am J Psychiatry 139:212–215, 1982

Tardiff K, Marzuk PM, Leon AC, et al: A prospective study of violence by psychiatric patients after hospital discharge. Psychiatr Serv 48:678–681, 1997a

Tardiff K, Marzuk PM, Leon AC, et al: Violence by patients admitted to a private psychiatric hospital. Am J Psychiatry 154:88–93, 1997b

Taylor PJ, Gunn J: Homicides by people with mental illness: myth and reality. Br J Psychiatry 174: 564–565, 1999

Taylor SP, Leonard KE: Alcohol and human aggression, in Aggression: Theoretical and Empirical Reviews, Vol 2. Edited by Green RG, Donnerstein EI. New York, Academic Press, 1983, pp 77–101

Tiihonen J, Hakola P, Eronen M, et al: Risk of homicidal behavior among discharged forensic psychiatric patients. Forensic Sci Int 79:123–129, 1996

Truscott D, Evans J, Mansell S: Outpatient psychotherapy with dangerous clients: a model for clinical decision making. Professional Psychological Research and Practice 26:484–490, 1995

Virkkunen M, Linnoila M: Serotonin in early onset, male alcoholics with violent behaviour. Ann Med 22:327–331, 1990

Volavka J: Neurobiology of Violence. Washington, DC, American Psychiatric Press, 1995

Volavka J, Tardiff K: Substance abuse and violence, in Medical Management of the Violent Patient: Clinical Assessment and Therapy. Edited by Tardiff K. New York, Marcel Dekker, 1999, pp 153–171

Wack RC: The ongoing risk assessment in the treatment of forensic patients on conditional release status. Psychiatr Q 64:275–293, 1993

Werner PD, Rose TL, Yesavage JA, et al: Psychiatrists' judgments of dangerousness in patients on an acute care unit. Am J Psychiatry 141:263–266, 1984

Widom CS: Does violence beget violence? A critical examination of the literature. Psychol Bull 114:68–79, 1989

Yesavage JA: Bipolar illness: correlates of dangerous inpatient behaviour. Br J Psychiatry 143:554–557, 1983

Yesavage JA, Werner PD, Becker JMT, et al: Short-term civil commitment and the violent patient. Am J Psychiatry 139:1145–1149, 1982

Yudofsky SC, Silver JM, Jackson W, et al: The Overt Aggression Scale: an operationalized rating scale for verbal and physical aggression. Am J Psychiatry 143:35–39, 1986

9

Evaluating Mental States Without the Benefit of a Direct Examination

Basic Concepts and Ethical and Legal Implications

Roy B. Lacoursiere, M.D.
Glen Weissenberger, J.D.
A. J. Stephani, J.D.

If psychiatrists could read minds, would it be admissible in court?

—*The chapter authors*

Mental health expert testimony for the courts usually may be proffered to describe the functioning of an individual—for example, at the time of an alleged criminal act—or may be more general scientific mental health knowledge, such as whether a certain type of pharmacological agent can help depression. In the former case the mental health professional's approach to the court's query requires evaluating the individual. In the latter case although the issue initially appears more as the "general science" and less as the "individually applied art" of the mental health field, the science of studying the therapeutic effects of an agent will have been based on the study of individuals who will have had evaluations of some sort to determine, inter alia, if each person was initially depressed and if the depression improved with the use of the agent. In this latter context the "art" and the "science" of mental health work will have been more commingled. In this chapter we emphasize contexts in which a mental health professional evaluation plays the outstanding role in gathering material for the proffered testimony. The methods for doing these evaluations are of interest to post-*Daubert* courts. Therefore, in this chapter we return to basics about evaluations of mental states so that issues such as evaluation methodology and diagnostic and other opinion reliability and validity can be examined "from the ground up" in reviewing mental health professional conclusions for testimonial purposes.

To explore certain limits and opportunities of data-gathering possibilities for mental health professional evaluations, we investigate the degree to which mental health professional diagnostic and other conclusions can be arrived at without a direct, face-to-face mental health professional examination (cf. Slovenko 2000a). We especially explore these non-face-to-face evaluations for retrospective assessments, but much of what is discussed has broader relevance. Although the emphasis is on non-face-to-face contexts, the overview of basics will allow the reader—mental health professional or non–mental health professional—to review the details of an evaluation in both face-to-face and non-face-to-face contexts to be better able to consider what the mental health field can accomplish in providing testimony for the courts when the issue concerns the functioning of an individual. Non-face-to-face methods for evaluations have certain potential advantages because these methods can reduce the subjectivity in the data analysis and allow for evaluations when they might not otherwise be feasible.

At times mental characteristics that fall short of a diagnosis will be useful, but the emphasis will be on situations in which diagnoses are reached or excluded. Diagnoses often provide the starting point for certain expectations of the course of behavior, and diagnoses often provide a window into the suspected mental state of the evaluee at the relevant time. For example, a mental state in which a defendant "knew" he or she was being controlled by the devil and told to perform certain acts is unlikely to exist or convince a mental health professional, or fact-finder, independent of a diagnosis such as schizophrenia or drug toxicity.

In this chapter *mental health professional* generally means a person in a mental health career capacity, such as a psychiatrist, psychologist, or social worker. However, a primary care physician or similar person who is doing mental health work may be considered a mental health professional for the sake of some of the materials herein. Generally forensic mental health professionals are psychiatrists or psychologists, but in some cases another mental health professional may be the forensic expert (e.g., if the work of a psychiatric nurse is under the court's scrutiny, a psychiatric nurse likely would be used as a mental health professional expert). Finally, it should surprise few that the law's use of various terms later in the chapter, such as *reliability*, is different from the mental health field's use of the same term.

A Mental Health Professional Evaluation

Evaluation is the more general term applied to gathering and assessing a range of data that are used to reach certain conclusions. In its broadest sense an evaluation applies to a rather comprehensive assessment used to reach a diagnosis and other conclusions (e.g., for functioning, treatment) under the conditions of the evaluation in question. In a narrower sense evaluation can be used to apply to portions of a comprehensive evaluation, such as to the mental status evaluation (MSE) or the physical evaluation, when a range of data is used to assess this portion of the broader evaluation. Such an evaluation can come from examining a patient's arm and an X ray and concluding that he or she has a fracture or watching a patient's behavior in the emergency department, asking the patient a few questions, and concluding that he or she has a psychotic disorder. In neither of these restricted examples will the evaluator know when the problem started, how it began, and so forth. *Examination* is a narrower term used when the part of the evaluation in question is directly reviewed, such as the patient's arm or general behavior. As is discussed in more detail later in this chapter, in the section "Evaluations (and Examinations) and Their Parameters," an examination may be essentially face-to-face or not; in the latter case, examinations can occur from observations in court or in public otherwise from a distance. Evaluations therefore typically include examinations, such as those of the mental status or functioning of the evaluee.

Data Categories for Evaluations

In a particular evaluation the precise information collected will vary with the issue(s), but general consensus exists as to the usual *categories* of data needed for an evaluation (Groth-Marnat 1999; Menninger 1962; Nicholi 1999). These data categories are incorporated into various standards, such as those of the Joint Commission on the Accreditation of Healthcare Organizations (1999) and those of the American Psychiatric Association (1995a) in their "Practice Guidelines for Psychiatric Evaluation of Adults," and in case law standards of care for a psychiatric evaluation (see, e.g., *Littleton v. Good Samaritan Hospital and Health Center* 1988). These types of evaluation data can be grouped into categories in the traditional clinical (and forensic) way as follows:

1. *Reason for the evaluation* (clinically often called the *chief complaint* and *history of the present problem*)—This data category comprises the presenting complaint or other reason for the evaluation (e.g., the person has been feeling down or depressed or is referred for a criminal responsibility evaluation) and the story of that complaint or reason. This data category is listed first because it determines to some considerable extent the details of what is pursued in the remainder of the evaluation data gathering. Information in this data category includes the onset and development or history of the reason for the evaluation and a relevant review of "systems" (mental and physical symptoms) associated with the situation. Forensically related evaluations may include the evaluee's version of what occurred and other versions, and various records may form part of this data pool. (Traditionally this data category was often considered the most important category for determining diagnosis and differential diagnosis, but current medical evaluations often quickly jump from a brief complaint and history to laboratory testing to make or exclude some diagnostic hypothesis [Braunwald et al. 2001; L. Goldman 1994; Isselbacher et al. 1994].)

2. *Background history*—This data category constitutes the full relevant background of the person from the perspective of his or her family, education, work history, legal history, health history, and so on. Besides background information gathered from the evaluee, this material may include information from family members, neighbors, employers, and others. When these background data are gathered contemporaneously during the evaluation, they may contain certain biases of recall, denial, dishonesty, and so forth, as, of course, may other evaluation information. Information for the background history also may be obtained from medical and related records, public records (e.g., criminal history, bankruptcy filings), videotapes of police interviews, and other records (e.g., employment and school records). Insofar as background history is reconstructed in a current evaluation, it is retrospective, but such history sometimes can be obtained or corroborated from prior contemporaneous records. (See Rogers, Chapter 10, this volume.)

3. *MSE*—This data category consists of the mental functioning as seen at

the time of the evaluation (e.g., cooperativeness, hallucinatory behavior, irritability, ability to do arithmetic, orientation). On the basis of various pieces of information, the mental health professional may attempt to essentially reconstruct the mental status for a prior time. The gathering of such MSE information for a prior time is part of the reason for the evaluation or of the background history above, but it also may be past information consistent with the current MSE, such as for a diagnosis of schizophrenia.

4. *Psychological testing*—This data category consists of more specific testing of mental or psychological functioning beyond that included in the MSE—for example, testing with the Minnesota Multiphasic Personality Inventory, 2nd Edition (MMPI-2; Butcher et al. 1989), or intelligence or neuropsychological testing (Groth-Marnat 1999).

5. *Physical and laboratory evaluation*—This data category includes a relevant physical examination with appropriate laboratory testing, which may include blood tests, X rays, and brain magnetic resonance imaging.

6. *Other data*—This category is for data not easily classifiable into any of the above categories. For example, this may include videotapes or audiotapes of interviews by law enforcement officers that may be relevant to the category "reason for the evaluation" and to the MSE.

Comment on Data Categories for Evaluations

Traditionally the data from all these parts of the evaluation fit together so that a certain reason for the evaluation was associated with a certain background history, particular MSE results, certain kinds of psychological testing data, and particular physical and laboratory evaluation findings. That is, this combined information formed an overall entity for a clinical diagnosis, such as for schizophrenia or antisocial personality disorder. The person with suspected schizophrenia would have a background with some expected interpersonal and other specific difficulties, certain findings on the MSE, certain psychological test results, noncontributory or healthy physical and laboratory evaluation findings, and so on. These findings would be different from the overall types of findings with the person with antisocial personality disorder, who would show a background with some "antisocial" problems in childhood and/or adolescence of a conduct disorder diagnostic nature and so on. That is, the evaluative material has some internal consistency and internal corroboration, and in this way it is tested as to its reasonableness.

This is not to suggest that this internal consistency and corroboration are always by any means unambiguous or that mental health professionals are always careful to know the range of backgrounds and behaviors that are part of the story of people with various diagnoses. In the simplest cases of diagnostic ambiguity, the ambiguity is resolved by common differential diagnostic questions such as bipolar disorder versus schizoaffective disorder or antisocial personality disorder versus narcissistic or borderline personality disorder. In more ambiguous cases we may have serious mental illness versus malingering or versus less serious mental illness, such as a personality disorder, as in the Hinckley case (Bonnie et al. 2000).

This traditional means of data gathering and then using all the data categories to reach conclusions about a diagnosis, ability to function, treatment recommendations, and so on is advocated in the American Psychiatric Association's (1995a) "Practice Guidelines for Psychiatric Evaluation of Adults" to some extent, for certain mental health settings by the Joint Commission on the Accreditation of Healthcare Organizations (1999), and to some degree in general clinical medicine (cf. Braunwald et al. 2001; Isselbacher et al. 1994). But this traditional approach to evaluation is no longer the case with DSM-III, DSM-III-R, DSM-IV, and DSM-IV-TR (American Psychiatric Association 1980, 1987, 1994, 2000) (besides the influence of managed care and other contemporary strictures on mental health professional practice, although these latter areas are not further discussed here [see Zatzick 1999]). Currently a significant body of mental health professionals (with an accepted methodology, a tested knowledge base, peer-reviewed publications, known error rates which may or may not be made explicit, and so forth) encourages diagnoses not especially without any such general, broad-based data gathering but with a very pronounced de-emphasis on such a broad approach. Furthermore, considerable diagnostically relevant data gathering may be done by non–mental health professionals, including at times by the patients themselves. (These matters are discussed in detail later in this chapter, especially in the sections "Diagnostic Reliability Without a Direct Examination: The Lifetime Diagnosis Study" and "The PRIME-MD Patient Health Questionnaire Study," but also passim.)

Evaluations (and Examinations) and Their Parameters

For the purposes of this chapter and the concepts herein of evaluating mental states without the benefit of a face-to-face examination, the word *examination* usually will be reserved for a direct, face-to-face contact between an evaluator and an evaluee in its personal and physically proximal sense. This face-to-face contact allows for a multisensorial (visual, auditory, olfactory, and often tactile, at least in a handshake) perceptual evaluation. The more specific meaning of this definition of examination will become clearer as the chapter progresses. (The degree to which telephonic, e-mail, and television/audiovisual data qualify as subspecies of face-to-face data will vary with the medium, the data that are being evaluated, and so on. A more complete discussion of this subject is beyond the scope of this chapter, but obviously important data can be collected within the limitations of these methods [see, e.g., Baer et al. 1995; Klein and Manning 1995].)

To shed light on retrospective evaluations without the benefit of a face-to-face examination compared with other evaluations, some additional aspects of mental health professional evaluations are discussed. These are general aspects of evaluations culled from clinical experience and the references above for data categories. These particular aspects of evaluations are 1) evaluation contexts of availability, cooperativeness, and credibility; 2) direct, face-to-face examination parts of the evaluation; 3) the individual wh the retrospective continuum of evaluations; 6) clinical versus forensic mental health professional evaluations; 7) miscellaneous evaluation parameters; and 8) the quality of mental health professional evaluations.

These various parameters or aspects of evaluations will allow for a court's more in-depth consideration of the "trustworthiness" (see below) of non-face-to-face mental health professional evaluations in comparison to the full picture of mental health professional evaluations. For example, a face-to-face evaluation of someone suspected of pedophilic behavior that accepts at face value what the evaluee says without other information will lack credibility and be less "trustworthy" than a non-face-to-face evaluation in such a case that is based on material that includes credible records and interviews of others. This chapter shows that in the context of what constitutes mental health professional evaluative work for certain diagnoses and settings, non-face-to-face evaluations will assist the court as much as, or at times more than, face-to-face evaluations.

Evaluation Contexts

Evaluation contexts will address the related evaluation parameters of degrees of availability, cooperation, and credibility. *Availability* refers to the actual physical availability of the evaluee. This availability at one extreme covers the continuum of the currently available evaluee to the other extreme of the completely unavailable evaluee for a variety of reasons, including that the evaluee is deceased or cannot be located, with gradations between these extremes. These availability gradations consider factors such as prior availability of the evaluee when a mental health professional evaluation had been done; without current availability various degrees of other information about the evaluee from other sources still can be used for an evaluation.

Cooperation is the usual understanding of this term and considers the degree to which an evaluee, at one extreme, conscientiously and insofar as possible takes an active and involved part in the evaluation, and, at the other extreme, refuses to be seen by the mental health professional. This cooperation also refers to not only giving or not giving information in various parts of the evaluation but also consenting or not consenting to the release of medical and other records. *Credibility* refers to the usual understanding of this term, with the extremes of highly credible to highly incredible information being provided for the evaluation, with all gradations in between.

These interrelated evaluation context parameters cover the range of 1) the available, cooperative, and credible evaluee who as well as possible gives all information requested, including access to records; 2) the available, less cooperative, and deceptive (e.g., malingering) person who talks with the evaluator; 3) the available person who will not or cannot talk with the evaluator (e.g., brain damaged), and there may be much or little other data available about the person; and 4) the unavailable person who is neither physically nor mentally present because of death or otherwise. In this last context there may be much or little information to evaluate in the way of medical records, interviews of family members, and so on.

The evaluation needs to be addressed in each of these contexts. However, as we will see, at times, high reliability and validity can be reached for diagnoses and other opinions in a non-face-to-face evaluation without either the cooperation or the presence of the evaluee. This can be the case, for example, with repeated sexual offenses against children when credible criminal and witness records are available. Some of these latter non-face-to-face evaluations may be for retrospective settings (e.g., for past sexual and other violence).

This evaluation context topic can be further elucidated by noting forensic settings in which a full evaluation with a face-to-face examination usually is done, such as cooperative evaluees in civil damages cases and competency to stand trial cases. In other settings a full evaluation with a face-to-face examination is seldom or never done, such as with testamentary capacity evaluations for decedents. In any setting in which an evaluation is done, there will, of course, be some information to evaluate regardless of whether a face-to-face examination occurs, and various aspects of these data availability possibilities will be explored.

Direct, Face-to-Face Examination Parts of the Evaluation

Discussion of which parts of the evaluation are or can be face to face is needed for the issue of what evaluation data and subsequent conclusions can be attained without such face-to-face examination data. Which aspects of an evaluation usually are obtained via a face-to-face examination will vary with the circumstances, but under many mental health professional evaluation circumstances, they are the reason for the evaluation, the MSE, and the physical and laboratory evaluation. In addition, psychological testing, when there is any, and the background history may be face to face. That is, the complete evaluation may be face to face.

However, as will be seen, there can be exceptions for some or all of these data categories as being face-to-face data in clinical and/or forensic settings. The reason for the evaluation and the background history may be given by others, such as family members. The MSE, insofar as it exists, may come from sources other than a mental health professional face-to-face examination, as is seen in detail later in this chapter (especially the sections "Diagnostic Reliability Without a Direct Examination: The Lifetime Diagnostic Study" and "The PRIME-MD Patient Health Questionnaire Study," but also passim). Although a current complete physical examination or laboratory data cannot be obtained without face-to-face interaction, some physical examination data can be provided otherwise (e.g., by observations in court or on videotape as obtained by an investigator), and past physical and laboratory evaluation data may be available in various records. Finally, although some psychological testing can hardly avoid being face-to-face data, much psychological test data can be obtained with minimal face-to-face interaction with the evaluee, such as with the popular MMPI-2. Furthermore, an evaluee who might attempt to present himself or herself as mentally retarded, for which face-to-face psychological testing would be required to meet DSM-IV diagnostic criteria, might be shown not to be mentally retarded by non-face-to-face data, such as in school or work records or by information from a reliable informant.

To further illustrate the preceding discussion about evaluation contexts and face-to-face parts of the evaluation, consider an acutely disturbed, previously unknown person who is brought to the emergency department by the police. The potential patient may refuse to give information on background history or reason for the evaluation, although the accompanying police officer may provide some such information. The patient, without cooperating in the evaluation, nonetheless takes part in some degree of a face-to-face MSE and physical examination performed by the psychiatrist on duty (e.g., speech is illogical, and all limbs are moved without apparent pain). The patient soon thereafter kills himself or herself or someone else. Subsequent forensic mental health professional questions might be as follows: Did the evaluation meet the standard of care under the circumstances? Could the suicidal or homicidal behavior have been predicted or prevented?

The Individual Who Gathers the Evaluation Data

There are many variations in who gathers the evaluation data. In many mental health professional practice settings, all the categories of the evaluation data will be gathered by the single mental health professional in question, including whatever physical examination and psychological testing are done. In other mental health professional settings, such as some specialized mental health programs, including specialized forensic evaluation and substance abuse treatment settings, the data gathering likely will be shared by several people. In the normal course of data gathering in such places, some background history may be gathered by a social worker from the family, by nurses from the patient, or by a recovered ("recovering") counselor for substance abuse questions. These social worker, nurse, and counselor mental health professionals also may gather reason for evaluation data and do whatever MSE is done. In some settings the evaluee may complete some of the information database herself or himself, such as for reason for evaluation and background history. All of these data can be pooled, and then they may be confirmed or not to varying degrees by the mental health professional(s) who render(s) the final diagnoses and other opinions (e.g., for treatment recommendations, civil commitment, or criminal responsibility).

The MSE, which might be considered the most face-to-face part of the evaluation, may be obtained by the primary mental health professional doing the evaluation. At times and in some settings there is hardly any MSE, or an evaluee may give his or her own symptoms and whatever "MSE" there is. As the mental health field has striven for higher reliability and progressively objectified diagnostic criteria in DSM-III, DSM-III-R, DSM-IV, and DSM-IV-TR, gratification has been taken in having apparently reliable diagnoses made not only by non–mental health professionals but also by patients themselves. (This work is reviewed later in this chapter, especially in the section "Diagnostic Reliability.")

Psychological testing data also may be gathered in many ways and by various people. Tests such as the MMPI-2 are self-report data with little interaction required between the evaluee and a mental health professional to acquire the test data; this is partly compensated for by various validity scales and other devices in this and some other tests. Conversely, intelligence testing, such as the individually administered Wechsler Intelligence Scale for Children—III and the Wechsler Adult Intelligence Scale—III (Groth-Marnat 1999), is given face to face and usually with a psychologist. This is similar with projective psychological testing, such as with the Rorschach test. But some psychological tests are administered by technicians with varying degrees of skills, and we would hesitate to consider some of these technicians mental health professionals. Increasingly psychological testing is being done with the evaluee at a computer terminal; at the least, a professional must ensure that the evaluee was appropriately attentive, could understand what was needed, and so on (Groth-Marnat 1999).

The physical evaluation may be performed by a physician, but it may equally likely be performed by a nurse practitioner or physician assistant, with varying degrees of confirmation by the overseeing physician when one is available. It is also obvious that various findings can be made about physical functioning from others' observations of the evaluee and without a regular physical examination, such as based on observations in public, including in court, or based on videotape material obtained by investigators.

There also may be important face-to-face aspects of laboratory data gathering. For example, under the most stringent conditions, urine samples to test for drugs of abuse are not accepted unless they have been collected under direct "eye on the urethra" observational conditions (Glezen and Lowery 1999). This helps to avoid the collection of fraudulent samples and allows for more credible results.

Information Sources for the Evaluation

Besides the obvious gathering of information directly from the evaluee when feasible, such as in a face-to-face context or from questionnaires, multiple other sources of information may be available for an evaluation. Various medical, school, employment, and similar records form another information source, primarily for background history material but possibly for prior MSE. Family members, friends, and neighbors can provide another source of information, primarily for background history, but also for reason for the evaluation and MSE (see studies reported later in this chapter, especially the sections "Diagnostic Reliability Without a Direct Examination: The Lifetime Diagnosis Study" and "Discussion of Diagnostic Criteria and Non-Face-to-Face Information Sources for Selected Diagnoses"). At times victims or alleged victims of the evaluee also may provide relevant information for different data categories for an evaluation, not neglecting biases that may be in the information.

Some of the sources of evaluation information may be public sources; some emphasis in this chapter is on public sources and the credibility of such information. Obvious public sources of information are criminal records and other court records, including transcripts, information from sexual offender registration, and some deed documents. In pursuing criminal records, the possibilities of pardons and expungement of criminal records in other ways should not be neglected (Wallace-Capretta 2000). (For a listing of some sources of information that can be obtained publicly, see White and Cawood 1998.) Other information not usually considered evaluation information can be publicly gathered, such as that collected by an investigator, courtroom observations, and data provided for testimonial hypotheticals.

For a particular evaluation there may be questions raised as to what information sources were or could have been available and which of these sources were used for the evaluation. The failure to use certain potentially relevant sources of information may lessen the credibility of the evaluation.

The Retrospective Continuum of Evaluations

The retrospective continuum of evaluations takes note of the fact that evaluations, whether fully retrospective or not, may well have considered much past data. Even at the extreme when mental health professionals conduct current evaluations with generally all of the usual requisite data, such as in competency to stand trial, personal injury, civil commitment, disability, and (current) witness competency evaluations, much past data will be considered. Although all of these mentioned evaluations assess current functioning (e.g., diagnosis), it would be rare that considerable past or retrospective data do not need to be considered in the evaluation. For example, does the apparently currently incompetent schizophrenic person have a history that is consistent with schizophrenia, or is she or he malingering? Is current psychiatric distress (e.g., diagnosis, impaired functioning) related to a past injury? (See also Chapter 10, this volume.)

Evaluations for posttraumatic stress disorder (PTSD) provide a special case of the past or retrospective evaluation of mental state for a usually current diagnosis of PTSD. For a traumatic experience to qualify as Criterion A for a PTSD diagnosis, not only a certain severity of a past traumatic event is required, but also the person's response to the event (his or her mental state at the time or soon after the trauma) must have "involved intense fear, helplessness, or horror" (American Psychiatric Association 2000, pp. 467). This past or retrospectively assessed mental state evaluation too often gets short shrift in nonforensic and sometimes forensic mental health professional diagnoses of PTSD. The person's presence at the traumatic event and to a lesser extent his or her mental state at the time of the trauma may come from non-face-to-face data. He or she may never have been in the combat zone as claimed, or others may describe his or her reactions in ways not consistent with "intense fear, helplessness, or horror."

In some evaluations the emphasis is on past behavior to opine on current or future functioning, such as in sexually violent predator evaluations, some sentencing evaluations, and most violence prediction/risk assessments, which may be for sentencing mitigation or aggravation, including in capital cases. For example, what is the past violent and other history of the person evaluated for sentencing? Although the decision has received considerable criticism, the United States Supreme Court approved the use of such non-face-to-face, evaluative information for the purpose of demonstrating aggravating circumstances in the sentencing phase of capital cases (*Barefoot v. Estelle* 1983). And violence risk assessments in employment settings may be done to some extent with past data without a face-to-face examination (cf. Resnick 1998). In each of these examples the degree to which the non-face-to-face data are prior data or are current data collected with a retrospective focus will vary. For example, a current evaluation that is not face to face may assess the degree to which past violence was at least partly a function of behavior related to antisocial personality disorder.

At the other end of the retrospective continuum are retrospectively oriented evaluations, usually done with a present examination, such as for criminal responsibility, competence to have waived Miranda rights, to determine whether a rape trauma syndrome is present, and to determine whether a child witness was "contaminated" in a sexual abuse evaluation. The types of retrospective evaluations that are or might be done without a face-to-face examination include, in addition to the familiar psychological autopsy and testamentary capacity evaluations, cases of the effects of a blood alcohol level on driving and other behavior, the quality of parental supervision (negligent?), the duty to warn and other release-related matters, the quality of a child sexual abuse investigation, and the quality of memories in a "recovered memories" case.

Clinical Versus Forensic Mental Health Professional Evaluations

Another parameter of mental health professional evaluations is whether they are primarily clinical (essentially for treatment purposes) or primarily undertaken for court-related or potentially court-related reasons, including for disability purposes (Strasberg et al. 1997). Clinical and forensic mental health professional evaluations differ from each other in various ways. For instance, as long as clinical evaluations are treatment related and ongoing, these evaluations can tolerate uncertainty as to diagnosis and other matters, such as 1) is the diagnosis a bipolar disorder? 2) do the symptoms respond to an antidepressant or to a mood stabilizer or both? and 3) is it "real" physically caused pain or a somatization disorder? Conversely, forensic evaluators are often called on to render more definitive conclusions (e.g., competent or not) at a time requested by the agency requiring the evaluation, underscoring the need to gather as much information as necessary so that adequate certainty can be achieved, if possible, when needed. But when the clinical evaluator crosses over into rendering similar, more definitive conclusions (such as whether the mental disorder symptoms are related to work or a motor vehicle accident), this clinical-forensic distinction is blurred (Strasburger et al. 1997). Also, it is obvious that evaluations for primarily clinical purposes may be used for court-related purposes, such as in helping to evaluate a decedent's testamentary capacity or suicidal intent, or evaluated directly for clinical standards, as in a malpractice case (Simon and Sadoff 1992).

For the purposes of this chapter and evaluations without a face-to-face examination, a forensic evaluation may have advantages in being at times more "black and white" than a "grayer" clinical evaluation. In certain forensic circumstances the diagnostic and opinion matters to be discussed lend themselves easier to the needed forensic mental health conclusions than to ongoing issues of treatment. For example, it is easier to state that a person has pedophilia and will be a danger to children than to determine what treatment the person may respond to and make ongoing treatment adjustments as needed. It is also easier to opine that a person had a psychotic breakdown and is currently evaluated as having not been criminally responsible rather than to manage the ongoing and more complex issues of continuing long-term treatment of such a person. But good forensic mental health professional work is premised on a good clinical mental health professional foundation; otherwise the complexities of disturbed human behavior would not be understood. And at times the forensic mental health professional needs to assess standard clinical issues such as whether the treatment changed the previously adjudicated sexually violent predator or violent schizophrenic person (i.e., is either now a candidate for release?).

Forensic mental health evaluations are often grouped into a small number of categories of the most frequent types of such evaluations (e.g., personal injury, criminal responsibility, testamentary capacity, and other types of cases) (American Academy of Psychiatry and the Law 1999). However, in practice forensic mental health professional evaluations may cover many types of situations. It is almost easier to consider that a forensic mental health professional may be involved in almost any type of case in which such an expert may "assist the trier of fact," as long as the evaluative material is admissible. Evaluations that are not admitted or whose admissibility is never tested may nonetheless be useful in a case, such as for plea negotiations or for other types of settlement purposes.

Miscellaneous Evaluation Parameters

Two miscellaneous parameters—temporal continuum and voluntariness continuum—should be considered. A *temporal continuum* exists between a current evaluation and an evaluation conducted at some time in the past when an answer to a question relative to functioning at present is needed but no present evaluation is available. This parameter overlaps with the retrospective continuum discussed earlier in this chapter (see "The Retrospective Continuum of Evaluations"), but here an evaluation is available. For example, a clinician needs to determine whether a patient with past sexual pedophilic offenses and a past evaluation has a significant continuing threat today for pedophilic behavior.

A *voluntariness continuum* exists at one extreme when an evaluee wants to be evaluated and noncoercively does so and at the other extreme when the evaluation is (legally) coerced (e.g., for competency to stand trial). Whether an evaluation is legally voluntary or coerced still leaves open the issues of cooperation and credibility discussed earlier. Mental health professionals routinely evaluate people who are coerced into the evaluation yet are essentially fully cooperative and adequately credible. (And sometimes beyond what counsel would wish!)

The Quality of Mental Health Professional Evaluations

The above discussion of the basics of mental health professional evaluations leaves unaddressed the issue or parameter of the quality of the evaluation that has been done; this should not be neglected. For myriad reasons an evaluation may be of poor quality—poor mental health professional training, inadequate skill, communication problems, and so forth. In some settings at times the workload or requirements of the working arrangements (e.g., managed care) do not allow the quality of evaluation that the task requires. And, of course, that may be the case whether it is a forensic or clinical mental health professional evaluation (Nicholson and Norwood 2000). Thus although optimal mental health professional evaluations are often considered here against which, for example, non-face-to-face evaluations are compared and tested, the reality may be quite different. It is, of course, the reality of the evaluation that the evaluee has to in some ways accept, as usually does the court if it accepts (admits) the evaluation at all. And non-face-to-face evaluations also can be of poor quality. Sometimes the quality of the evaluation will be an important aspect of the forensic mental health professional opinion.

Physical Evaluation Considerations in Diagnosis

Aspects of the evaluation relative to the physical and laboratory evaluation require comment. If the mental health professional in question is not a psychiatrist, or has not worked with some other physician or physician extender, then the potential physical and laboratory evaluation aspects of the evaluation may have received inadequate attention. This is not to assume that psychiatrists routinely carefully address this issue, but it is an explicit psychiatric evaluative consideration that should be attended to as noted above in discussing evaluation standards (e.g., American Psychiatric Association 1995a). And for the multiplicity of DSM-IV-TR diagnoses requiring the exclusion of a medical or physical cause, a medical assessment cannot be avoided for a valid diagnosis, such as for a major depressive disorder (MDD) (American Psychiatric Association 2000).

Conclusions From an Evaluation

In most settings the first conclusion from an evaluation will be an opinion about a diagnosis, which, often with other data, will lead to additional opinions about a certain act or level of functioning. (In this chapter the word *opinion* often is reserved for nondiagnostic opinions such as capacity and functioning level.) Therefore, various issues relating to diagnoses must be considered, such as their reliability and validity.

Before examining diagnostic reliability, it is useful to note the degrees of clinical certainty in diagnoses as reflected in diagnostic manuals such as DSM-IV-TR. A *definitive diagnosis* is made with the highest degree of clinical certainty (such as reasonable medical or psychological certainty or probability, which generally means at least more than "clinical speculation"; Rappeport 1985). Such a definitive diagnosis may be for schizophrenia or bipolar disorder. This high level of certainty is followed by diagnoses of a *not otherwise specified (NOS)* particular disorder, such as depressive disorder NOS (311) or personality disorder NOS (301.9). These are followed by less particular, broader diagnostic disorders NOS, such as nonpsychotic disorder NOS (300.9) or psychotic disorder NOS (298.9), in which the general nature of the disorder as being nonpsychotic or psychotic is certain but not more than this. The next level of diagnostic certainty is a *provisional* diagnosis, such as of schizophrenia, when data are inadequate to make a more definitive diagnosis. Also, *deferred* diagnoses (799.9), *rule-out* diagnoses, and an *incomplete evaluation* all imply that further information would complete the evaluation and lead to a more definitive diagnosis.

A diagnosis can be *excluded* after an evaluation is conducted for that particular diagnosis. For example, alcoholism (e.g., alcohol dependence, abuse) can be excluded when no evidence for such a diagnosis is found after careful investigation; this type of evaluation might be conducted with someone for whom such a diagnosis would affect his or her employability (Lacoursiere 1989). An evaluation could exclude a diagnosis of pedophilia when no or insufficient evidence is found, such as when a diagnosis of pedophilia is relevant to sexually violent predator laws (Lacoursiere, in press) or otherwise. In these and related instances of establishing a negative, one should more accurately state that evidence for making the diagnosis was not found, but at times this will be a distinction without a difference. Finally, some diagnoses are excluded on fictitious grounds after an evaluation—for example, finding a factitious disorder (e.g., 300.19) such as Munchausen's syndrome or identifying malingering (V65.2) for a particular diagnosis (an attempt to present as having, for example, schizophrenia or PTSD [Lacoursiere 1993]) or more generally (an attempt to present with a vague mental illness).

Comment on Mental Health Professional Evaluations

Having laid the general foundation for evaluations, an exploration of various aspects and studies of evaluations will progressively lead to a general consideration of non-face-to-face evaluations. This exploration will place non-face-to-face evaluations in the context of the broader mental health professional evaluation field for the mental health professional and non–mental health professional reader.

Diagnostic Reliability

Having discussed the basics of what constitutes a mental health professional evaluation so that a mental health professional can make a diagnosis, we now discuss diagnostic reliability and validity. For decades psychiatrists and other mental health professionals have been justifiably concerned about diagnostic reliability because diagnoses were not reliable (Grove et al. 1981). Several types of reliability exist. Because mental disorders do change, test-retest reliability or reliability over time likely has been least problematic. Intertester (interevaluator) reliability, in which two or more evaluators evaluate the same person ostensibly for the same diagnostic condition, has been more problematic (as to a lesser degree has been intratester reliability, in which the same evaluator evaluates different persons and ostensibly uses the same diagnostic criteria in each case). Interevaluator reliability was especially problematic, with large discrepancies in the number of diagnoses of many conditions when different evaluators performed evaluations on apparently similar patient groups. Such reliabilities greatly improved beginning with DSM-III, when specific and detailed criteria were established for each psychiatric disorder.

Another consideration in diagnostic reliability is that of each person using the same database to reach diagnostic conclusions. This usually is not a reasonable approach to diagnosis except in research settings, but this approach is used to some extent when groups such as forensic psychiatric boards jointly interview an evaluee. This issue of the use of the same or at least a very similar database to reach diagnoses is itself an important question that will be largely sidestepped here. (For a discussion of some reliability studies that provide the evaluators with the same database, see, e.g., Matarazzo 1983 and studies discussed later in this chapter in the sections "Diagnostic Reliability Without a Direct Examination: The Lifetime Diagnosis Study" and "The PRIME-MD Patient Health Questionnaire Study.")

Coefficient of Agreement: κ

The steps entailed in getting to the specific diagnostic criteria in DSM-III, DSM-III-R, DSM-IV, and DSM-IV-TR are not reviewed here (see American Psychiatric Association 2000; Matarazzo 1983). But this history entailed describing specific diagnostic criteria that evaluators could agree on to achieve better intertest reliabilities than had previously been obtained. The statistical expression for one of the most common of these reliabilities is the *coefficient of agreement*, expressed by κ, a statistic that corrects for chance agreement. Generally a κ statistic of 0.70 or better is considered a good level of agreement for mental health professional diagnoses and within the range of what can be achieved, with values in the 0.60s often being acceptable. (At times values less than this are also useful; see, e.g., the discussion of the different diagnostic criteria for the diagnosis of schizophrenia in DSM-IV in Andreasen and Flaum 1994.)

Note is also made of two other statistics: the *weighted* κ statistic allows for partial agreements between evaluators; the *intraclass correlation coefficient* statistic can be used when not every person is evaluated by every evaluator, a statistic that is generally equivalent to κ (Grove et al. 1981; see also Cohen 1968; Fleiss and Cohen 1973; Spitzer et al. 1967). These latter statistics are encountered in some reliability studies, including research cited below—for example, in the section "Opinion Reliability."

The actual meaning in practice of a particular κ statistic will depend on several factors, including the incidence of the condition in the population or group being studied (e.g., the incidence of schizophrenic or malingering evaluees in the population evaluated), the sensitivity of the evaluative process for correctly detecting the condition (schizophrenia or malingering), and the specificity of the process (the correctness of "diagnoses" of noncases of schizophrenia or malingering) (Cohen 1960; Matarazzo 1983; Sackett 1992). This is by no means the full story of the meaning of reliability information, but this will suffice for purposes here.

The Individual Who Makes the Diagnosis

It will be instructive to examine who makes the diagnoses with a "good" coefficient of agreement and how this is done. Such information will be helpful in considerations by the courts or otherwise for the admissibility of mental health professional diagnostic conclusions with and without a face-to-face examination. In achieving this level of agreement, diagnostic categories have had their criteria relatively objectively specified (operationally defined when feasible) so that trained technicians can make acceptably reliable diagnoses that are adequately sensitive (percentage of cases correctly identified), specific (percentage of noncases correctly identified), and valid (satisfactory agreement with diagnoses made by mental health professionals as a common validity standard). Trained technicians can make these acceptable diagnoses for most DSM diagnostic categories (see a review of earlier work in Matarazzo 1983). The validity issue is addressed more later in this chapter (see the section "Diagnostic Validity"), but of note is that non–mental health professionals can make diagnoses with acceptable levels of reliability agreement, that is, consistency in using the diagnostic criteria.

To further explicate the DSM diagnostic process we review material for the DSM-IV diagnostic instrument, the Structured Clinical Interview for DSM-IV Axis I Disorders, Clinician Version (SCID-CV; First et al. 1997). The opening paragraph of the manual for this instrument is illustrative of DSM reliability work of the last several years. This paragraph notes that the SCID diagnosis made by a psychiatric nurse was both more accurate and more comprehensive than the diagnosis made by a clinician who used an unstructured clinical interview, ostensibly to some degree the type of psychiatric evaluation discussed earlier in this chapter. The SCID-CV requires an initial clinical interview and advises the use of all available sources of information about the patient. The test manual suggests various ways the instrument might be used, such as conducting a usual interview and then using a portion of the SCID-CV to confirm a suspected diagnosis. Not counting the initial interview, the review of data from other sources, and the possible administration of the personality disorder version (Structured Interview for DSM-IV Personality [SIDP-IV]; Pfohl et al. 1997), the SCID-CV requires 45–90 minutes for a full administration. For accuracy (reliability) of diagnosis, we will see below how necessary are the general interview and reviewing of other data (sometimes not very necessary).

Although an initial interview and the use of all data sources are advised in reaching a SCID-based diagnosis, a computer-administered patient self-report screening version of the SCID is available. This version "does *not* [emphasis in original] make diagnoses but instead produces a report indicating the diagnoses that are suggested (or unlikely) based on the patient's responses" (First et al. 1997, p. 47).

The SIDP-IV for personality disorder diagnoses discusses training for interviewers. The authors "have obtained good results with interviewers whose minimum training consists of an undergraduate degree in the social sciences plus 6 months previous experience in interviewing psychiatric patients. A person with this level of experience generally takes about 1 month of training to become a competent interviewer" (Pfohl et al. 1997, p. vii).

Reliability, Validity, and Gold Standards

Not only are reliable diagnoses wanted, but we want to reliably diagnose actual disorders, that is, valid psychiatric conditions that different raters state are present. For example, height can be reliably measured, but if height is used for an assessment of intelligence, it will have very limited validity (i.e., it will not be a valid measure). In discussing the validity of the reliable SCID-CV instrument, First et al. (1997, p. 46) stated that, "Unfortunately, a gold standard for psychiatric diagnosis remains elusive." It is suggested later in this chapter (see the section "Diagnostic Validity Standards in General") that this lack of a gold standard for diagnosis is not the case for some diagnoses (and opinions) for which such gold standards do essentially exist.

Example of a κ Statistic of 0.73

To show some of the significance of and a type of error rate for the coefficient of agreement as a measure of reliability, an example is provided of a κ statistic of 0.73. A κ statistic of 0.73 is generally considered a good coefficient of agreement and within the range of what can be achieved by mental health professionals. In evaluations in which up to 25% of 100 evaluees are diagnosed with the condition, a κ statistic of 0.73 could be achieved with one mental health professional (professional A) finding the condition (e.g., antisocial personality disorder or a schizophrenic disorder) in 25 patients and another mental health professional (professional B) finding this same condition in 16 of the patients. (The issue of the validity of the diagnoses in this example is nonetheless open, as it is in such circumstances; i.e., which, if any, of the 25 or 16 patients actually have the disorder under discussion.)

Although this degree of agreement in diagnosis would be considered a good level of agreement and what mental health professionals can achieve, what does this mean for testifying purposes? If the issue requires a beyond-reasonable-doubt standard of proof, such as for sentencing augmentation, and professional A finds 56% more cases of the diagnosis ($25-16=9$; $9/16 \times 100 = 56\%$) than does professional B, is professional A's opinion of the presence of antisocial personality disorder and high risk for violence admissible in capital sentencing augmentation if professional A testifies for the state and professional B testifies for the defendant? Is the evaluation of professional A reliable enough and valid under these circumstances? Is the error rate of the difference in making the diagnosis too high?

There are other error rates, such as the errors in the 25 and 16 diagnoses that were made and if these mental health professionals would make the same number of such diagnoses in another similar group of evaluees. This alludes to the error of measurement for the individual evaluator (e.g., professional A, who under similar conditions of 100 evaluees sometimes diagnoses as few as 20 or as many as 30 people with the condition, but on average diagnoses 25). When *Daubert* states that the error rate for the methodology needs to be considered, it is likely that any of these error rates, and others, can and sometimes should be considered (see below, especially the sections "Other Error Sources in Evaluations" and "The Effect of Daubert/Kumho on Expert Testimony Admissibility," but also passim).

Using the same reliability example, will the diagnoses be admissible in a criminal responsibility case in which professional A finds schizophrenia and nonresponsibility for the defendant compared with no such finding by professional B for the state? Will the court view these matters of reliability, error rate, and validity differently when the benefit will go for instead of against the defendant? Should a gatekeeper decide, especially when we cannot know which evaluator is correct (valid), that, given the presence of professional A and professional B and the reported reliabilities, the mental health professionals' testimony must be excluded? And if this is nonetheless the best that can be done, how will the questions of criminal responsibility and violence prediction then be evaluated by the court? (We address these matters below, in the section "Legal Admissibility Issues for Non-Face-to-Face Evaluations," but for now we suggest that admission may well be the court's decision, with the trier of fact determining credibility.)

Although we may generally know achievable reliabilities and related error rates from peer-reviewed research studies, in the usual clinical and forensic practice this will be a different matter. It may be difficult or impossible for particular mental health professionals, or the courts, to have the information necessary to calculate reliabilities for the mental health professionals for the evaluations or settings under consideration, such as an evaluator's diagnostic rate in this setting and whether the diagnoses are valid or accurate.

Diagnostic Reliability Without a Direct Examination: The Lifetime Diagnosis Study

We summarize a study that is directly relevant to the question of reliable diagnoses without a face-to-face examination. Leckman and colleagues

(1982) studied 1,878 individuals with diagnoses that could have been made at any time over their lifetimes (lifetime diagnoses). Two clinicians (an M.D. and an M.A. mental health professional) made the diagnoses based on data from relatives, as well as from medical records when they were available, which was about two-thirds of the time. About 40% of the time they also had a face-to-face diagnostic interview with the individual based on the Schedule for Affective Disorders and Schizophrenia, Lifetime Version (SADS-L), which was then used to make Research Diagnostic Criteria (RDC) diagnoses; these latter instruments are precursors of the current SCID-CV and DSM-III, DSM-III-R, DSM-IV, and DSM-IV-TR diagnostic criteria (see Matarazzo 1983). This study allowed for the determination of reliability coefficients (κ) for several diagnoses based on data that included the direct face-to-face interviews versus data that did not have such an interview of the person. To make the diagnoses in these latter cases, the clinicians used only information from relatives and from medical records the two-thirds of the time that these were available.

Of note for this chapter from the study is that clinically satisfactory mental health professional level reliabilities similar to those currently achieved with recent DSM-based diagnoses could be achieved for several diagnoses without the additional benefit of a face-to-face examination. The diagnoses most relevant for this chapter and their κ reliabilities with and without a face-to-face interview are, respectively, as follows: major depression, 0.86 and 0.66; alcoholism, 0.81 and 0.88; drug abuse, 0.89 and 0.60; antisocial personality, 0.76 and 0.66; and never mentally ill, 0.73 and 0.82. For several diagnoses, this diagnostic methodology—in which information from relatives and available medical records only was used without a face-to face examination—did not work as well, several diagnoses occurred too rarely for a determination of the methodology's reliability, and some diagnoses were not evaluated.

The PRIME-MD Patient Health Questionnaire Study

Some information was presented on the level of mental health professional involvement needed to make DSM-IV diagnoses in the earlier discussion on the use of the SCID-CV or SIDP-IV (First et al. 1997; Pfohl et al. 1997). Information also is available that for some diagnostic categories using self-administered assessment forms, a technician may not be necessary, or, as will be seen, even the clinician may hardly be necessary in arriving at diagnoses (Spitzer et al. 1999). This Primary Care Evaluation of Mental Disorders (PRIME-MD) Patient Health Questionnaire (PHQ) (Spitzer et al. 1999) instrument is for diagnosing selected DSM-IV disorders in primary care physician settings based on how the patients fill in the diagnostic instrument. These selected disorders include MDD with a κ of 0.54 up to a κ of 0.80 for panic disorder, with these values achieved partly at the cost of some minor adjustments in diagnostic criteria. This diagnostic instrument was validated by having a Ph.D. clinical psychologist or a senior psychiatric social worker conduct a telephone interview of the patient. (Note the nature of the validating evaluations and the degree to which these validating interviews might or might not be considered face-to-face examinations.)

As is true of other DSM-based diagnostic instruments, not much attention is paid here to an overall story or history or to the range of data suggested earlier in this chapter and by the American Psychiatric Association's (1995a) "Practice Guidelines for Psychiatric Evaluation of Adults." Rather, the emphasis is essentially restricted to the description of various symptoms and their duration. With the PRIME-MD PHQ a further question of dysfunction is optional, although this or some other equivalent effect of the symptoms is required or implied for the existence of a psychiatric disorder according to DSM-IV-TR criteria. But the final word has not been said on whether such a dysfunctional or "clinical significance" criterion is needed for all psychiatric diagnoses (Kendler 1999; Spitzer and Wakefield 1999). Overall, 15% of the sample of 3,000 medical patients were found by means of this instrument to have psychiatric diagnoses (Spitzer et al. 1999).

The clinician's involvement in confirming these PHQ diagnoses based on information self-reported by the patients was less than 1 minute for 42% and 1–2 minutes for 43% of the patients. The physicians did not make much use of these diagnoses. Of the 74 patients in the study with a newly found diagnosis of MDD, only 22% were given follow-up appointments, only 10% were prescribed antidepressant medication, and only 5% were given a referral to a mental health professional (Spitzer et al. 1999).[1] Nonetheless, this study illustrates that for some disorders reliable diagnoses can be achieved with non-face-to-face, essentially self-report data. (Again, see the section "Specific Criteria and Information Sources for a Diagnosis" later in this chapter.)

Recall that the United States Supreme Court's opinion in *Daubert v. Merrell Dow Pharmaceuticals, Inc.* (1993) expressly condoned the use of peer

---

[1]This study and some of its results were played out at a continuing medical education presentation on the PHQ attended by the first author (R.B.L.) (Smith 1999). The presenter enthusiastically presented the ease of making the diagnoses, how little time it took to do so, and how easy it was to treat the identified disorders. The largely internist and primary care physician audience decried not having even this amount of time to do such diagnosing and treating.

review and publication in determining the evidentiary reliability of proffered expert testimony. However, judged from the perspective of a validity consideration of clinical relevance (a type of criterion validity), this PRIME-MD PHQ study suffers, and therefore such data might not warrant a gatekeeper's admission under a *Daubert/Kumho* analysis (see the section "The Effect of *Daubert/Kumho* on Expert Testimony Admissibility" later in this chapter). It will be obvious that a patient's chart with such a PHQ diagnosis could come under court scrutiny, such as in a malpractice case in which it was alleged that a patient was not properly treated for depression.

Additional Comments Regarding Reliability

This emphasis on reliabilities and their attainment helps to underscore several points. DSM-III and later diagnostic manual disorders are considerably objectified so that little mental health professional evaluation may be required for a reliable diagnosis, also helping to open the door to nonexaminational data sources for diagnoses. Also open are many ancillary questions, such as when are non–mental health professional diagnoses real *diagnoses* and when are they "diagnoses," as apparently was the case to some extent in the PRIME-MD PHQ study (Spitzer et al. 1999), in which the "diagnoses" were largely ignored. And considering evaluations done by methods with little professional involvement, whether by mental health professionals or otherwise, how are validity factors such as malingering considered? What is the level of dysfunction, disability, or related impairment that is considered as required to diagnose a disorder with DSM-IV-TR criteria, especially when it is not explicit in the diagnostic criteria for the disorder that such dysfunction, disability, or related impairment is present? (See, e.g., Kendler 1999; Spitzer and Wakefield 1999.)

If such non–professionally obtained diagnoses are used, how does one evaluate the relation of the diagnosed disorder to any etiological factor(s), such as a work injury or general tortious action? Such questions lead to the obvious comment that more is usually required than reliable diagnoses, with which few readers will take serious issue. Nonetheless, a diagnosis often is an important starting point in much of our work, including for opinions that at least partly grow from diagnoses.

Diagnostic Validity

Mental health professionals have achieved what are considered acceptable diagnostic reliabilities. These reliabilities have been achieved at times with the progressively less necessary involvement of mental health professionals themselves, or at least of the most thoroughly trained mental health professionals, psychiatrists, psychologists, psychiatric social workers, psychiatric nurses, and such. To explore further the nature of diagnoses, diagnostic validity must be considered.

Diagnostic Validity Standards in General

What is a validity standard and a validity gold standard for a diagnosis from a methodology that produces a diagnosis and purports to accurately diagnose a real or "valid" condition? If a diagnostician uses a methodology and says that this is a case of *X*, is it really a case of *X*? If a neurosurgeon diagnoses a brain mass as cancerous and provides a biopsy from the brain mass to a neuropathologist who reports it as neoplastic brain tissue, we have a validity standard and essentially a so-called gold standard for the diagnosis of brain cancer. Conversely, if the neuropathologist reports that the biopsy is nonneoplastic, we have a gold standard for the diagnosis of noncancer. (However, questions remain as to whether the sample was from the cancerous area of the brain and from the correct patient, whether the pathologist is competent, and so on.) This example, of course, still leaves open the myriad questions about how the patient is currently functioning and so forth, which the gold standard valid diagnosis alone does not answer.

Psychiatry and the mental health field overall have a paucity of gold standards for diagnostic validity purposes, but some essentially gold standards do exist. And some of these gold standards come not from face-to-face data or from what often would be standard clinical data, but may come from public and non-face-to-face examinational data. Partly this is a function of how various diagnostic conditions are defined and understood. For example, if a person has multiple criminal convictions for sexual offenses against children, the chance for an accurate (and valid) diagnosis of pedophilia (meeting DSM-IV-TR diagnostic criteria) is very high, as it is for a diagnosis of antisocial personality disorder (with DSM-IV-TR criteria) with repeat juvenile (if records are available) and adult criminal convictions, and for alcoholism (of some form) with multiple convictions for driving under the influence. And each of these diagnoses—pedophilia, antisocial personality disorder, and alcoholism—will be consistent with generally agreed on conceptions of the disorders (i.e., valid). Repeated sexual behavior with children that leads to problems (convictions) is consistent with our conception of pedophilia, repeated behavior that leads to criminal convictions is consistent with our conception of antisocial personality disorder, and repeated alcohol use that leads to problems is consistent with our conception of alcoholism. Conversely, a diagnosis of PTSD may be excluded if it can be shown that the person was not exposed to the suspected or claimed trauma, for example, that the person was never in Vietnam (and the diagnosis may be malingering). As long as there is general consensus in the mental health professional field that such disorders exist, then the diagnoses noted above may achieve essentially the same degree of validity as that with the brain cancer example in the previous paragraph. The carefully conducted brain biopsy with an adequate and appropriate tissue sample and specimen analysis usually will be valid, the carefully conducted pedophilia evaluation with an adequate data source and analysis usually will be valid, and so on. (See also the section "Specific Criteria and Information Sources for a Diagnosis" later in this chapter and passim for more on these gold standard issues.)

No such gold standard for making or excluding a diagnosis exists for many psychiatric diagnoses, and what can be examined for validity data may include factors such as the course of the disorder's or condition's history, including the treatment response (see, e.g., Kendell 1989; Robins 1985). For example, if patients have an expected clinical course for a type of depression and respond to antidepressant medication, the likelihood is increased that their condition is or was a valid depressive disorder.

A less vigorous way to examine validity is by looking at diagnostic agreement between a non–mental health professional and a mental health professional for a diagnosis, assuming that the latter is accurate (i.e., valid, as in the PRIME study above) (Spitzer et al. 1999). The more that diagnoses are at least reliable, the more we can say that at least the evaluators are diagnosing the same thing. However, the "thing" that they are diagnosing remains uncertain. To take an example from recent years, the dexamethasone suppression test may have generally high reliability, but exactly what it diagnoses is less clear. It is not the regularly valid diagnosis of depression as was initially thought because, among other reasons, the test is confounded by alcohol intake (Morihisa et al. 1999). Also, use of even reliable mental health professional conclusions about a diagnosis to state that that it is the valid diagnosis has the risk of being tautological in that it becomes "the diagnosis is what it is because the mental health professional says it is."

DSM-IV-TR Diagnostic Validity Standards

The DSM-IV task forces and work groups for the developing manual considered various kinds of data relative to validity (Widiger et al. 1994, 1996, 1997, 1998b). Because certain diagnostic conditions are considered in some detail below (see the section "Specific Diagnostic Criteria and Information Source Possibilities for Selected Diagnoses"), these same conditions and PTSD are discussed briefly here relative to their DSM-IV-TR diagnostic validities. DSM-IV-TR alcohol dependence and abuse diagnoses correlate with certain courses over time after diagnosis and with certain differential problem severities for dependence versus abuse (e.g., job loss or drunken driving convictions) corresponding to generally accepted conceptions of these conditions (Helzer 1994). The conception of pedophilia (American Psychiatric Association 2000; see also the section "Pedophilia" later in this chapter) as recurrent sexual behavior relative to children that is problematic is largely a matter of definition, and the condition's validity is confirmed in studies of the past and then future behavior of the individuals with this diagnosis.

PTSD's validity as a disorder has been largely validated by the finding of the existence of a certain symptom pattern after various traumatic events, as has been shown in many studies (Davidson and Foa 1993; Scrignar 1996). Although there are issues about the nature of the symptom pattern, enough consensus indicates that it is a valid disorder. A diagnosis conceptualized as occurring after a severe trauma can be excluded by the gold standard datum of lack of exposure to the claimed trauma, as may be documented with nonexaminational data. This lack of exposure to the required trauma is a PTSD erroneous diagnosis problem that affects some 5% of the Vietnam veteran–related diagnoses (Lacoursiere 1993; Resnick 1997).

The DSM Work Group on Antisocial Personality Disorder reflected two different conceptions of the disorder having emphases on characteristics of callousness and lack of remorse (as exemplified in the clinical work of Cleckley [1941, 1988]) or on specific, more behavioral criteria, including antisocial and criminal behavior (Widiger et al. 1998a). The latter emphasis prevailed in the diagnostic manual (Widiger et al. 1998a). This disorder is validated by the existence of the defined symptomatic construct of a history of antisocial behavior and by the continued similar behavior of individuals so diagnosed. This conception of the disorder means, as is seen in the section "Antisocial Personality Disorder" later in this chapter, that public records such as criminal conviction records essentially can be used to diagnose antisocial personality disorder. (The alternative conception of antisocial personality is embodied within the Psychopathy Checklist—Revised (PCL-R) instrument discussed in the "Psychopathy Checklist—Revised" section later in this chapter [Hare 1991].)

Specific Criteria and Information Sources for a Diagnosis

In this section, we investigate a method to determine what information might be used to reach selected diagnoses. This includes reviewing what publicly available information might be so used and overall the degree to which these selected diagnoses might be made without a face-to-face examination. Within the limits of the chapter, only selected diagnoses of frequent interest to forensic mental health professionals are examined: two Axis I disorders, alcohol (or drug) dependence (and by implication abuse) and pedophilia, and one Axis II disorder, antisocial personality disorder (see Tables 9–1, 9–2, and 9–3). To the extent that public and nonexaminational information is emphasized, these retrospectively focused evaluations allow an evaluator to state, when appropriate, whether a diagnostic condition existed at a prior time. (Whether the condition still exists will be an independent matter, depending on the disorder, what has intervened, and so on.)

It is somewhat of a coincidence, but not one to be ignored, that the conditions examined here are ones in which evaluees regularly downplay or outright deny the symptoms and problems from these disorders. This, of course, renders the use of non-face-to-face data all the more helpful in these conditions. Later in this chapter other disorders in which non-face-to-face diagnoses can be made without such downplaying and denial (e.g., depression) are discussed.

Specific Diagnostic Criteria and Information Source Possibilities for Selected Diagnoses

Tables 9–1, 9–2, and 9–3 show along the top row the various information sources that can be used to reach a diagnosis, with public sources and medical and nonmedical records being nonexaminational sources, and for simplified illustrative purposes here, face-to-face examinational sources being considered for the standard clinical data categories (reason for the evaluation, background history, MSE, psychological testing, and physical and laboratory evaluation), although, of course, public sources, medical records, and so forth can provide material for these standard clinical data categories, as discussed earlier in this chapter. The left column in the tables lists the required DSM-IV-TR diagnostic criteria for the condition under consideration.

Alcohol (Drug) Dependence or Abuse

A diagnosis of alcohol dependence requires within a 12-month period the presence of at least three of the seven diagnostic criteria listed in the left column of Table 9–1. As can be seen, data for the diagnosis could be found for an individual exclusively in public records or from these and other nonexaminational data. Without attempting to fill in many of the cells of the table, other generally noncurrent, nonexaminational data sources for a di-

Table 9–1. Diagnostic criteria and information sources for diagnosing alcohol (drug) dependence[a]

Criteria for diagnosis	Information source							
	Public information	Medical record	Nonmedical record	Background	Reason for evaluation	Mental status	Psychological testing	Physical and laboratory evaluation
1. Tolerance	DUI BAC level	?						
2. Withdrawal		?						
3. More intake than intended								
4. Unsuccessful desire to decrease amount taken								
5. Much time spent in the use activity	Public observations							
6. Important social, occupational, or recreational acts decreased	DUI, possession charge		Work (and marital) record					
7. Continued use despite problems from use	>1 DUI?	?	Work record					?

Note. DUI=driving under the influence and related terms; BAC=blood alcohol concentration.
Without making a diagnosis such as alcoholism, medical records may show illnesses, symptoms, or laboratory results that are highly alcohol related; this also may occur with drug dependence or abuse. (See, e.g., Lacoursiere 1989; Skinner et al. 1986).
[a]Three of seven criteria required within 12 months.

Table 9–2. Diagnostic criteria and information sources for diagnosing pedophilia[a]

Criteria for diagnosis	Public information	Medical record	Nonmedical record	Background evaluation	Reason for evaluation	Mental status	Psychological testing	Physical and laboratory evaluation
				Information source				
A. Recurrent, intense sexually arousing fantasies, urges, or behavior regarding sex with child	Appropriate crime conviction(s)							Phallometric or similar data
B. These cause clinically significant problems in social, occupational, or other functioning	Appropriate crime conviction(s)		Jobs lost, marital record?					
C. The person is at least age 16 years and 5 years older than child in criterion A	Appropriate crime conviction(s)							

Note. Phallometric and similar interest or arousal data are listed to note that such data can provide significant diagnostic information that may be contrary to an examinee's history.

[a]A 6-month history is required.

Table 9–3. Diagnostic criteria and information sources for diagnosing antisocial personality disorder[a]

Criteria for diagnosis	Information source							
	Public information	Medical record	Nonmedical record	Background	Reason for evaluation	Mental status	Psychological testing	Physical and laboratory evaluation
1. Repeated grounds for arrest	Repeated arrest							
2. Repeated lies, aliases, or conning for personal gain	NSFs for checks; aliases							
3. Impulsive and does not plan ahead								
4. Aggressiveness seen in repeat fights/assaults	Repeated arrest	Injured in fights						
5. Reckless disregard for self and others' safety	DUIs; speeding tickets	Injured in MVAs						
6. Consistent irresponsibility in work or money obligations	Unpaid bills; bankruptcy		?					
7. Lack of remorse in indifference to hurting, mistreating, or stealing from others								

Note. DUI=driving under the influence and related terms; NSFs=nonsufficient funds; MVAs=motor vehicle accidents.
The table highlights primarily only public and nonexaminational sources of data. The Psychopathy Checklist—Revised, which may be scorable essentially from records, adds further nonexaminational information toward a diagnosis of antisocial personality in emphasizing some of the diagnostic criteria; see text.
[a]Three of seven criteria required.

agnosis of alcohol dependence also have been suggested, such as laboratory and alcohol-related illness information in past medical records, regardless of whether these records ever contained a diagnosis of alcoholism or of a related condition (see, e.g., Allen et al. 2000; Lacoursiere 1989; Levine 1990; Reynaud et al. 2001; Salaspuro 1999; Skinner et al. 1986; cf. Sobell et al. 1999). When a diagnosis of alcohol dependence cannot be made in these public record and other nonexaminational ways, it may sometimes still be feasible to make the generally more restrictive diagnosis of alcohol abuse. Various diagnoses of drug dependence or abuse also might be made in these ways, although this will not be feasible as often because of the broader range and generally less specificity of possible medical complications from drugs of abuse, the greater difficulty of detection of some of these drugs in a driving under the influence context, and so on.

It is appropriate to ask if this non-face-to-face examinational diagnosing methodology is of little practical use because the criteria data noted, for example, in public records, are apt to be found too seldom. Information on this question can be garnered from a *DSM-IV Sourcebook* study of the data found primarily in alcohol dependence but also in some alcohol abuse diagnoses in 460 male veterans (average age=45 years) (Schuckit 1998). In reporting if they ever had problems related to alcohol, 38%–59% of these men reported automobile accidents, 60%–79% reported more than one driving under the influence conviction, 24%–49% reported public intoxication offenses, and 41%–66% reported being in jail. From driving while intoxicated data, of the estimated 513,200 offenders on probation or in jail in 1997, they had, respectively, 0.19 and 0.24 g/dL blood alcohol concentration levels at arrest (a blood alcohol concentration level of 0.08 usually is presumptive driving impairment, and levels to 0.24 indicate some alcohol tolerance); 8.3% and 34.3% had three or more prior convictions for driving while intoxicated, 59.7% and 55.2% had histories of being in alcohol or drug treatment, and 23.8% and 37.7% had to have a drink in the morning, an indication of alcohol dependence, overall adequate data to make records-based diagnoses of alcohol dependence or abuse in many of these individuals (U.S. Department of Justice 1999). From a community sample of 628 at-risk drinkers, the diagnosis of alcohol abuse was most often made with the single criterion of recurrent, hazardous alcohol use, which usually was manifested as driving after drinking too much, something done on average 4.5 times per year by these drinkers (Hasin and Paykin 1999). Of the alcohol-intoxicated patients admitted to emergency services, 80% showed laboratory values for γ-glutamyltransferase (GGT) or carbohydrate-deficient transferrin (CDT) indicative of more than casual alcohol consumption (Reynaud et al. 2001; see also references regarding these tests for alcohol consumption excess, e.g., Salaspuro 1999).

Pedophilia

A diagnosis of pedophilia needs information to meet all three of the diagnostic criteria given in Table 9–2. All the necessary information for such a diagnosis could come from criminal records. If a person is arrested for certain sex crimes, such as indecent liberties with a child in a nonincest context, the chances are high that other, often many, similar incidents have occurred that were not detected (Abel and Osborn 1992). Therefore, reasonable *clinical* conclusions often can be drawn regarding the recurrence and intensity of certain urges and behaviors, even if the person may have only one to two convictions for relevant sexual offenses; obviously the more of these convictions, the more certain is the diagnosis. Phallometric or other sexual arousal or interest laboratory data are included in the table to help underscore that even with an evaluee's blatant denial about sexual interest, other information may lead a mental health professional to suspect otherwise.

In terms of the practicality of the ability to make a diagnosis of pedophilia, with the current sexually violent predator laws, several states are evaluating many hundreds of felons who have committed crimes against children to determine whether these offenders might meet criteria for diagnoses such as pedophilia (Lacoursiere, in press; Winick and LaFond 1998). These evaluees obviously have criminal records that can be reviewed.

Antisocial Personality Disorder

The diagnosis of antisocial personality disorder in Table 9–3 requires that three of the seven listed criteria be met from behavior since age 15 years for a person now at least 18 years old. Again public records might provide all the data needed for a suspected diagnosis in an adult. The current DSM-IV-TR diagnostic criteria also require that evidence of conduct disorder be present with onset before age 15. Although this is not shown in a table, evidence of illegal behavior in certain categories again can largely be used. Because of protected records at times, such information may not be accessible, but at other times the court will make the juvenile records available. Even when the juvenile records are unavailable or no evidence for a childhood conduct disorder is found so that an adult antisocial personality disorder diagnosis cannot be made, adequate data may be available to diagnose a personality disorder NOS, with antisocial traits. The latter diagnosis may be helped with the scoring from records of the PCL-R (Hare 1991; see "Psychopathy Checklist—Revised" section later in this chapter), another possible nonexaminational procedure.

The number of people potentially meeting the criteria for a diagnosis of antisocial personality disorder based largely on criminal records is large when one considers the size of the prison population and that a very sizable percentage of imprisoned felons meet the criteria for such a diagnosis (Kaplan and Sadock 1998). More relevant for purposes here, a study of some 400 nonincarcerated sexual offenders found that more than 50% met the criteria for antisocial personality disorder, and these diagnoses were made by reviewing the persons' files for the criteria for the disorder (Hanson and Harris 1998).

Discussion of Diagnostic Criteria and Non-Face-to-Face Information Sources for Selected Diagnoses

The previous section indicates that certain psychiatric disorders, such as alcohol dependence, pedophilia, and antisocial personality disorder, may be diagnosed without a face-to-face examination and with information with which one can achieve high diagnostic reliability and validity. Certain diagnoses can similarly be excluded without a face-to-face examination, or a diagnosis of malingering might be made in the context.

Without going into the same details, other diagnoses might be made (or strongly suspected) largely from public information, such as dementia (see below in this section). At the risk of being "politically incorrect," the repeated observation of a coughing smoker outside a business in the cold of winter probably would be adequate data for a diagnosis of nicotine dependence. (This frivolous example brought to mind a workers' compensation evaluation in which, although of limited probative value regarding credibility, the evaluee had obtained reduced health insurance rates by claiming to be a nonsmoker, which was not the case.)

For many other disorders, such as schizophrenia, the attempt to make a diagnosis from public information and from other non-face-to-face data is more difficult and complex, and the diagnosis is not as easily made and its validity is not as easily verified. This does not mean that schizophrenia cannot be diagnosed with a high likelihood of reliability and validity without a face-to-face examination. This might be the case, for example, when credible, extensive, and repeated public observations are made by workers in programs for homeless people or by others or when an extensive prior evaluative and treatment record exists. However, such records also must not be accepted too glibly. Most forensic mental health professionals with experience reviewing extensive sets of records for evaluations have been involved in cases in which repeatedly recorded histories, and examinations, of "hallucinations," "suicidal ideation," "sexual abuse," "posttraumatic" symptoms, and so forth do not stand up to careful scrutiny.

The data required for each of the various DSM-IV-TR diagnoses need to be evaluated diagnosis by diagnosis for disorders that are of note in a particular context when certain data may or may not be available. This brings to mind the particularized, case-by-case gatekeeping admissibility function of the courts noted in *Daubert*. Furthermore, it can be reiterated that mental health evaluations that do not study certain data, such as extant criminal records, may run a risk of missing important information and of serious evaluative error.

The ability to reach a reliable and at times explicitly valid diagnosis without a face-to-face examination can have broad forensic implications. When such non-face-to-face data are available and relevant to a particular situation, an evaluation with a face-to-face examination cannot be done, and doing the evaluation is nonetheless appropriate within its limits, mental health professionals may provide diagnostic data and other opinions of use for the court and otherwise. For example, the defendant in a capital crime may refuse to be examined for mitigation purposes, or the capital defendant may refuse an examination for competency to be executed.

In applying the use of public data sources to a usual retrospective forensic evaluation such as a psychological autopsy without an examination, only rarely will public data help in the evaluation. The public circumstances of a suicide may be relevant. There may be public data such as an arrest, which may or may not have diagnostic significance (e.g., for alcoholism or general criminal behavior), or may stand on its own as a stressor that contributed to the suicide. But other public data also may be noteworthy, such as a recent real estate purchase.

If a person can essentially self-diagnose an MDD, can a family member also do so for him or her, especially a spouse or other partner, and do so with adequate accuracy? The Lifetime Diagnosis study described earlier noted that this can be done (Leckman et al. 1982). It is understood how a spouse or other partner may well be able to "diagnose" MDD when one examines the criteria for MDD in DSM-IV-TR or in the PRIME-MD PHQ (Spitzer et al. 1999). MDD includes criteria such as "depressed mood" that could be "indicated by... observation made by others (e.g., appears tearful)," "markedly diminished interest or pleasure" that can be "indicated by... observation made by others," "psychomotor... retardation nearly every day (observable by others)," sleeping problems, and other possibly publicly observable behaviors (American Psychiatric Association 2000, p. 356). If a significant other can "diagnose" or provide reliable diagnostic information for MDD and maybe other depressions, then this person can be interviewed for gathering information in psychological autopsies, and the obtained data can be examined relative to the reliability estimates found in the nonexaminational studies above (Leckman et al. 1982; Spitzer et al. 1999). If a significant other can provide reliable diagnostic information, then undoubtedly close co-workers also can do so to some extent. Nevertheless, the information provided and reliabilities may change in a forensic context when personal interest may be considerable.

Regarding testamentary capacity evaluations, although no particular direct relation exists between any diagnosis and testamentary capacity, the greater the dementia, the less likelihood for testamentary capacity. And the DSM-IV-TR criteria for dementia are considerably observable and reportable by family members (e.g., "impaired ability to learn new information or to recall previously learned information" and at least one of the following: "language disturbance," "impaired ability to carry out motor activities despite intact motor function," "agnosia," or "disturbance in executive functioning" [American Psychiatric Association 2000, p. 168]). Similarly, severity criteria for dementia are considerably observable. Furthermore, for testamentary capacity evaluees who had been admitted to nursing facilities, the federally mandated Minimum Data Set (Rantz et al. 1999) contains considerable information on dementia and related matters, and this information has been used to develop functional dementia severity ratings correlating with instruments such as Folstein's Mini-Mental State Exam (Folstein et al. 1975; see, e.g., Hartmaier et al. 1994, 1995; Morris et al. 1994).

Interim Summary: Diagnoses

We have reviewed the collection of data usable to make diagnoses, with some emphasis on retrospectively oriented evaluations, non-face-to-face data sources, and particular diagnoses of special forensic mental health professional interest. The reliabilities of diagnoses—their consistency between evaluators, for example—that can be achieved in practice still may vary considerably between evaluators. These achievable levels of reliability may be obtained by nonclinicians (Spitzer 1983) or largely by patients themselves under certain conditions. Such diagnoses arrived at with instruments such as the SCID-CV (First et al. 1997) and PRIME-MD PHQ (Spitzer et al. 1999) emphasize current and recent symptoms, often with little or no attention to traditional, broader evaluation methods of diagnosis. Also, non-face-to-face methods can achieve levels of reliability similar to those of face-to-face methods for several diagnoses.

We discussed validity standards for diagnoses, again emphasizing certain diagnoses that could be of special interest in forensic mental health professional contexts. Mental disorder diagnoses rarely have gold standards for validity, but when they do these validity standards may come from nonexaminational methods, including sources such as public records.

From Diagnoses to Other Opinions

So far this chapter has focused on diagnoses, very often the initial conclusion and first threshold issue from forensic mental health professional evaluations and for subsequent postdiagnostic opinions: competence to stand trial, criminal responsibility, damage in personal injury cases, disability, and so on. When any retrospectively focused diagnoses are based on non-examinational data that are used to reach other opinions, these other opinions will necessarily be based partially or even fully on non-face-to-face examinational data. Such postdiagnostic opinions may include the presence of criminal intent or "sanity" if a suicide was the result of a mental disorder or if mental damage (a diagnosis) was the result of an allegedly tortious act.

Mental health professionals may give certain retrospectively oriented opinions that are less dependent on a specific DSM diagnosis for their rendering. Such opinions may be given, for example, if alcohol consumption of a certain amount (a sort of "diagnosis" that may be short of a diagnosis of alcohol intoxication) would have impaired driving in a particular person or if some level of parental supervision was inadequate under the circumstances (negligent supervision). And such non–diagnostically dependent opinions also might result from non-face-to-face evaluation methods; for example, from reviewing records of the motor vehicle accident and blood alcohol concentration levels.

General or sexual violence and whether it may or may not occur or re-occur is a frequent mental health professional opinion. Violence in the past is one of the best predictors of violence in the future (e.g., for aggravation in sentencing or in parole release considerations). And violence in the past, whether sexual or not, often may most credibly come from nonexaminational materials such as criminal conviction records and police reports. (The literature on violence prediction and risk assessment is extensive; see, e.g., Borum 1996; Ferris et al. 1997; Monahan 1996; Sreenivasan et al. 2000.)

Standards for Opinions

Although it is difficult enough to have adequate standards such as reliability and validity for diagnoses, at least diagnoses are limited in number, even including their severity ratings and other modifiers, and have generally agreed-on criteria. Nondiagnostic opinions are often much more complicated, as accordingly will be issues, for example, of reliability, validity, and error rates. Although the criteria for certain opinions are somewhat delineated, these criteria are rarely as defined and operationalized as recent DSM diagnostic criteria, making the determination of opinion standards more difficult. In this context, examples of criteria for opinions that are difficult to carefully delineate in practice are those for criminal responsibility and whether a mental disorder is disabling. For other types of opinions that are frequently given by forensic mental health professionals, there is more information available to examine the reliability, validity, and other characteristics of these opinions, such as is the case for competency to stand trial or fit to proceed opinions. (This discussion continues with consideration of opinion validity and then proceeds to what reliability can be achieved with opinions that are valid for their purposes.)

Opinion Validity

Opinions are given for a wide variety of matters and contexts. Sometimes opinions are given to help resolve a conflict when no clear external standard for validity exists. Instead a settlement is reached between the parties, as in many testamentary capacity cases and some insurance disability cases. At other times some degree of an external standard can be agreed on, although it is not a gold standard in the sense of medical diagnostic gold standards and some psychiatric gold standards. In retrospective criminal responsibility evaluations there may be only a state's evaluation or this and a private evaluation of the defendant. The concurrence of a single evaluation with the court's decision or of each side's mental health professional evaluation with the other and then with the court's decision provides some degree of validation of such evaluation opinions (not ignoring that the evaluators and the court all could be in error). Janofsky and colleagues (1989, 1996) presented some concurrence data for criminal responsibility opinion decisions. For these decisions a coefficient of agreement between the opinions of the state's mental health professional evaluators and the court's decisions can be calculated from their data (Janofsky et al. 1989). Of the 51 defendants with full evaluations by the state's evaluators, 37 were opined to be criminally responsible with 36 of these defendants so found by the court, and 14 were opined to be not responsible with 13 so found by the court. These data yield a κ statistic of 0.90, higher than for most diagnostic reliabilities that can be achieved in the mental health field.

Validity in the usually non–retrospectively oriented competency to stand trial evaluations can be assessed in a manner similar to that for criminal responsibility. Again when there is one mental health professional evaluation, this evaluation and the court may agree; if there are evaluations on both sides, both sides' mental health professionals may agree, and the court may concur.

At times, opinions regarding sexual recidivism or general violence potential have an external standard, such as when an evaluation for such recidivism is low for a particular person, and follow-up confirms this. But this validation for this individual's evaluation opinion usually would be available only after significant time and often not when a known, valid opinion on this individual was wanted, such as at sentencing. If the methodology yielded generally valid results in such cases, and the current case is similar, then the similarly derived opinion in the instant case may, by extension, be considered to have some validity. However, if an opinion is for high violence recidivism and an intervention ensues, such as incarceration or placement in a sexually violent predator treatment program or the execution of a death sentence, then the intervention interferes with the chance of the event to recur (sexual recidivism, for instance). This intervention also interferes with the ability to determine whether the opinion on its own was accurate.

For the validity of certain opinions, the more peer-reviewed consensus, at times reflected in consensus statements or in the proliferation of guidelines (see, e.g., American Medical Association 1996; BMJ Publishing Group 2000), the higher the likelihood for some degree of validity about these opinions. This applies, for example, to the nature of investigations in child sexual abuse cases in which, based on considerable study, the consensus is that information gathered in certain ways may be reliable but is not valid as representing what actually happened to the child (American Academy of Pediatrics 1991; Jenkins and Howell 1994). A similar situation occurs in recovered memory matters (see, e.g., American Medical Association 1994; American Psychiatric Association 1993; Canadian Psychiatric Association 1996). Additionally, the qualitatively worse the initial work being evaluated retrospectively—such as the child sexual abuse investigation and the circumstances of obtaining the "recovered memories"—and the more the forensic mental health professionals on each side are knowledgeable about relevant standards, the easier it is for the mental health professionals to conclude, for example, that the investigation or "memories" were likely contaminated or incredible. In such cases it also will be easier for courts to agree with the mental health professionals and conclude that the mental health professionals' opinions on the quality of the child sexual abuse investigation or on the quality of the "recovered memories" are *valid* or *trustworthy* (or some other term the courts use) and therefore admissible. (See the section "Legal Admissibility Issues for Non-Face-to-Face Evaluations" later in this chapter.)

Opinion Reliability

As suggested in the previous subsection, sometimes evaluators on both sides in certain mental health professional evaluations will agree in their opinions, such as in some criminal responsibility cases, providing reliability data. Undoubtedly more often, for many reasons, including whom an attorney might seek out and hire in a case and the advocacy nature of most forensic mental health work, the mental health professionals on opposite sides of the case will not be in agreement on various aspects of their evaluations, including opinions. Nonetheless, for certain kinds of evaluations some reliability data for opinions will be available. Within the limits of the type of data, the state forensic conference board in the Janofsky et al. (1989) study found that the board was unanimous in its criminal responsibility opinion 96% of the time.

Although not retrospective or non-face-to-face data, when competency to stand trial evaluations are based at least partly on various assessment instruments, these instruments generally have had reliabilities such as intertester reliability measured. Instruments such as the Competency Screening Test and the Georgia Competency Court Test have reliabilities in the 0.90s. (For a summary of this work see Rogers and Mitchell 1991, pp. 100–105.)

The more concurrence there is in the literature about the nature of the opinion in question (e.g., recovered memories), the more likely it is that well-informed forensic mental health professionals will agree (i.e., that reliability will be higher between evaluators for this type of retrospective opinion). The more the recovered memories appear incredible, the greater the likelihood that forensic mental health professional evaluators will be in agreement. The expected long-term effect of this agreement is that the more mental health knowledge and mental health professionals agree, it is hoped that fewer attempts will be made to "recover" such memories, and subsequently the chance for mental health professionals to show their agreement in this area will wane. We are a long way from such a time.

The DSM-IV-TR Axis V, Global Assessment of Functioning (GAF) Scale (American Psychiatric Association 2000; see also H.H. Goldman et al. 1992), is a general, single measure of overall functional level from 0 (worst) to 100 (best) derived from anchored points, usually in psychological, social, and educational/occupational domains. The GAF Scale can be used not only as a single measure for an opinion on overall functioning at the time of an evaluation but also to compare an evaluee at different times or to compare opinions between evaluators. The GAF Scale therefore provides an overall measure of an evaluator's opinion of an evaluee's ability or impairment (cf. American Medical Association 2000). (The GAF Scale is referred to again in examining the first author's [R.B.L.'s] forensic practice work.)

A Veterans Affairs GAF reliability study (Edson et al. 1997; Tracy et al. 1997) used 23 written patient vignettes. Ten raters gave a GAF rating based on these vignettes, and an intraclass correlation coefficient of 0.90 was obtained (Edson et al. 1997), excellent overall agreement. Nonetheless, 3 of these 10 raters gave ratings significantly higher or lower than did the others (Edson et al. 1997). Videotaped interviews were used as the main data source in another reliability study of the GAF Scale (Hilsenroth et al. 2000) in which an intraclass correlation coefficient of 0.86 was obtained. This study's outpatient population presented a restricted range of GAF scores, aiding in getting such a high coefficient. (To examine validity, this study used patient self-ratings and found these significantly correlated with GAF scores.) The use of standardized materials for rating in these studies likely gave higher agreement than having each rater independently gather the data to rate for the GAF.

Hall (1995) used the intake histories and discharge summaries of 16 hospitalized patients with major depression as the information sources for 2 groups of 12 professional raters from various mental health disciplines who each used either the regular version or a more detailed version of the earlier GAF Scale from DSM-III-R. This earlier version of the GAF Scale has a range of 1 to 90. These raters used the regular and their modified versions of this GAF and obtained intraclass correlation coefficients of 0.62 and 0.81, respectively, for the admission GAF and 0.90 and 0.95, respectively, for the discharge GAF, quite good reliabilities, especially for the discharges. To test the validity of the modified GAF Scale, it was compared with the original GAF Scale and also with patients' self-ratings of their GAF scores, and it was highly and significantly correlated, especially with the original GAF Scale. Note that both of these GAF studies were based on non-face-to-face data.

Also of interest is a study on the Global Assessment Scale (GAS; Endicott et al. 1976), a precursor to the GAF Scale that is very similar to it and that provides some additional reliability information. "The information needed to make the rating can come from any source, such as a direct interview of the patient, a reliable informant, or a case record" (Endicott et al. 1976, p. 767). Reliability studies under various conditions obtained intraclass correlation coefficients for adult patients of 0.69–0.91, with the lower values coming from research assistants reviewing medical records. The coefficient for GAS ratings based on information from parents relative to their children was 0.61 (Endicott et al. 1976).

As a final opinion reliability comment, and to reiterate, the more that the opinion under consideration is one that is frequently rendered by forensic mental health professionals, the more likely that there will be a database allowing for some calculation of reliability for such an opinion.

Psychopathy Checklist—Revised

The PCL-R is an instrument that alone or with other factors has received considerable use in predictive evaluations (opinions) (Hare 1991; Hart et al. 1988). Over several years Hare and colleagues developed instruments to assess psychopathy as derived from the historical conception of antisocial (psychopathic) personality, emphasizing a lack of conscience and remorse, lack of empathy, a grandiose sense of self-worth, and so on (Cleckley 1941, 1988). This work led to the PCL-R, a 20-item instrument with reliabilities in the upper 0.80s and better (Hare 1991) and yielding a total psychopathology score. The instrument usually is scored from a record review and an interview of the person, but if the records are adequate, it can be scored from the records alone (Harris et al. 1991; Wong 1984; but see also Freedman 2001; Serin 1993). (The use of the PCL-R is noted below.)

Opinions Using Actuarial Assessment Instruments

To use the most relevant data and avoid inaccuracies about base rates and various biases in strictly clinically based predictions, several statistically and actuarially based instruments have been developed to help in rendering opinions. (For a general discussion of this clinical versus actuarial issue, see Dawes et al. 1989; Grove and Meehl 1996; Meehl 1954; Quinsey et al. 1998; and Sreenivasan et al. 2000.) The idea is to use optimally objective items that statistically can maximally predict some criterion behavior, such as violent recidivism as measured by a rearrest for violent crime. In view of the high objectivity of the data used with some of these instruments, they can achieve high interrater reliabilities and other favorable measures of the quality of the assessments. As a measure of predictive accuracy, some of these devices use a statistic called the relative operating characteristic (ROC) of the instrument, a statistic that considers a combination of factors, including base rates, sensitivity, and specificity (see Quinsey et al. 1998, pp. 43–54). Generally in predictive accuracy an ROC of 0.20 would be a small effect, 0.50 a moderate effect, and 0.80 a large effect in predicting a certain event or events (Quinsey et al. 1998, p. 54; cf. Mark 2001, p. 11), with ROCs in the upper 0.60s and higher being optimal.

Noteworthy among currently available actuarial instruments are ones for assessing violence and sexual recidivism risk, particularly in prison and parole release and sexually violent predator contexts. In general the instruments use from no to little information that needs to be collected from the evaluee in a face-to-face examination. These devices generally compute a score or rating based on data that are correlated with the occurrence or not of the respective recidivism at a level of accuracy (predictive validity) that often exceeds what standard clinical evaluations, including face-to-face examinations, can achieve. Actuarial instruments are under constant development for various purposes (e.g., Hanson and Harris 2000; Hanson and Thornton 1999), and we present only a sample of these; the user of these instruments needs to watch the literature, including that on the World Wide Web (some of the Web sites are included in the references—e.g., see Epperson et al. 2000 and several Hanson references).

The simplest of these instruments to be discussed, the Rapid Risk Assessment for Sexual Offense Recidivism (RRASOR; Hanson 1997), serves as an introduction to this field. The RRASOR uses only prior sex offenses (not including the index offense), age at release (current age), victim sex, and offender relationship to victim to predict the recidivism rate. This test was developed from a meta-analysis of information on some 29,000 sex offenders and then replicated on a sample of 2,592 sex offenders; the test has an ROC of 0.71, considered at least satisfactory for screening purposes for sexual recidivism (Hanson 1997). This instrument already has been superseded by the Static-99 (Hanson and Thornton 1999) and the Minnesota Sex Offender Screening Tool—Revised (Epperson et al. 2000); space precludes further discussion of these instruments here.

Two other recently developed and related instruments are the Violence Risk Appraisal Guide (VRAG) and the Sex Offender Risk Appraisal Guide (SORAG; Quinsey et al. 1998), which use considerable common data sources. The VRAG, developed on some 800 offenders, has been studied more and has reported ROCs of 0.73–0.82, which are moderate to large predictive effects, with violent, including sexually violent, reoffending (Quinsey et al. 1998). The test has an interrater reliability correlation coefficient of 0.90. (This is different from the κ statistic but can be interpreted in approximately the same way [see Sackett 1992].) The SORAG has been studied less, but it is expected to have similar predictive power for violent reoffending that includes sexual violence but a lower ROC of 0.62 for predicting only sexually violent reoffending in view of the greater difficulty of confirming sexual reoffending (Quinsey et al. 1998).

The VRAG and SORAG use 12 and 14 items, respectively, to obtain scores that are then checked against actuarial tables for the respective recidivism risks. Five or six of these items related to criminal behavior and the victim(s) are apt to be available in offense and prison record data; marital status and alcohol problem information are likely in the records; the Hare PCL-R score can be obtained from the records if these are sufficiently complete; living with both parents to age 16 (absent death of a parent) may be in the records; and school adjustment may be noted in other records or in the school records if these are available. This totals 10 items for the VRAG and 11 for the SORAG, leaving only items for personality disorder and schizophrenia for the VRAG and these plus phallometric testing for the SORAG. Some data relevant to one personality disorder may be obtained from the PCL-R score, but more extensive data for personality disorder and schizophrenia may be in prior mental health records, leaving, depending on the nature of available records, only one or more items unscored if no face-to-face examination is performed at the time of the evaluation (including for phallometric testing). Furthermore, the scores on both the VRAG and the SORAG can be prorated if not too many data are missing (Quinsey et al. 1998). And one or more missing item scores may not have a notable effect if a total score would not be significantly or at all affected in its predictive ability by the lack of the scored items—the score is otherwise low enough or high enough that the score(s) for the additional item(s) would not make a realistic predictive difference. To summarize, these predictions can be made with the VRAG and the SORAG without a direct face-to-face examination.

Although research shows that for some predictions clinical methods may not only not enhance the predictive accuracy but also actually detract from it (see Quinsey et al. 1998, pp. 62–65), clinicians may well prefer to combine actuarial and nonactuarial (clinical) methods (Dvoskin and Heilbrun 2001; Hanson 1997; Lacoursiere, in press; Sreenivasan et al. 2000). When the person being evaluated and the conditions of the evaluation do not closely enough approximate the conditions of the actuarial studies, a mental health professional not only is justified in combining methods but in more idiosyncratic cases also may be required to exclude or ignore actuarial results, such as with a first-time violent offender with a low prediction for recidivism who realistically and convincingly states that he or she will similarly reoffend. Also, the actuarial methods emphasize "static" variables like age and number of past offenses without generally giving much weight to "dynamic" variables like changes with completed treatment, which the evaluator often needs to consider as well as can be done. With time and study we will learn more about the limits and clinical complementarity of these actuarial methods.

Interim Summary: Opinions

Some opinions can be largely given without benefit of a face-to-face examination, such as some violence recidivism risk opinions. And such opinions based on actuarial methods may be made with as much or more accuracy than is usual clinically, including with face-to-face examinations.

Other Error Sources in Evaluations

Besides the sources of error already noted in matters such as differences in diagnoses by different mental health professionals, issues related to reliability and validity of diagnoses, and opinions and related matters that are an inherent part of the "error rate" of the mental health methodology, we briefly mention other sources of error. At times medical records are outright falsified, which may not be detected, making them less dependable as a source for the history of an evaluee's prior problems (Dwyer and Shih 1998; Jesilow et al. 1991; Prosser 1992). The recent number of reversals of convictions, including of capital cases, as a result of DNA findings underscores the issue of erroneous criminal convictions that may occur in criminal records. Also, at times various research "findings" have been fabricated (Korenman et al. 1998; Youngner 1998), adding an additional concern to one's evaluation of the scientific literature. Some of this work is later publicly retracted in journals, but it is not easy for mental health professionals to become aware that such previously accepted "peer review and publication" has been retracted (Budd et al. 1998). Accordingly, it is difficult for the court to be so informed, often unless a testifying expert so informs them.

These and other related sources of error are likely to affect the admissibility less than the credibility of evaluative testimony; the underlying scientific methods of testing the work should remain sound. But these matters are noted here because with non-face-to-face evaluations the evaluee is not available to contradict potentially erroneous information, which can be especially problematic when single sources of records that are not otherwise corroborated are heavily relied on for data. This is not to ignore that an evaluee's avowal of material in records as erroneous is always itself accurate or that there may not be other sources of correction for errors, but this is more of a problem with non-face-to-face evaluations than with face-to-face evaluations and should be considered in one's conclusions.

Forensic Practice Information and Interim Summary: Evaluations Without Benefit of a Direct Face-to-Face Examination

To illustrate and then summarize the above material, in this section we first review some actual forensic practice data. Rather than select cases that are usually not face to face, such as testamentary capacity cases, or cases that may not be face to face because the evaluee refused to be seen, as in a recent sexually violent predator evaluation, more routine forensic work is examined to consider the contribution of non-face-to-face material to such evaluations.

Forensic Practice: Information Sources and Evaluation Parameters

A sample of the first author's (R.B.L.'s) forensic psychiatric practice records were examined to view from another perspective information sources actually used for forensic mental health professional evaluative conclusions. This material is very preliminary information on this subject in view of the small numbers of cases involved, the lack of external raters, and the lack of reliability and external validity of the evaluations; these were not cases with a high degree of agreement by mental health professional evaluators on both sides. Nonetheless, this work illustrates a method of examining mental health professional evaluative data and the application of the method to selected types of forensic cases.

Forensic practice records were examined for homogeneous groups of evaluations; in a private general forensic psychiatric practice a broad range of issues are evaluated, and some issues are evaluated only a few times, which contrasts, for example, with state forensic mental health facilities where hundreds or even thousands of similar evaluations for competency to stand trial or criminal responsibility are conducted. From the author's groupings of certain homogeneous types of cases and referral sources, the evaluation report for each case was examined; these reports usually included an extensive records review section. The report was examined for information from each of the data categories discussed earlier in this chapter: reason for the evaluation, background history, MSE, psychological testing, and physical and laboratory evaluation data, all as only face-to-face data, and also examined for whether information for such categories may have come from the non-face-to-face sources of public information (e.g., witness statements for crimes), medical records, or nonmedical records (see Table 9–4). A determination was made separately for each diagnosis and the most relevant other opinion(s); for example, for criminal responsibility, what percentage of the conclusion for that diagnosis or other opinion arose from each of these three non-face-to-face and five face-to-face information sources? All the face-to-face data were gathered by the forensic mental health professional (R.B.L.). (No attempt was made in this work to determine what degree of information in the usual face-to-face data categories of reason for the evaluation, background history, MSE, psychological testing, and physical and laboratory evaluation data may have come from face-to-face *and* from some non-face-to-face sources, such as medical records.

The emphasis in this study as opposed to in the actual reports was in giving priority to the non-face-to-face versus the face-to-face data and determining the degree that non-face-to-face data contributed to the various conclusions.) Ten cases of person felonies for which retrospective evaluations of criminal responsibility were performed at the request of the defense were examined in this way.

Table 9–4 shows that public records contributed to 13% of the diagnosis and to 26% of the criminal responsibility opinion, and overall public information and medical and nonmedical records (non-face-to-face material) contributed to 31% of the diagnosis and to 41% of the responsibility opinion. In contrast, the most face-to-face part of the evaluations, the MSE, contributed only 17% to each of these areas of diagnosis and criminal responsibility opinion.

For comparison with the criminal responsibility cases, a sample of 10 workers' compensation cases evaluated at the request of the same insurer were similarly reviewed to identify information sources for diagnosis, level of functioning or disability (as seen via the GAF Scale), and the cause of the dysfunction. Among other ways, this latter issue was evaluated by examining functioning at the time of the evaluation and retrospectively to immediately after the work injury, at the time of the injury, and before the injury. (These are all Kansas cases; in that jurisdiction a physical injury is required for psychiatric injury to be work related [*Followill v. Emerson Electric Co.* 1984]. No table is provided for this material.) These patients came for a forensic evaluation generally only after considerable prior medical and sometimes psychiatric evaluation and/or treatment; therefore medical records were extensive. With these workers' compensation cases, public records contributed less than 1%, medical records 26%–34%, and nonmedical records 5%–9% of the overall conclusions, and on average 40% of the conclusions were derived from non-face-to-face sources.

In another review five homogeneous alleged sexual harassment cases examined for harassment-related damages were considered.[2] From this review various non-face-to-face sources contributed only 20% overall to the conclusions, and the three face-to-face data categories—reason for the evaluation, background history, and MSE—each contributed approximately 25%, or 75% total overall, of the information for the conclusions regarding harassment damages. (Unlike the workers' compensation cases, these cases had generally fewer prior medical or psychiatric records.)

---

[2]No table is provided for this material. For a discussion of *Daubert/Kumho* aspects of such cases, see Jorgenson and Wahl 2000.

Table 9–4. Information source contribution percentages for diagnoses and opinions in forensic practice criminal responsibility cases (see text)

Type of opinion rendered	Public information	Medical record	Non-medical record	Background	Reason for evaluation	Mental status	Psychological testing	Physical and laboratory evaluation	Total (%)
Diagnostic opinion	13	13	5	20	20	17	8	4	100
Criminal responsibility opinion	26	9	6	13	22	17	7	0	100
Average percent of contribution to opinion from that data source	20	11	5	17	21	17	7	2	100

From these limited forensic practice reviews, the tentative conclusions are that when the forensic evaluation question deals more with a retrospective situation or opinion, the more (past) records and non-face-to-face data will contribute to the conclusion, and for criminal matters these evaluations will include significant public records that are, of course, non-face-to-face data. Conversely, when the forensic evaluation question deals more with current damages, particularly as in the sexual harassment cases, the less such records and the more face-to-face data will be relevant to the conclusions.

It is also unknown from these forensic evaluations if the same diagnoses and other opinions could or would have been reached without the overall databases that were used. As noted initially in this chapter, the forensic evaluator examines the overall data for internal consistency, and one part of the evaluation helps corroborate another. Therefore, for example, the fact that certain public records were assessed as making a certain contribution to the conclusions only holds in this context when all the various sources of data were available and used in reaching the conclusions. And it is not denied that at times opposing, equally qualified experts "see" different things in various parts of similar databases.

Among additional limitations to such a methodology, and of forensic mental health professional evaluations in general, are that in a particular case a relatively small amount of the overall available information may contribute a very large effect to the evaluation. For instance, a brain tumor and seizure disorder may be found on the physical evaluation, a high likelihood of malingering may be determined on psychological testing, or armed forces records may fail to substantiate claimed service in Vietnam in a Vietnam veteran PTSD evaluation context. The data available in a case depend on several factors, with public information being routinely available in criminal cases, investigators' material being available in workers' compensation cases only if it is sought, and so forth.

To illustrate the parameters of evaluation (examination) discussed earlier in this chapter in the section "Evaluations (and Examinations) and Their Parameters," we briefly review the person felony evaluations, noting the application of these parameters to these evaluations overall, although this usually would be a case-by-case consideration.

- The contexts of the evaluations were that all the evaluees were available and (adequately) cooperative and provided generally credible information for their reasons for the evaluation, background histories, and related matters but somewhat less so for the crimes with which they were charged, but this varied.
- All parts of the evaluation from reason for the evaluation to physical evaluation were face to face.

- The first author gathered all of these data, including usually some psychological testing, and supplemented limited personally collected physical evaluation data with material from the medical records.
- The information sources used were noted earlier in the chapter.
- These evaluations were retrospectively focused in view of their purpose to determine criminal responsibility at the time of the alleged crime.
- These evaluations were forensic and not clinical, and the evaluator had never had a treatment relationship with these evaluees, although recommendations for treatment might have been made in the evaluation report when appropriate.
- The evaluator was board certified in forensic psychiatry and had some years of forensic psychiatric experience.
- The evaluations were done at about the time of request pretrial, and the evaluees voluntarily participated in the process.

Interim Summary: Evaluations Without Benefit of a Direct Face-to-Face Examination

In practice the forensic mental health professional evaluator does retrospective evaluations completely without the benefit of a direct examination primarily in cases in which the evaluee is unavailable because of death, as in testamentary capacity and psychological autopsy cases. But as this chapter has shown, nonexaminational information can contribute major data to various evaluative conclusions, and at times such data will be conclusive.

Practice and Ethics Issues in Evaluations Without Direct Face-to-Face Examinations

There are some practice matters to discuss relative to evaluations without a face-to-face examination. The first issue to consider is whether this idea of non-face-to-face evaluating is primarily theoretical and of negligible practical use, because it is rare in practice that things such as a diagnosis can be reached without a face-to-face examination. As noted in the discussion on the diagnosis of alcoholism earlier in this chapter, the various nonexaminational diagnostic criteria often may be present. Depending on the examination population a mental health professional is working with, that can be true of other diagnoses also, such as pedophilia and antisocial personality disorder. The application to other diagnoses such as depression and dementia also was mentioned. The limits of application of such nonexaminational evaluation remain to be determined.

Another practice issue is whether such non-face-to-face evaluative work is mental health professional work. There has been discussion of diagnoses by non–mental health professionals and nonexaminational data, but to be of relevance in a legal case or treatment context, such evaluations would require the overall application of the knowledge and clinical skills of a mental health professional and could not feasibly be done without such expertise. That is, although we saw that technicians could be trained to make diagnoses, for instance, in an actual case the question(s) will be more than only the diagnosis under most circumstances; there will also be questions such as whether the person is likely to reoffend, has been given the proper treatment, and has used the treatment—that is, questions requiring the use of professional expertise. If such is the case, then it appears that these non-face-to-face evaluations should be covered by one's medical or other malpractice insurance, although it is easy to imagine scenarios in which the insurance company would argue that in doing non-face-to-face evaluation one has performed unethical work and that therefore the work is not within the practice of the covered profession (see below in this section; case law has not been reviewed on this matter).

A further practice issue is whether such non-face-to-face diagnoses and opinions are given with reasonable medical or similar certainty. It depends on the diagnosis, opinion, context, and perhaps other factors, but at times some level of certainty is lost. In these cases one may speak of *clinical opinion* or some such term, but at times this will be a distinction without a difference. At other times one can have a high degree of certainty in a diagnosis or opinion without a face-to-face examination (e.g., with multiple convictions for child molestation) and reach reasonable certainty on the basis of the material reviewed.

Although the above matters have ethical implications, a more usual ethical issue regarding evaluations without examinations is with the American Psychiatric Association's so-called Goldwater rule, an ethical guideline developed after many psychiatrists commented for a magazine article on then–presidential candidate Goldwater's alleged psychiatric status. The subsequent ethical guideline states that

> On occasion psychiatrists are asked for an opinion about an individual who is in the light of public attention, or who has disclosed information about himself/herself through public media. It is unethical for a psychiatrist to offer a professional opinion unless he/she has conducted an examination and has been granted proper authorization for such a statement. (American Psychiatric Association 1998, Section 7.3, p. 9)

This two-sentence proscription that is meant to be read as a unit contains many qualifiers (American Psychiatric Association 1995b). Note is taken of "in the light of public attention," "through public media," "conducted an examination," and "been granted proper authorization." This proscription is easy to attend to in the "normal" course of business, but it does not appear to be one that tests one's mettle if it is not applied under various special circumstances. Such special circumstances could be—to cite only a couple of examples—1) the suspected, publicly known terrorist about whom a mental health professional is being consulted by a government agency charged with public safety, or 2) a president of the United States with known unusual behavior for whom the vice president requests consultation (which he or she has the authority to request according to the Twenty-Fifth Amendment to the United States Constitution, but is this "proper authorization?") when the president and his or her spouse refuse to allow an examination (Toole et al. 1997). It appears that this is an ethical rule at times meant to be honored in the breach, underscoring at the same time that the examples given for "in the breach" are not frivolous. It is also ironically noted in this context that this ethical proscription is part of the American Medical Association's code section 7, "A physician shall recognize a responsibility to participate in activities contributing to an improved community" (American Psychiatric Association 1998, p. 9).

The American Academy of Psychiatry and the Law ethical guideline related to the Goldwater rule is one that is more consistently applicable and honored in forensic psychiatric work. This guideline states that

> Honesty, objectivity and the adequacy of the clinical evaluation may be called into question when an expert opinion is offered without a personal examination. While there are authorities who would bar an expert opinion to an individual who has not been personally examined, it is the position of the Academy that if, after earnest effort, it is not possible to conduct a personal examination, an opinion may be rendered on the basis of other information. However, under such circumstances, it is the responsibility of forensic psychiatrists to assure that the statements of their opinions and any reports of [sic] testimony based on those opinions, clearly indicate that there was no personal examination and the opinions expressed are thereby limited. (American Academy of Psychiatry and the Law 1999, p. xii)

The material presented in this chapter does not generally encourage giving psychiatric diagnoses or opinions without a full evaluation, including a face-to-face examination, when that can be done. There is always the possibility of unknown, unexpected, and maybe never before encountered extenuating circumstances or conditions. But when such an evaluation cannot be done, we are also not without considerable diagnostic and opinion-rendering skills, and, to reiterate, at times the non-face-to-face data will be more accurate and persuasive.

Legal Admissibility Issues for Non-Face-to-Face Evaluations

We are now ready in this lengthy endeavor to consider *Daubert* and other legal admissibility issues for non-face-to-face evaluations. How difficult this admission via *Daubert* hearings will be is uncertain; in one compilation of various types of federal circuit court cases applying these standards, more experts were excluded than admitted (22 admitted and 38 excluded out of 60 cases; Agrimonti 1995); in a wrongful death case dealing with nuclear power, the court held 6 days of hearings and received 71 exhibits and 14 affidavits regarding admissibility matters and then concluded that the expert medical and other testimony on causation was inadmissible (*Whiting v. Boston Edison Co.* 1995); however, more recent studies show that *Daubert* hearings for behavioral and social science evidence have "not resulted in changes in the admissibility of that kind of evidence" (Slovenko 2000b, p. 436).

Relevancy and Allied Restrictions on Admissibility

Proof of past and current mental states may be adduced either through the testimony of fact witnesses under Federal Rules of Evidence 602 and 701 (the 1975 codification to provide for a unitary but not exhaustive federal system of evidence; the cognate state evidentiary rules are typically numbered in identical fashion) or through the testimony of a witness qualified as an expert under Federal Rule of Evidence 702. Although fact witness and expert witness testimony differ markedly in many respects, each method of proof must satisfy the basic requirement of relevancy under Federal Rule of Evidence 401: "'Relevant evidence' means evidence having any tendency to make the existence of any fact that is of consequence to the determination of the action more probable or less probable than it would be without the evidence" (Federal Rule 401).

Although the relevancy threshold usually is crossed for most evidence attorneys wish to present, it may operate to legally differentiate mental health professionals' assessments of past mental states from their opinions about the likelihood of present or future mental states or behavior. For example, in this context, a past mental disorder without a present mental disorder can be distinguished from a continuing or otherwise current mental disorder. In cases such as competency to stand trial determinations, involuntary civil commitments, and guardianship petitions, determination of an individual's past mental state or disorder that is not a continuing matter is less likely to be legally relevant and admissible than is a current mental state or disorder, which may be more relevant to the issue for which the mental health professional's expert opinion is sought.

There is also the issue of circumscription of expert testimony to those subjects for which the expert is qualified to testify. The nature of this circumscription should, as a preliminary matter, depend on the particular bases set forth in Federal Rule 702 on which a witness may be qualified as an expert: "If scientific, technical, or other specialized knowledge will assist the trier of fact to understand the evidence or determine a fact in issue, a witness qualified as an expert by knowledge, skill, experience, training, or education, may testify thereto in the form of an opinion or otherwise" (Federal Rule 702). An expert witness qualified largely on the basis of experience alone generally should be limited to testifying to those matters that the expert has encountered with sufficient frequency to be able to render an opinion of acceptable quality, such as from a technician who has administered tests of sexual arousal and interest testifying on the manner of administering the tests or a technician who has conducted structured DSM diagnostic interviews testifying on the usual manner of conducting these interviews. However, an expert qualified on the basis of knowledge, skill, training, education, *and* experience should be permitted greater latitude in testifying on issues within the broader subject matter for which the witness has proven expertise, which may, for example, constitute the broad field of the practice of adult psychiatry.

After determining the universe of potential issues on which the expert is qualified to testify, the specific factual questions at issue and the nature of the proffered expert testimony should be assessed. The factors that will affect a particular legal question typically will encompass separate factual questions, any one (or all) of which may be an appropriate candidate for expert testimony (Hutchinson and Blend 1994; Krauss and Sales, 1999). To take a usually retrospective and non-face-to-face evaluative example, the legal question of testamentary capacity encompasses several separate questions, including knowledge of the person's usual natural heirs, awareness of one's assets, and information that one is making a will (e.g., Spar and Garb 1992). Expert testimony that does not bear directly on the specific factual questions presented should be excluded, and the scope of admitted expert testimony should be limited to the factual questions for which the testimony is relevant. Mental health professional testimony on only one or two of these factual matters standing alone may not rise to the level of allowing an opinion on the broader, overall issue of testamentary capacity, which requires evaluation of each of the factual matters on which this opinion is based.

Furthermore, as commentators have noted: "Offering [an] opinion on an issue for which there is no relevant data is not an appropriate professional or scientific task" (Shuman and Sales 1999, p. 10). But "lawyers are typically happy to have their experts reach conclusions on the witness stand that support their client's position, even if it goes beyond the bounds of the witness' expertise" in the case (Shuman and Sales 1999, p. 11). And judges frequently embrace expert testimonial overreaching as well. We add in this context that the court may need to appoint nonagreeing experts to obtain information on the issue of whether any and adequate "relevant data" for the evidentiary area in question exist, as Federal Rule of Evidence 706(a) authorizes a court to do.

The circumscription of expert testimony to a specific issue or issues is an aspect of a heightened admission standard for expert witnesses. This heightened standard, which the *Daubert* court conceded "goes primarily to relevance," is articulated in Federal Rule 702's mandate that the testimony must "assist the trier of fact." The *Daubert* court explained the standard as presenting a question of the requisite connection between the pertinent legal issue and the subject matter of the expert testimony; although termed the *helpfulness* test, the *Daubert* court approvingly cited a lower court description of the standard as one of "fit." This standard raises the bar for the admission of expert testimony by requiring somewhat more than "mere relevancy," or merely "*any* tendency to make the existence of any fact…more probable or less probable than it would be without the evidence" (Federal Rule 401; emphasis added). Instead, as the *Daubert* court made clear, the "helpfulness" standard requires that the testimony be "*sufficiently* tied to the facts of the case that it will aid the jury in resolving a factual dispute" (*Daubert v. Merrell Dow Pharmaceuticals, Inc.* 1993, at 589, citing *United States v. Downing* 1985; emphasis added).

The degree of "fit" between the legal issue and the subject matter of an expert's testimony that will be "sufficient" to "assist the trier of fact" also alludes to the standard expert testimony requirement that the testimony be beyond the scope of knowledge of the trier of fact. Additionally, the proffered testimony should not be prejudicial to the fact-finder's task, such as can occur when juries give an aura of "infallibility" and excessive credibility to testifying experts (Imwinkelried 1994). When considering the admissibility of non-face-to-face evaluations of retrospective mental states, this standard could operate to admit such testimony only when its reliability is shown to be equal to that of face-to-face evaluative data or when more reliable testimony is unavailable. Expert testimony from an unreliable, non-face-to-face evaluation in this situation could distract instead of assist the trier of fact in a proper consideration of the issue(s), even though the testimony might arguably be "relevant." Similarly, actuarial assessments that do not adequately apply to the person in question may be more prejudicial than helpful and could be excluded on this basis.

Finally the question of "fit" also may depend on a determination of the extent to which the expert testimony is sufficiently "reliable" to merit admission. A review of the United States Supreme Court cases of *Daubert v. Merrell Dow Pharmaceuticals, Inc.* (1993) and *Kumho Tire Co. v. Carmichael* (1999) is necessary to understand this legal concept of "reliability" in relation to the admissibility of expert testimony.

The Effect of *Daubert/Kumho* on Expert Testimony Admissibility

The 1993 case of *Daubert v. Merrell Dow Pharmaceuticals, Inc.*, is crucial in modern evidentiary doctrine in the area of admissibility of expert scientific testimony, and descriptions of the case are presented throughout this volume. However, a brief recounting of legal concepts from *Daubert* and its 1999 companion, *Kumho*, is helpful for understanding the additional restrictions on expert opinions that the court imposed in these cases and for our discussion of these restrictions on non-face-to-face mental health professional opinions. The *Daubert* court explained that the adoption of the Federal Rules of Evidence replaced the Frye (*Frye v. United States* 1923) "general acceptance" test for the admissibility of scientific evidence with a more flexible and more complicated standard. Under *Daubert*, trial judges must play a heightened "gatekeeping" function to ensure that scientific testimony meets a sufficient threshold of "reliability," in addition to screening out evidence that does not meet the preliminary standard of relevancy or that would be excessively prejudicial to the fact-finder.

The court reasoned that "the adjective 'scientific' implies a grounding in the methods and procedures of science" (*Daubert*, at 590) and then concluded that an expert opinion must be derived by the scientific method to be regarded as scientific "knowledge" and qualify for admission under Federal Rule 702. This determination of "scientific method" establishes the standard of evidentiary reliability under Federal Rule 702 and not the simplified general acceptance inquiry from *Frye*.

Noting that courts also must determine whether the proffered testimony will "assist the trier of fact to understand or determine a fact in issue," the question of "fit" described above, *Daubert* set forth a nondefinitive checklist for courts to use in determining whether the "reliability" and "fitness" standards have been met before scientific expert testimony can be admitted. A proper application of this checklist allows courts to engage in "a preliminary assessment of whether the reasoning or methodology underlying the testimony is scientifically valid and of whether that reasoning or methodology properly can be applied to the facts in issue" (*Daubert*, at 592–593). Accordingly, from *Daubert*, areas of inquiry are whether

1. The theory or technique on which the testimony is based is subject to empirical testing and may be falsified.
2. The theory or technique has been subjected to scrutiny through peer review and publication.
3. The theory or technique's known or potential rate of error is within acceptable limits.
4. Adequate standards exist for controlling the operation of the theory or technique.
5. The theory or technique has achieved a sufficient degree of general consensus within the relevant scientific community.

A sixth area of inquiry has been distilled from the case—namely whether "the proposed theory [has] been tested using valid and reliable procedures, and with positive results" (Grove and Barden 1999). Emphasizing that the application of these inquiries must be sufficiently flexible to accommodate the range of proffered scientific testimony, the court concluded that the "overarching subject [of the standard] is the scientific validity—*and thus the evidentiary relevance and reliability*—of the principles that underlie a proposed submission" (*Daubert*, at 594–595; emphasis added).

The court expanded the reach of *Daubert* in the 1999 case *Kumho Tire Co. v. Carmichael*. On its surface, *Kumho* extends *Daubert's* core gatekeeping obligation of trial courts to ensure the reliability of expert testimony to such testimony based on "technical" or "other specialized" knowledge, not simply expert testimony based on "scientific" methods. The *Kumho* court clarified that the function of the trial court with respect to expert witnesses is the same regardless of the underlying nature of the testimony: to determine the reliability of the testimony and to admit proffered testimony when in the court's discretion, in addition to meeting the threshold of relevancy, it meets a sufficient threshold of reliability.

Kumho underscores the limits of the holdings of *Daubert* when applied to generally nonscientific expert testimony (i.e., to technical and other specialized experts). The *Kumho* court declined to limit the trial court's determination of the reliability of expert testimony to the list of factors set forth in *Daubert* and also said that an application of those *Daubert* factors was not necessary in every case. After *Kumho* it is clear that factors other than those listed in *Daubert* may be considered by trial courts in determining the evidentiary reliability of proffered testimony, and certain *Daubert* factors may simply be inapplicable to certain kinds of expert testimony. The *Kumho* court stated that "the relevant reliability concerns may focus upon personal knowledge or experience [rather than upon a scientific foundation]" (*Kumho*, at 1175). At several points in the opinion, the *Kumho* court gave examples of the kinds of testimony in which the scientific foundation for the testimony (or, by implication, an examination of the methodological process through which the *Kumho* court's expert's knowledge—i.e., opinion—was produced) may be less important than the personal experience of the expert (or, in certain cases, totally inapplicable), such as in criminal modus operandi, handwriting analyses, and agricultural practices.

Although portions of *Kumho* appear to disclaim any distinction between the trial court's admissibility determination for scientific expert testimony and for "technical, or other specialized" expert testimony, the reasoning of the court implicitly acknowledges differences in the underlying subject matter of proffered testimony, which affects the course of the court's admissibility determination. In each case, the function of the court in determining the reliability of the testimony remains the same, although the analysis used in doing so will vary depending on the subject matter of the testimony.

It is clear that the reliability with which the law of evidence is concerned is not synonymous with various scientific notions of reliability. *Daubert* and *Kumho* use the term *reliability* in a distinctly legal sense (although, e.g., *Kumho* [at 1177] also uses the term as synonymous with scientific *validity*, such as would be used for the validity of DSM criteria for a particular diagnosis as discussed earlier). The *Daubert* court made this definitional point explicit in its striking footnote 9:

> We note that scientists typically distinguish between "validity" (does the principle support what it purports to show?) and "reliability" (does application of the principle produce consistent results?). Although "the difference between accuracy, validity, and reliability may be such that each is distinct from the other by no more than a hen's kick," our reference here is to *evidentiary* reliability—that is, trustworthiness....In a case involving scientific evidence, *evidentiary reliability* will be based upon *scientific validity*. (*Daubert*, at 590 note 9; citations omitted, emphasis in original.)

Daubert suggests connections between standards regulating the admission of expert testimony and the familiar kinds of reliability issues raised by the testimony of fact witnesses. As a preliminary matter, the reliability of eyewitness testimony is minimally assured by the requirement contained in Federal Rule 602 that the testimony be based on firsthand knowledge of the event or fact in question. For experts there is no such requirement, although a rough proxy for the minimal assurance of evidentiary reliability in Federal Rule 602 is contained in Federal Rule 702's requirement that the expert must be qualified as such before being permitted to testify:

> Presumably, this relaxation of the usual requirement of firsthand knowledge—a rule which represents "a 'most pervasive manifestation' of the

common law insistence upon 'the most reliable sources of information,' is premised on an assumption that the expert's opinion will have a reliable basis in the knowledge and experience of his discipline. (*Daubert*, at 592, citing the Advisory Committee's Notes on Federal Rule 602)

The reliability of eyewitness testimony is subject to scrutiny through the familiar impeachment techniques expressly authorized in Article VI of the Federal Rules of Evidence and implicitly sanctioned as a matter of traditional cross-examination procedures. Although expert testimony is not subject to the Federal Rule 602 requirement of firsthand knowledge, it remains subject to the impeachment techniques. Accordingly, the exposure of the traditional testimonial defects—such as in "sincerity" of the opinion (as opposed to being given, e.g., for remuneration "only"), accurate "memory" for what the expert actually did, "narration" or explication of the evaluation and opinion as applying to this situation, and accurate "perception," such as of the circumstances under which the opinion was formed—is also a component of assuring the evidentiary reliability of expert testimony. Although at times these traditional methods of exposing testimonial defects may pertain to the scientific, technical, or other specialized knowledge reliability or validity of the subject matter of the expert's testimony, they may be more likely invoked to reveal other defects, such as in "sincerity" in always applying the scientific testimony to only defendant's or to only plaintiff's cases.

Although *Daubert* rather paradoxically makes clear that the evidentiary reliability of scientific evidence will be based on scientific validity, the lesson of *Kumho* is that evidentiary reliability may actually almost equate with the scientific or general empirical concept of reliability in the methods (methodology) or techniques used in assessing the tire's failure, and the court considered the method used as not very reliable. (The interested reader can review the presentation of the tire expert's method in *Kumho*.) A threshold level of legal reliability is obtained simply through the requirement in Federal Rule 702 that experts be qualified as such before they testify, as discussed earlier. Ostensibly, the training, skill, knowledge, experience, or education of an expert witness guarantees some minimal degree of (scientific or general empirical) reliability for the matter on which the expert will offer testimony. The *Daubert* court's assumption that an expert's opinion will have a "reliable basis in the knowledge and experience of his discipline" (at 592) would appear to mean that there is a conferring of general reliability on the expert's opinion as a function of this basic level of "knowledge and experience" of the discipline involved. And when the notion of scientific validity is inapplicable, such as with expert testimony on land valuation, handwriting analysis, and the like, "the relevant reliability concerns may focus upon personal knowledge or experience [rather than upon a scientific foundation]" (*Kumho*, at 1175).

An understanding and reconciliation of the methods of assuring the evidentiary reliability of various kinds of expert testimony as set forth in *Daubert* and *Kumho* can be obtained by considering the factual contexts of those cases and the nature of the proffered expert knowledge (opinion) along an epistemological continuum. At one end of the continuum lies testimony based on knowledge that is regarded as primarily scientific, based largely on general scientific methodology with empirical testing methods, such as that which may be heard on issues of causation in whether a drug or toxin causes certain teratogenic or other deleterious effects (as was the case in *Daubert*). In such cases an application of the factors set forth in *Daubert* that ensure the scientific *validity* of the theory or process(es) in question will be most appropriate because here the scientific validity is the touchstone of the knowledge that helps to elucidate the evidence or a fact in issue. These *Daubert* factors include the falsifiability or testability of the theory or technique, the known or potential (and acceptable) rate of error, the adequacy of the standards controlling the operation of the theory or technique, peer review and publication, and whether the proposed theory has yielded positive results with valid procedures.

When the knowledge basis involved is further along the epistemological continuum toward knowledge that is based less on general scientific methodology and more on technical skills and experience, as in technical and other specialized knowledge, including in engineering, the importance of consistency of the data gathering and its validity for the purpose proposed (e.g., testing tire failure proclivity, showing that a way of analyzing handwriting is applicable to a case dealing with forgery) will increase. At this end of the epistemological continuum lies testimony based on knowledge that one might consider especially experience based as opposed to scientific methodology based, not that scientific methodology may be outright ignored. The reliability of the knowledge in question at this end of the epistemological continuum will be partly secured by qualifying the expert with such "specialized knowledge." Highly specialized knowledge, such as the modus operandi of a drug dealer, should be the subject of testimony only by experts who have been specifically qualified to testify on such a matter.

The *Kumho* court implicitly supported the existence of this epistemological continuum and the role of expert qualification in determining the scientific or general empirical reliability, and thus the evidentiary reliability, of the subject matter: "In other [non-scientific] cases, the relevant reliability concerns may focus upon personal knowledge or experience… '[t]he factors identified in *Daubert* may or may not be pertinent in assessing reli-

ability, depending on the nature of the issue, the expert's particular expertise, and the subject of his testimony'" (*Kumho*, at 1175, quoting Brief for
United States as curiae, at 19). In addition, the *Kumho* court acknowledged
that some of the *Daubert* factors did not address the issue of *scientific* validity
exclusively: "[S]ome of *Daubert's* questions can help to evaluate the reliability *even* of experience-based testimony" (*Kumho*, at 1176; emphasis added).

Miscellaneous Admissibility Considerations for Mental Health Professional Opinions

We note miscellaneous admissibility considerations for mental health professional testimony. Mental health professionals may not necessarily be
permitted to provide an opinion on an ultimate issue, which is specifically
proscribed in Federal Rule of Evidence 704(b). In 1983 the Insanity Defense Reform Act added Federal Rule 704(b) to the Federal Rules of Evidence. This rule states that

> No expert witness testifying with respect to the mental state or condition
> of a defendant in a criminal case may state an opinion or inference as to
> whether the defendant did or did not have the mental state or condition
> constituting an element of the crime charged or of a defense thereto. Such
> ultimate issues are matters for the trier of fact alone.

An additional consideration regarding admissibility is that from the
perspective of the courts' requirements for and scrutiny of evaluations; they
may establish higher standards for more strictly forensic evaluations, such
as for criminal responsibility or sexual predator evaluations, than for more
strictly clinical evaluations. At times this might be feasible. At other times
these clinical and forensic types of evaluations will be commingled, such as
when a forensic criminal responsibility decision makes extensive use of
prior clinical evaluative material or the clinical mental health professional
proffers testimony on the criminal issue or when a clinical evaluation is itself the matter in issue, such as the standard of care in a malpractice or
wrongful death case.

Although courts might want to apply a higher standard for admissibility to forensic as opposed to clinical mental health professional evaluations,
they may find it more difficult to evaluate forensic mental health professional work from the perspectives of scientific reliability, validity, error
rates, and so forth. Available data on these issues for various aspects of the
evaluation may apply to clinical settings for patients coming for treatment
(or coming to participate in a research study!) and may not apply equally
well to forensic settings for evaluees presenting for other reasons, such as
for criminal responsibility or sexual predator evaluations.

"Reliability" Restrictions on
Admissibility of Non-Face-to-Face-Based Testimony

For admissibility non-face-to-face testimony must be "relevant," "fit" the case, and not unduly prejudice the fact-finder, but these threshold "gates" are not belabored. Rather we look at the nature of non-face-to-face mental health professional testimony for admissibility purposes.

From the preceding discussion, a step in determining evidentiary restrictions on the admissibility of non-face-to-face evaluative testimony lies in the placement of mental health professional evidence generally along the epistemological continuum between more scientific-methodology–based knowledge and more experience-based knowledge that is less dependent on a scientific knowledge base. The progressively objectified diagnostic criteria in DSM-III, DSM-III-R, DSM-IV, and DSM-IV-TR and the proliferation of carefully conducted studies of treatment outcome, among other matters, will push mental health professional evidence toward the more purely scientific pole of the continuum. Accordingly, mental health professional expert witnesses in general should be familiar with the research relating to the scientific validity of the subject matter in question (e.g., evaluations to reach diagnostic and other opinions), the scientific methodology used to develop reliable and valid diagnoses (as discussed earlier, especially in the sections "Diagnostic Reliability" and "Diagnostic Validity"), the testability and falsifiability of the methodology, the error rates, and so on.

Whether the absence of a face-to-face examination will place the consequent expert testimony any differently on the epistemological continuum occupied by mental health professional evidence in general must be determined. This, in part, depends on the particular kind of evaluation performed and the purpose for which the evaluation is offered. As this chapter has indicated, scientific or general empirical validity (diagnostic and other opinion reliability and validity) need not be sacrificed, and may be enhanced, in the absence of a face-to-face examination in some kinds of evaluative contexts. The reasoning in *Daubert* and *Kumho* would appear to require the existence of a methodology for diagnoses and other opinions that is "trustworthy" or, in more usual behavior science terms, has acceptable validity and reliability measures before the gatekeeper's admission of the proffered evidence based on a non-face-to-face evaluation.

To speculate, some the difficulty of establishing diagnostic validity criteria for certain kinds of mental health professional evaluations, such as for a diagnosis of premenstrual dysphoric disorder or factitious disorder by proxy, might currently suggest a placement of that knowledge toward the "*Kumho*" pole of the continuum. The more flexible and somewhat liberal standards for admissibility under *Kumho* might be welcomed by some members of the mental health professional community if one did not mind the reduced "status" of being considered "less scientific." Or maybe certain mental health workers, such as recovering (nonprofessionally trained) counselors and bachelor's level social workers and psychologists would have their proffered testimony examined under *Kumho*, but psychiatrists and Ph.D. psychologists would testify under *Daubert*.

The lack of laboratory confirmation for many mental illnesses might suggest that this negates the possibility that a particular mental health professional diagnosis can be falsified, but this depends on the diagnosis and "falsifying" methods. The validity of some diagnoses can be falsified by finding that the appropriate diagnostic criteria have not been met for a variety of reasons, including that the condition is actually a manifestation of a medical condition. At other times it will be a question of not only the diagnostic criteria for validity but also the "validity" of the very existence of the "disorder," such as for homosexuality.

Last in this context, the function of other, nonexpert evidence in determining the evidentiary reliability of non-face-to-face evaluative data should not be ignored. In this sense the nonexpert evidence serves as a unique source of extrinsic confirmation (at times a validity of sorts) for the expert testimony. Incongruence between the credible testimony of a lay witness and the testimony of an expert witness could cast doubt on the evidentiary reliability of the expert opinion. For example, expert mental health professional testimony formulated by a method that opines that the deceased lacked the requisite testamentary capacity may be insufficiently reliable in the face of credible eyewitness accounts that the deceased took care of her or his own finances and deliberated in a rational manner on the day that the will was signed. (Of course the skilled forensic mental health professional doing this non-face-to-face retrospective evaluation will have been previously aware of and considered such evidence in the evaluation.)

Other Restrictions on Admissibility of Non-Face-to-Face-Based Testimony

Besides the evidentiary relevancy and reliability restrictions placed on non-face-to-face (and other) mental health professional evaluative testimony, Federal Rule 703 provides another potential admissibility restriction: whether the sources of data used for performing a particular evaluation are "reasonably relied upon by experts in the particular field in forming opinions or inferences upon the subject" (Federal Rule of Evidence 703). If the data sources do not meet this "reasonably relied upon" evidentiary standard, then only those facts or data that are perceived by or made known to the expert at or before the hearing and that would otherwise be admissible as evidence may be used in forming an opinion.

Regarding the use of non-face-to-face data, it must be established that the data are "reasonably relied upon" or that the non-face-to-face data are otherwise admissible. The mental health professional expert must be aware of these restrictions and anticipate potential problems. For example, Federal Rule 703 may operate to exclude non-face-to-face testimony on those components of an examination that customarily rely primarily on a face-to-face examination, such as the MSE, the physical evaluation, and some kinds of psychological testing. The rationale for the potential exclusion is not that the absence of a face-to-face examination per se will render the opinion inadmissible but that the non-face-to-face bases of knowledge on which a mental health professional will ostensibly rely in rendering an evaluative opinion may not be customarily relied on by other experts in the field.

But this customary practice restriction may be overcome. As we showed with various diagnoses, such as antisocial personality disorder, the diagnosis requires little (or no) face-to-face MSE data, which is also the case with several other DSM diagnoses when the criteria are examined. The customary practice issue of using non-face-to-face data may be easily dealt with in testamentary capacity evaluations on decedents. This issue may be more difficult with the non-face-to-face use of an investigator's videotape in a claimed disability case, but the mental health professional may show, for example, that orthopedic disability evaluators often surreptitiously view their evaluees' physical functioning, such as in the office parking lot. Obviously the post-*Daubert/Kumho* "shopping for experts" may need to include shopping for those experts who use similar methods and data sources so that they may testify at admissibility hearings.

In regard to the data used for one's work, the determination of the "particular field" also is important. If the "particular field" is considered the clinical context of mental health professional examinations, then the absence of a face-to-face examination may exclude certain non-face-to-face evaluative data or grant them lowered probative value because in some contexts a clinical evaluation for treatment would not be meaningful in the absence of some face-to-face examinations. But if the "clinical evaluation for treatment" was in a sexually violent predator case (e.g., the Sexual Predator Act 1994, in Kansas; Lacoursiere, in press), then such an evaluation when the suspected predator refused to be examined might be very admissible.

In contrast, if the "particular field" is limited to the forensic context of mental health professional evaluations, the "basis of knowledge" restriction could impose undue restrictions if clinical standards were followed. Because the purpose of any forensic field is to aid in the judicial fact-finding process by providing knowledge that will assist the trier of fact in understanding the evidence or in determining a fact in issue, forensic mental health professionals can establish standards within their "particular field," including for the use of non-face-to-face data. Therefore, the extrinsic admissibility restrictions applied to the use of certain data sources in forming opinions or inferences within a variety of particular fields, such as the usual practice of clinical psychiatry, may not be applicable in the forensic mental health professional context, including when non-face-to-face data are used.

An appropriate proxy for this data source admissibility restriction may need to be formulated so that highly questionable data sources are not used. The American Academy of Psychiatry and the Law (1999) guideline excerpted earlier in the "Practice and Ethics Issues in Evaluations Without Direct Face-to-Face Examinations" section may provide some help in the requirement that an evaluator make an "earnest effort" to conduct a face-to-face examination and disclose when no face-to-face examination has occurred.

Barefoot and *Daubert/Kumho* Considerations for Admissibility

In *Barefoot v. Estelle* (1983) the United States Supreme Court upheld the admissibility of a psychiatrist's expert testimony on the expected future dangerousness of Mr. Thomas Barefoot. This expert testimony was admitted without the psychiatrist having performed a face-to-face examination (except what might ostensibly have occurred in the courtroom), but on the basis of a hypothetical question. And the court admitted the opinion in spite of objections in the amicus brief of the American Psychiatric Association that such future dangerousness could not be predicted. The court noted that such objections went to credibility and not admissibility (at 898–899). Unfortunately for Mr. Barefoot, the jury found the evidence adequately credible, and he was executed long ago.

The *Barefoot* case is cited here primarily to note at least its historical relevance to non-face-to-face mental health professional evaluations and opinions. We also note that *Daubert/Kumho* do not per se preclude testimony based on hypothetical questions.

Conclusions From Legal Restrictions on Non-Face-to-Face Evaluations

A court's view of and gatekeeping function regarding non-face-to-face mental health professional evaluative material will depend appropriately on the case (legal question) and the nature and circumstances of the evaluation. Once relevance and "fit" restrictions to admissibility are met, then other *Daubert/Kumho* matters can be considered. Many of these matters were discussed throughout the course of this chapter for non-face-to-face evaluations and are only briefly noted here. (For a more detailed admissibility analysis, particularly for primarily psychometric data based on instruments such as the PCL-R, see Marlowe 1995. For an illuminating judicial perspective, see Gless 1995.)

The *Daubert* factor of empirical testing and falsifiability of the methodology for reaching diagnostic and other opinions has been noted. For diagnoses a variety of falsifying methods are available, such as in a failure to meet DSM diagnostic criteria and a diagnosed condition that does not follow the course for the suspected diagnosis.

The *Daubert* factor of scrutiny through peer review and publication is noted in the publication in peer-reviewed journals of the many studies cited herein. A pre-*Daubert* survey of judges ($N=10$) found that 40% considered publications by a testifying expert "unimportant" (Champagne et al. 1991); will judges still consider publications "unimportant" in this post-*Daubert* era of admissibility hearings even if the publications reflect on the expert's methodology?

The *Daubert* factor of "error rate" and its acceptable level often is not as explicit as could be in mental health professional data, but it can be made so in various ways, as in the earlier discussion of a κ statistic of 0.73 (see the section "An Example of a κ Statistic of 0.73"). In this regard courts are constrained somewhat in that the best that mental health professionals can do still may have significant error rates, yet there may well be nothing better available to "assist the trier of fact." If this imperfect knowledge is the best available, and not unduly prejudicial, it will often warrant admission, and then its credibility can be weighed.

The *Daubert* factor of standards for controlling the operation of the theory or technique is found in the mental health professional and related literature showing that various procedures are acceptable, such as for reaching opinions (e.g., clinical and actuarial procedures for assessing the risk for violence, evolving assessment methods for neuropharmacological changes in certain mental disorders). These procedures are always evolving, as this chapter shows, regarding diagnoses and opinions. And as the *Daubert* and *Kumho* decisions note, the too-rigid application of admissibility review factors would be detrimental.

The *Daubert* factor of achieving a sufficient degree of general consensus within the relevant community was mentioned earlier in this chapter. We noted that the most "relevant scientific community" for purposes of this chapter is the community of forensic mental health professionals, and forensic mental health professionals can have a significant role in this consensus setting.

The additional distillation of a sixth *Daubert* factor (Grove and Barden

1999) of valid and reliable testing with positive results has been repeatedly noted herein with positive results for various diagnoses and other opinions reached by non-face-to-face methods. That is, with non-face-to-face methods, diagnoses and other opinions can be reliably and validly ("trust-worthily") reached under certain circumstances.

With some retrospective, non-face-to-face evaluations, such as the testamentary capacity of a decedent, no other evaluation or expert opinion may be available for the court's assistance and admissibility consideration. In other cases there may be situations in which face-to-face evaluations are the usual consensus, and there could be a need for the expert who uses non-face-to-face data to show how and why the non-face-to-face methods used meet standards for scientific validity (i.e., *Daubert's* "reliability" and trustworthiness). This expert must illustrate that the methods used to achieve the diagnoses are replicable or testable and refutable, such as when no adequate data are available for a particular non-face-to-face diagnosis.

From the earlier review in this chapter, the informed forensic mental health professional using non-face-to-face data should be able to help the court examine the *Daubert* and/or *Kumho* factors and hopefully pass through the admissibility gate. Any expert who gets this far—that is, has determined that the evaluation is adequate to proffer it to the court—can at this stage, when feasible, advocate for the non-face-to-face evaluation's merits as to a methodology and as to reliable and valid conclusions within its limits. At other times the non-face-to-face data that have been used may be too sparse to let the mental health professional expert evaluator proffer the testimony or try to pass the gate.

Forensic Mental Health Professional Conclusions and Recommendations for Non-Face-to-Face Evaluations

In this chapter we have presented what can be considered an introduction to the subject of non-face-to-face or indirect mental health professional evaluations. Some diagnoses and opinions were examined in detail, but the vast majority of psychiatric disorders, and types of opinions, have not been considered from this perspective of what can be reliably and validly done via indirect or non-face-to-face examination methods. The careful consideration of other disorders such as dementias, pathological gambling, and borderline personality disorder awaits further work. And the conditions examined within this chapter, such as pedophilia, of course warrant much more study as to when and what types of non-face-to-face data can be available, when these data are not adequately credible for various reasons, and so on.

Although the emphasis in this chapter has been on forensic applications of this non-face-to-face, indirect, evaluative material, it is obvious that this approach need not be limited to such uses and to considerations for a court's admissibility. Much of this material has clinical applications, such as in helping a worried person (such as a primary care physician's patient) determine whether his or her spouse may have a significant depressive disorder and one that could be associated with suicidal risk, whether a spouse might be developing dementia and be at serious risk for financial exploitation or otherwise for mismanaging the family's finances, or whether a child has depression and may be suicidal. The wider potential applications of non-face-to-face methods await continued exploration.

Several specific recommendations regarding non-face-to-face evaluations are as follows:

1. Forensic mental health professional centers with large case pools could study the limits of non-face-to-face data uses. This study could include when apparently accurate non-face-to-face diagnoses are not so accurate for whatever reasons, such as when apparent antisocial personality disorder is really a bipolar or schizophrenic disorder that is more treatable or when ostensibly credible records are not credible and cannot be relied on.

2. Men with a potential for violence, such as those arrested in domestic disturbance calls, could be evaluated via non-face-to-face methods to more carefully assess their violence potential and follow-up studies conducted. For example, the public records of such men could be examined for the possibility of antisocial personality disorder diagnoses and alcohol-related and other violence-related assessments to help determine those men most in need of intensive intervention services.

3. The beginning study here of the types of data (e.g., public records, medical records) that lead to diagnostic and other conclusions (opinions) in various types of cases (see the section "Forensic Practice: Information Sources and Evaluation Parameters") could be pursued further with larger, appropriately homogeneous collections of cases in various forensic contexts. This could help establish whether, in areas with a majority of the conclusion contribution coming from non-face-to-face data, similar conclusions could be reached if there were no additional face-to-face data; and, in such a context, which types of non-face-to-face data make conclusory differences and how often and under what circumstances such credible data are found.

4. Large bodies of literature on the effects of other non-face-to-face accessible data regarding an individual's expected functioning can be relevant to mental health professional conclusions about that person (e.g.,

Bowlby 1980; Gilbert 1992; Kerr and Bowen 1988; Toman 1976). These effects are based on information such as losses and the ages at which they occurred from infancy to the elderly years; sibling position; and other information on family constellation that can be gleaned from birth, death, marriage, and divorce data of the individual and his or her parents, siblings, and spouse(s). There are also the effects of serious crimes on victims who later might be the focus of a mental health professional evaluation for other reasons (Kilpatrick and Resnick 1993). The systematic exploration of these non-face-to-face data mines for forensic purposes remains for future study.

> Well, a psychiatrist can sometimes read minds, like the mind of a person wanting alcohol or of a person wanting a sexual encounter with a child. And courts sometimes admit such mind reading. But if we could read the court's mind, then that would really be something!
>
> —*The chapter authors*

References

Abel GG, Osborn C: The paraphilias: the extent and nature of sexually deviant and criminal behavior. Psychiatr Clin North Am 15:675–687, 1992

Agrimonti LM: The limitations of *Daubert* and its misapplication to quasi-scientific experts: a two year case review of *Daubert v. Merrell Dow Pharmaceuticals, Inc.*, 113 S. Ct. 2786 (1993). Washburn Law Journal 35:134–156, 1995

Allen JP, Litten RZ, Fertig JB, et al: Carbohydrate-deficient transferrin, gamma-glutamyltransferase and macrocytic volume as biomarkers of alcohol problems in women. Alcohol Clin Exp Res 24:492–496, 2000

American Academy of Pediatrics: Guidelines for the evaluation of sexual abuse of children. Pediatrics 87:254–259, 1991

American Academy of Psychiatry and the Law: Ethical Guidelines for the Practice of Forensic Psychiatry. Bloomfield, CT, American Academy of Psychiatry and the Law, 1995

American Academy of Psychiatry and the Law: Forensic Psychiatry Review Course. Bloomfield, CT, American Academy of Psychiatry and the Law, 1999

American Medical Association: Council on Scientific Affairs: Reports on Memories of Child Abuse. Chicago, IL, American Medical Association, 1994

American Medical Association: Directory of Practice Parameters: Titles, Sources, and Updates. Chicago, IL, American Medical Association, 1996

American Medical Association: Guides to the Evaluation of Permanent Impairment, 5th Edition. Chicago, IL, American Medical Association, 2000

American Psychiatric Association: Diagnostic and Statistical Manual of Mental Disorders, 3rd Edition. Washington, DC, American Psychiatric Association, 1980

American Psychiatric Association: Diagnostic and Statistical Manual of Mental Disorders, 3rd Edition, Revised. Washington, DC, American Psychiatric Association, 1987

American Psychiatric Association: Statement on Memories of Sexual Abuse. Washington, DC, American Psychiatric Association, 1993

American Psychiatric Association: Diagnostic and Statistical Manual of Mental Disorders, 4th Edition. Washington, DC, American Psychiatric Association, 1994

American Psychiatric Association: American Psychiatric Association Practice Guidelines: Practice Guidelines for Psychiatric Evaluation of Adults. Am J Psychiatry 152 (suppl):66–77, 1995a

American Psychiatric Association: Opinions of the Ethics Committee on the Principles of Medical Ethics: With Annotations Especially Applicable to Psychiatry. Washington, DC, American Psychiatric Association, 1995b

American Psychiatric Association: The Principles of Medical Ethics: With Annotations Especially Applicable to Psychiatry. Washington, DC, American Psychiatric Association, 1998

American Psychiatric Association: Diagnostic and Statistical Manual of Mental Disorders, 4th Edition, Text Revision. Washington, DC, American Psychiatric Association, 2000

Andreasen N, Flaum M: Characteristic symptoms of schizophrenia, in DSM-IV Sourcebook, Vol 1. Edited by Widiger TA, Frances AJ, Pincus HA, et al. Washington, DC, American Psychiatric Association, 1994, pp 351–392

Baer L, Cukor P, Jenike MA, et al: Pilot studies of telemedicine for patients with obsessive-compulsive disorder. Am J Psychiatry 152:1383–1385, 1995

Barefoot v Estelle, 463 US 880, 103 SCt 3383 (1983)

BMJ Publishing Group: Clinical Evidence. London, England, BMJ Publishing Group, June 2000

Bonnie RJ, Jefferies JC, Low PW: A Case Study in the Insanity Defense: The Trial of John W. Hinckley, Jr. New York, Foundation Press, 2000

Borum R: Improving the clinical practice of violence risk assessment: technology, guidelines and training. Am Psychol 51:945–956, 1996

Bowlby J: Attachment and Loss, Vol 3: Loss: Sadness and Depression. New York, Basic Books, 1980

Braunwald E, Fauci AS, Kasper DL, et al: The practice of medicine, in Harrison's Principles of Internal Medicine, 15th Edition. Edited by Braunwald E, Fauci AS, Kasper DL, et al. New York, McGraw-Hill, 2001, pp 1–5

Budd JM, Sievert ME, Schultz TR: Phenomena of retraction: reasons for retraction and citations to the publications. JAMA 280:296–297, 1998

Butcher JN, Dahlstrom WG, Graham JR, et al: Minnesota Multiphasic Personality Inventory—2 (MMPI-2) Manual for Administration and Scoring. Minneapolis, MN, University of Minnesota Press, 1989

Canadian Psychiatric Association: Position Statement: Adult Recovered Memories of Childhood Sexual Abuse. Ottawa, ON, Canadian Psychiatric Association, 1996

Champagne A, Shuman D, Whitaker E: An empirical examination of the use of expert witnesses in American courts. Jurimetrics Journal 31:375–392, 1991

Cleckley H: The Mask of Sanity. St. Louis, MO, Mosby, 1941

Cleckley H: The Mask of Sanity, 5th Edition. Augusta, GA, Emily S Cleckley, 1988

Cohen J: A coefficient of agreement for nominal scales. Educational and Psychological Measurement 20:37–46, 1960

Cohen J: Weighted kappa: nominal scale agreement with provision for scaled disagreement or partial credit. Psychol Bull 70:213–220, 1968

Daubert v Merrell Dow Pharmaceuticals, Inc., 509 US 579, 113 SCt 2786 (1993)

Davidson JRT, Foa EB (eds): Posttraumatic Stress Disorder: DSM-IV and Beyond. Washington, DC, American Psychiatric Press, 1993

Dawes RM, Faust D, Meehl PE: Clinical versus actuarial judgment. Science 243:1668–1674, 1989

Dvoskin JA, Heilbrun K: Risk assessment and release decision-making: toward resolving the great debate. J Am Acad Psychiatry Law 29:6–10, 2001

Dwyer J, Shih A: The ethics of tailoring the patient's chart. Psychiatr Serv 49:1309–1312, 1998

Edson R, Lavori P, Tracy K, et al: Interrater reliability issues in multicenter trials, part II: statistical procedures used in Department of Veterans Affairs Cooperative Study #394. Psychopharmacol Bull 33:59–67, 1997

Endicott J, Spitzer RL, Fleiss JL, et al: The Global Assessment Scale: a procedure for measuring the overall severity of psychiatric disturbance. Arch Gen Psychiatry 33:766–771, 1976

Epperson DL, Kaul JD, Huot SJ, et al: Minnesota Sex Offender Screening Tool Revised (MnSOST-R). St. Paul, MN, Department of Corrections, 2000. Available at: http://psych-server.iastate.edu./faculty/epperson/mnsost_download. Accessed December 18, 2001

Ferris JE, Sandercock J, Hoffman B, et al: Risk assessments for acute violence to third parties: a review of the literature. Can J Psychiatry 42:1051–1060, 1997

First MB, Spitzer RL, Gibbon M, et al: User's Guide for the Structured Clinical Interview for DSM-IV Axis I Disorders, Clinician Version, SCID-I. New York, Biometrics Research, New York State Psychiatric Institute, 1997

Fleiss JL, Cohen J: The equivalence of weighted kappa and the intraclass correlation coefficient as measures of reliability. Educational and Psychological Measurement 33:613–619, 1973

Followill v Emerson Electric Co., 234 Kan 791, 674 P2d 1050 (1984)

Folstein MJ, Folstein S, McHugh PR: Mini-Mental State: a practical method for grading the cognitive state of patients for the clinician. Psychiatry Res 2:189–198, 1975

Freedman D: False predictions of future dangerousness: error rates and Psychopathy Checklist—Revised. J Am Acad Psychiatry Law 29:89–95, 2001

Frye v United States, 293 F 1013 (DC Cir 1923)

Gilbert RM: Extraordinary Relationships: A New Way of Thinking about Human Interactions. Minneapolis, MN, Chronimed Publishing, 1992

Gless AJ: Some post-Daubert trial tribulations of a simple country judge: behavioral science evidence in trial courts. Behav Sci Law 13:261–291, 1995

Glezen LA, Lowery CA: Practical issues of program organization and operation, in Methadone Treatment for Opioid Dependence. Edited by Strain EC, Stitzer ML. Baltimore, MD, Johns Hopkins University Press, 1999, pp 223–250

Goldman HH, Skodol AE, Lave TR: Revising Axis V for DSM-IV: a review of measures of social functioning. Am J Psychiatry 149:1148–1156, 1992

Goldman L: Quantitative aspects of clinical reasoning, in Harrison's Principles of Internal Medicine, 13th Edition. Edited by Isselbacher KJ, Braunwald E, Wilson JD, et al. New York, McGraw-Hill, 1994, pp 43–48

Groth-Marnat G: Handbook of Psychological Assessment, 3rd Edition. New York, Wiley, 1999

Grove WM, Barden RC: Protecting the integrity of the legal system: the admissibility of testimony from mental health experts under *Daubert/Kumho* analyses. Psychology, Public Policy, and Law 2:224–242, 1999

Grove WM, Meehl PE: Comparative efficiency of informal (subjective, impressionistic) and formal (mechanical, algorithmic) prediction procedures: the clinical-statistical controversy. Psychology, Public Policy, and Law 2:293–323, 1996

Grove WM, Andreasen NC, McDonald-Scott P, et al: Reliability studies of psychiatric diagnosis: theory and practice. Arch Gen Psychiatry 38:408–413, 1981

Hall RCW: Global assessment of functioning. Psychosomatics 36:267–275, 1995

Hanson RK: The Development of a Brief Actuarial Risk Scale for Sexual Offense Recidivism (User Report 97-04.) Ottawa, ON, Department of the Solicitor General of Canada, 1997

Hanson RK, Harris A: Dynamic Predictors of Sexual Offense Recidivism (Document JS42-82/1998-01E). Ottawa, ON, Department of the Solicitor General of Canada, 1998. Available at: http://www.sgc.gc.ca/epub/corr/e199801b/e19801b.htm. Accessed June 2, 2000

Hanson RK, Harris A: The Sex Offender Need Assessment Rating (SONAR): A Method for Measuring Change in Risk Levels (Document JS42-88/1999E). Ottawa, ON, Department of the Solicitor General of Canada, 2000. Available at: http://www.sgc.gc.ca/Epub/Corr/e200001b/e200001b.htm. Accessed June 2, 2000

Hanson RK, Thornton D: Static 99: Improving Actuarial Risk Assessments for Sex Offenders (Document 1999-02). Ottawa, ON, Department of the Solicitor General of Canada, 1999. Available at: http://www.sgc.gc.ca/Epub/Corr/e199902/e199902.htm. Accessed June 29, 2000

Hare R: The Hare Psychopathy Checklist—Revised Manual. Toronto, ON, Multi-Health Systems, 1991

Hart SD, Kropp PR, Hare RD: Performance of male psychopaths following conditional release from prison. J Consult Clin Psychol 56:227–232, 1988

Harris GT, Rice ME, Cormier CA: Psychopathy and violent recidivism. Law Hum Behav 15:625–637, 1991

Hartmaier SL, Sloane PD, Guess HA, et al: The MDS Cognition Scale: a valid instrument for identifying and staging nursing home residents with dementia using the Minimum Data Set. J Am Geriatr Soc 42:1173–1179, 1994

Hartmaier SL, Sloane PD, Guess HA, et al: Validation of the Minimum Data Set Cognitive Performance Scale: agreement with the Mini-Mental State Examination. J Gerontol A Biol Sci Med Sci 50A:M128–M133, 1995

Hasin D, Paykin A: Drinkers in the community. J Stud Alcohol 60:181–187, 1999

Helzer JE: Psychoactive substance abuse and its relation to dependence, in DSM-IV Sourcebook, Vol 1. Edited by Widiger TA, Frances AJ, Pincus HA, et al. Washington, DC, American Psychiatric Association, 1994, pp 21–32

Hilsenroth MJ, Ackerman SJ, Blagys MD, et al: Reliability and validity of DSM-IV Axis V. Am J Psychiatry 157:1858–1863, 2000

Hutchinson CT, Blend JE: Preclusion of scientific evidence after *Daubert*. Shepard's Expert and Scientific Evidence 1:673–697, 1994

Imwinkelried EJ: The next step after *Daubert:* developing a similarly epistemological approach to ensuring the reliability of nonscientific expert testimony. Cardozo Law Review 15:2271–2294, 1994

Isselbacher KJ, Braunwald E, Wilson JD, et al: The practice of medicine, in Harrison's Principles of Internal Medicine, 13th Edition. Edited by Isselbacher KJ, Braunwald E, Wilson JD, et al. New York, McGraw-Hill, 1994, pp 1–6

Janofsky JS, Vandewalle MB, Rappeport JR: Defendants pleading insanity: an analysis of outcome. Bulletin of the American Academy of Psychiatry and the Law 17:203–211, 1989

Janofsky JS, Dunn MH, Roskes EJ, et al: Insanity defense pleas in Baltimore City: an analysis of outcome. Am J Psychiatry 153:1464–1468, 1996

Jenkins PH, Howell RJ: Child sexual abuse examinations: proposed guidelines for a standard of care. Bulletin of the American Academy of Psychiatry and the Law 22:5–17, 1994

Jesilow P, Geis G, Pontell H: Fraud by physicians against Medicaid. JAMA 266:3318–3322, 1991

Joint Commission on the Accreditation of Healthcare Organizations: SBHC: 1999–2000 Standards for Behavioral Health Care. Oakbrook Terrace, IL, Joint Commission on the Accreditation of Healthcare Organizations, 1999

Jorgenson LM, Wahl KM: Psychiatrist as expert witnesses in sexual harassment cases under *Daubert* and *Kumho.* Psychiatric Annals 30:390–396, 2000

Kaplan HI, Sadock BH: Synopsis of Psychiatry: Behavioral Sciences/Clinical Psychiatry. New York, Williams & Wilkins, 1998

Kendell RE: Clinical validity, in The Validity of Psychiatric Diagnosis. Edited by Robins LN, Barrett JE. New York, Raven, 1989, pp 305–323

Kendler KD: Setting boundaries for psychiatric disorders. Am J Psychiatry 156:1845–1848, 1999

Kerr ME, Bowen M: Family Evaluation: An Approach Based on Bowen Theory. New York, WW Norton, 1988

Kilpatrick DG, Resnick HS: Posttraumatic stress disorder associated with exposure to criminal victimization in clinical and community populations, in Posttraumatic Stress Disorder: DSM-IV and Beyond. Edited by Davidson JRT, Foa EB. Washington, DC, American Psychiatric Press, 1993, pp 113–143

Klein SR, Manning WL: Telemedicine and the law. Journal of Healthcare Information Management 9:35–40, 1995

Korenman SG, Berk R, Wenger NS, et al: Evaluation of the research norms of scientists and administrators responsible for academic research integrity. JAMA 278:41–47, 1998

Krauss DA, Sales BD: The problem of "helpfulness" in applying *Daubert* to expert testimony: child custody determinations in family law as an exemplar. Psychology, Public Policy, and Law 5:79–99, 1999

Kumho Tire Co. v Carmichael, 119 SCt 1167 (1999)

Lacoursiere RB: Excluding a psychoactive substance use disorder in forensic psychiatric evaluations. J Forensic Sci 34:64–73, 1989

Lacoursiere RB: Diverse motives for fictitious posttraumatic stress disorder. J Trauma Stress 6:137–145, 1993

Lacoursiere RB: Sexually violent predator evaluations: the practical practice. Psychology, Public Policy and Law (in press)

Leckman JF, Sholomskas D, Thompson D, et al: Best estimate of lifetime psychiatric diagnosis: a methodological study. Arch Gen Psychiatry 39:879–883, 1982

Levine J: The relative value of consultation, questionnaires and laboratory investigation in the identification of excessive alcohol consumption. Alcohol Alcohol 25:539–553, 1990

Littleton v Good Samaritan Hospital and Health Center, 39 Ohio St 3d 86 (1988)

Mark DB: Decision making in clinical medicine, in Harrison's Principles of Internal Medicine, 15th Edition. Edited by Braunwald E, Fauci AS, Kasper DL, et al. New York, McGraw-Hill, 2001, pp 8–14

Marlowe DB: A hybrid decision framework for evaluation psychometric evidence. Behav Sci Law 13:207–228, 1995

Matarazzo JD: The reliability of psychiatric and psychological diagnosis. Clin Psychol Rev 3:103–145, 1983

Meehl PE: Clinical Versus Statistical Prediction. Minneapolis, University of Minnesota Press, 1954

Menninger KA: A Manual for Psychiatric Case Study, 2nd Edition. New York, Grune & Stratton, 1962

Monahan J: Violence prediction: the last 20 years and the next 20 years. Criminal Justice and Behavior 23:107–120, 1996

Morihisa JM, Rosse RB, Cross CD, et al: Laboratory and other diagnostic tests in psychiatry, in The American Psychiatric Press Textbook of Psychiatry, 3rd Edition. Edited by Hales RE, Yudofsky SC, Talbott JA. Washington, DC, American Psychiatric Press, 1999, pp 281–314

Morris JN, Fries BE, Mehr DR, et al: MDS Cognitive Performance Scale. J Gerontol A Biol Sci Med Sci 49:M174–M182, 1994

Nicholi AM: History and mental status, in The Harvard Guide to Psychiatry, 3rd Edition. Edited by Nicholi AM. Cambridge, MA, Belknap Press, 1999, pp 26–39

Nicholson RA, Norwood S: The quality of forensic psychological assessments, reports, and testimony: acknowledging the gap between promise and practice. Law Hum Behav 24:9–24, 2000

Pfohl B, Blum N, Zimmerman M: Structured Interview for DSM-IV Personality: SIDP-IV. Washington, DC, American Psychiatric Press, 1997

Prosser RL: Alteration of medical records submitted for medicolegal review. JAMA 267:2630–2631, 1992

Quinsey VL, Harris GT, Rice ME, et al: Violent Offenders: Appraising and Managing Risk. Washington, DC, American Psychological Association, 1998

Rantz MJ, Zwygart-Stauffacher M, Popejoy LL, et al: The Minimum Data Set: no longer just for clinical assessment. Annals of Long-Term Care 7:354–360, 1999

Rappeport JR: Reasonable medical certainty. Bulletin of the American Academy of Psychiatry and the Law 13:5–15, 1985

Resnick PJ: Malingering of posttraumatic disorders, in Clinical Assessment of Malingering and Deception. Edited by Rogers R. New York, Guilford, 1997, pp 130–152

Resnick PJ: Risk assessment for violence. Course presented at the 151st annual meeting of the American Psychiatric Association, Toronto, ON, Canada, May 30–June 4, 1998

Reynaud M, Schwan R, Loiseaux-Meunier MN, et al: Patients admitted to emergency services for drunkenness: moderate alcohol users or harmful drinkers? Am J Psychiatry 158:96–99, 2001

Robins LN: Epidemiology: reflections on the testing the validity of psychiatric interviews. Arch Gen Psychiatry 42:918–924, 1985

Rogers R, Mitchell CN: Mental Health Experts and the Criminal Courts. Scarborough, ON, Canada, Carswell, 1991

Sackett D: A primer on the precision and accuracy of the clinical examination. JAMA 267:2638–2644, 1992

Salaspuro M: Carbohydrate-deficient transferrin as compared to other markers of alcoholism: a systematic review. Alcohol 19:261–271, 1999

Schuckit MA: DSM-IV criteria for abuse and dependence: basis for a field trial, in DSM-IV Sourcebook, Vol 4. Edited by Widiger TA, Frances AJ, Pincus HA, et al. Washington, DC, American Psychiatric Association, 1998, pp 69–84

Scrignar CB: Post-Traumatic Stress Disorder: Diagnosis, Treatment and Legal Issues, 3rd Edition. New Orleans, LA, Bruno Press, 1996

Serin RC: Diagnosis of psychopathy with and without an interview. J Clin Psychol 49:367–372, 1993

Sexual Predator Act, Kan Stat Ann 59-29a01–59-29a14, 1994

Shuman DW, Sales BD: The impact of Daubert and its progeny on the admissibility of behavioral and social science evidence. Psychology, Public Policy, and Law 5:3–15, 1999

Simon RI, Sadoff RL: Psychiatric Malpractice: Cases and Comments for Clinicians. Washington, DC, American Psychiatric Press, 1992

Skinner HA, Holt S, Sheu WJ, et al: Clinical versus laboratory detection of alcohol abuse: the alcohol clinical index. BMJ 292:1703–1708, 1986

Slovenko R: Psychiatric opinion without examination. Journal of Psychiatry and Law 28:103–143, 2000a

Slovenko R: From *Frye* to *Daubert* and beyond. Journal of Psychiatry and 28:411–444, 2000b

Smith NL: Who gets sick the most? The role of stress, depression and anxiety in physical illness. Paper presented at Kansas Medical Education Foundation Combined Grand Rounds, Topeka, KS, November 6, 1999

Sobell LC, Agrawal S, Sobell MB: Utility of liver function tests for screening "alcohol abusers" who are not severely dependent on alcohol. Subst Use Misuse 34:1723–1732, 1999

Spar JE, Garb AS: Assessing competency to make a will. Am J Psychiatry 149:169–174, 1992

Spitzer RL: Psychiatric diagnosis: are clinicians still necessary? Compr Psychiatry 24:399–410, 1983

Spitzer RL, Wakefield DSW: DSM-IV diagnostic criterion for clinical significance: does it help solve the false positives problem? Am J Psychiatry 156:1856–1864, 1999

Spitzer RL, Cohen J, Fleiss JL, et al: Quantification of agreement in psychiatric diagnosis. Arch Gen Psychiatry 17:83–87, 1967

Spitzer RL, Kroenke K, Williams JBW, et al: Validation and utility of a self-report version of PRIME-MD: the PHQ Primary Care Study. JAMA 282:1737–1744, 1999

Sreenivasan S, Kirkish P, Garrick T: Actuarial risk assessment models: a review of critical issues related to violence and sex-offender recidivism assessments. J Am Acad Psychiatry Law 28:438–448, 2000

Strasburger LH, Gutheil TG, Brodsky A: On wearing two hats: role conflict in serving as both psychotherapist and expert witness. Am J Psychiatry 154:448–456, 1997

Toman W: Family Constellation: Its Effects on Personality and Social Behavior, 3rd Edition. New York, Springer, 1976

Toole JF, Link AS, Smith JH: Disability in US presidents report: recommendations and commentaries by the Working Group. The Working Group on Presidential Disability. Arch Neurol 54:1256–1264, 1997

Tracy K, Adler LA, Rotrosen J, et al: Interrater reliability issues in multicenter trials, part I: theoretical concepts and operational procedures used in Department of Veterans Affairs Cooperative Study #394. Psychopharmacol Bull 33:53–57, 1997

United States v Downing, 733 F2d 1224 (3d Cir 1985)

U.S. Department of Justice: Bureau of Justice Statistics Special Report: DWI offenders under correctional supervision (Document No NCJ 172212). Washington, DC, U.S. Department of Justice, June 1999

Wallace-Capretta S: Pardoned Offenders in Canada: A Statistical Analysis. Ottawa, ON, Canada, Department of the Solicitor General of Canada, 2000

White SG, Cawood JS: Threat management of stalking cases, in The Psychology of Stalking: Clinical and Forensic Perspectives. Edited by Meloy JR. San Diego, CA, Academic Press, 1998, pp 295–315

Whiting v Boston Edison Co., 891 F Supp 12 (D Mass 1995)

Widiger TA, Frances AJ, Pincus HA, et al (eds): DSM-IV Sourcebook, Vol 1. Washington, DC, American Psychiatric Association, 1994

Widiger TA, Frances AJ, Pincus HA, et al (eds): DSM-IV Sourcebook, Vol 2. Washington, DC, American Psychiatric Association, 1996

Widiger TA, Frances AJ, Pincus HA, et al (eds): DSM-IV Sourcebook, Vol 3. Washington, DC, American Psychiatric Association, 1997

Widiger TA, Cadoret R, Hare RD, et al: DSM-IV antisocial personality disorder field trial, in DSM-IV Sourcebook, Vol 4. Edited by Widiger TA, Frances AJ, Pincus HA, et al. Washington, DC, American Psychiatric Association, 1998a, pp 907–936

Widiger TA, Frances AJ, Pincus HA, et al (eds): DSM-IV Sourcebook, Vol 4. Washington, DC, American Psychiatric Association, 1998b

Winick BJ, LaFond JQ (eds): Special theme: sex offenders: scientific, legal and policy perspectives. Psychology, Public Policy and Law 4:1–570, 1998

Wong S: The Criminal and Institutional Behavior of Psychopaths (Report 1984–87). Ottawa, ON, Canada, Ministry of the Solicitor General of Canada, 1984

Youngner JS: The scientific misconduct process: a scientist's view from the inside. JAMA 279:62–64, 1998

Zatzick DF: Managed care and psychiatry, in The American Psychiatric Press Textbook of Psychiatry, 3rd Edition. Edited by Hales RD, Yudofsky SC, Talbott JA. Washington, DC, American Psychiatric Press, 1999, pp 1645–1654

10

Validating Retrospective Assessments

An Overview of Research Models

Richard Rogers, Ph.D., A.B.P.P.

A fundamental misassumption is that clinical evaluations are easily separable into current and retrospective time perspectives. This artificial dichotomy gives rise to false comfort for current assessments and exaggerated concerns for retrospective assessments. Current assessments are supposed to be easily confirmed by clinical observations and collateral sources. In direct contrast, retrospective assessments are presumed to be fraught with temporal distortions and the lack of observable data. Although intuitively appealing, this dichotomic conceptualization belies the multiple-time perspective of most clinical evaluations.

What are putative current clinical assessments? In the realm of symptoms and memories, *current* refers specifically to *past* experiences. Depending on the time framework, a current assessment may reflect a person's functioning during an indefinite (e.g., prior episode) or arbitrary (e.g., the last month or week) period. Past experiences are central to current assessments. Certainly, many mental health professionals would question diagnostic data based simply on the past day, likely doubting the adequacy of their sampling and the stability of their findings.

Circumscribed exceptions do occur in which current assessments are limited to *current* abilities. Especially in intellectual and neuropsychological evaluations, testing provides a contemporaneous appraisal of cognitive functioning. Even in these cases, psychologists and other mental health professionals often seek retrospective information to confirm whether these appraisals are representative of general functioning. As an example of the potential dangers in overreliance on current evaluations, Carnes et al. (1987) found important diurnal variations in patients with dementia.

What about supposedly retrospective assessments? Retrospective evaluations typically encompass current data via systematic comparisons and clinical observations. Parallel inquiries about past and current episodes provide a standardized method of evaluating retrospective symptoms and their correlates. In the context of retrospective insanity evaluations, Rogers (1986; Rogers and Shuman 2000) recommended that mental health professionals systematically compare past (i.e., the time of the alleged offense) and current symptoms to better understand retrospective presentations. Even without systematic comparisons, mental health professionals scrutinize the reporting of past episodes with respect to the patients' current sincerity and present emotions about their past symptoms.

Redefining Time Perspectives for Clinical Assessments

The past-current dichotomization appears to have limited value in describing the temporal dimensions of clinical and forensic evaluations. As an alternative, I propose a tripartite conceptualization of time that considers duration (i.e., whether the evaluation concerns an episode or an occurrence) and observability (i.e., whether currently observable). The three alternatives are composed of the following:

1. *Ongoing episode*, in which psychopathology or impairment extends from the past to the current time
2. *Prior episode*, in which psychopathology or impairment is limited to a defined past period and does not extend to the current time
3. *Prior occurrence*, in which specific past experience has a very limited duration

The tripartite model encompasses most temporal dimensions found in clinical evaluations. A useful distinction is made between episodes and occurrences. Episodes typically entail a diagnosable mental disorder or definable syndrome in which symptom patterns can be evaluated and corroborated. In contrast, an occurrence focuses on a specific event that is typically very circumscribed and may not be associated with psychological impairment. In operationalizing these terms, a prior occurrence is reserved for a noteworthy event that does not result in a prior episode. For example, a sexual assault may be designated as a prior occurrence or prior episode depending on whether the resulting impairment constitutes a recognized pattern of symptoms and associated features.

Ongoing episodes, prior episodes, and prior occurrences pose different challenges for clinicians. Ongoing episodes have substantial advantages in the availability of symptoms for clinical observation and testing. However, evaluations of ongoing episodes are complicated by variations in the episodes and reactions to external events or stressors. Appraisals of prior episodes are dependent on the quality of contemporaneously recorded data (e.g., past hospital records) and retrospective accounts. Prior occurrences (e.g., intoxication or a traumatic experience) are often challenging because of the typically poor documentation and reliance predominantly on retrospective reporting. Especially under stressful conditions, the comprehensiveness of the retrospective accounts is likely diminished.

In this chapter, I provide an overview of different research models for validating retrospective evaluations.[1] I limit its focus by emphasizing clinical applications for the accurate appraisal of psychological impairment and mental disorders. The chapter is intended to serve both seasoned practitioners and applied researchers. For practitioners the chapter provides a framework for estimating the clinical value of different methods of retrospective evaluations. For researchers the chapter presents research paradigms, delineating their respective strengths and limitations.

Research Models for Retrospective Assessments

I have categorized four research models that are used in retrospective clinical studies. Two paradigms (i.e., corroborative model and analogue model) have been researched extensively. The remaining two paradigms (i.e., time-lapse model and biological-marker model) are innovative approaches with unrealized research opportunities. For each model, I provide 1) a description, 2) recent examples of forensic or clinical research, and 3) a critique of its relative strengths and weaknesses.

---

[1]The term *retrospective evaluations* is used in this chapter to describe assessments of prior episodes and prior occurrences.

Corroborative Model

Description

The bulk of clinical research on retrospective evaluations relies on the corroborative model. The primary focus of the corroborative model is the collection of independent sources to confirm or disconfirm retrospective accounts by the evaluatee. The concept of *independent sources* requires explication. In most studies family members are enlisted to provide their observations and reports. However, family members may simply be reiterating what the evaluatee told them about specific symptoms (e.g., hallucinations). In this case, we are studying the evaluatee's consistency rather than providing truly independent corroboration. Both researchers and practitioners should carefully discriminate three categories of data: 1) behavioral observations (e.g., staying awake all night or attempting suicide), 2) inferences based on behavior (e.g., locking bedroom door, which suggests paranoid thoughts), and 3) derivative reports (e.g., recounting what the evaluatee told the informant[2] about symptoms or treatment). Within this schema, behavioral observations are likely to be more independent than are derivative reports; inferences are typically unwarranted.

An der Heiden and Krumm (1991) provided an excellent overview of the corroborative model and its relevance to retrospective evaluations. They observed that efforts toward establishing lifetime diagnoses tended either to assume the accuracy of patients' recall or to apply the corroborative model. The corroborative model typically involves either informant interviews or record reviews.

The corroborative model has been used extensively to develop specific measures of retrospective functioning. Clinical examples include the following:

- The Wender Utah Rating Scale (Ward et al. 1993) was developed for retrospectively diagnosing attention-deficit/hyperactivity disorder (ADHD) in adults. On ratings of behaviors spanning more than two decades, correlations between parents and adults with ADHD were in the low to moderate range ($r=0.41$).
- The Biographical Personality Interview (BPI; von Zerssen et al. 1998) compared interview notes from an unstructured interview (BPI) with

---

[2]Utterances from the evaluatee may be either behavioral observations or derivative statements. As an example of behavioral observation, a person with major depression may exclaim, "I cannot stand it anymore." As an example of a derivative statement, the same person may report, "I have been taking my Prozac every day."

case notes from the patients' records. The unstandardized nature of the BPI militates against standard comparisons.

- The Interview for the Retrospective Assessment of the Onset of Schizophrenia has been extensively studied to examine the onset of symptoms during the first episode of schizophrenia (see Maurer and Hafner 1995). Problems were observed in confirming patients' accounts via informants, with most symptoms achieving only modest κ coefficients (<0.40).

The corroborative model is likely to offer intuitive appeal in gathering as much clinical data as possible from multiple sources. The corroborative model is similar to Spitzer's (1983) Longitudinal Expert Evaluation Using All Data (LEAD) paradigm, except that it focuses on retrospective assessment. Like the LEAD, its inherent limitation is the establishment of truly independent sources of clinical data.

Examples in Forensic Research

In forensic evaluations, the corroborative model has served as the standard for assembling relevant data from a variety of sources. In the context of retrospective insanity evaluations, Rogers and Shuman (2000) recommended that corroborative data (i.e., collateral interviews and records) should constitute the standard of forensic practice. Surprisingly, this emphasis on the corroborative model for forensic practice has not led to its widespread use in forensic research.

A major research effort has been validation of the Psychopathy Checklist (PCL; Hare 1985) and its revised edition (PCL-R; Hare 1991) for both the categorization of offenders and the determination of their risks for further violence and recidivism. The PCL-R requires the use of collateral information, especially records, in its administration. However, its original validation also relied on comparisons with independent sources of data. For example, the PCL was tested against interview and case history information (R. D. Hare, "The Psychopathy Checklist," unpublished manuscript, University of British Columbia, Vancouver, BC, 1985) and achieved a high correlation ($r=0.80$). In addition, Wong (1988) compared PCL ratings with extensive file information and found that the two sources of data had a moderately high correlation ($r=0.74$). More recently, Grann et al. (1998) found a high intraclass correlation (ICC=0.89) between interview and file data on 40 male offenders. As expected, the correlations were higher for antisocial behaviors (ICC=0.89) than for core personality traits (ICC=0.69).

Rogers and Wettstein (1985) administered the Schedule for Affective Disorders and Schizophrenia—Change Version (SADS-C; Spitzer and Endicott 1978b) to forensic outpatients, most of whom had been found not guilty by reason of insanity (NGRI). Multiple SADS-C interviews compared its results to symptom ratings (Symptom Checklist-90—Revised) and file information. Longitudinal data were gathered over an 18-month period with the focus on forensic patients' functioning during the past 3 months. As a study of ongoing episodes, the results suggested a moderate convergence between measures but with considerable variability across time periods.

Critique

A key issue in using the corroborative model is whether high levels of agreement are achievable from different data sources. It is instructive to examine the research findings for personality disorders, which are presumed to be both stable and observable. Comparisons of patient and informant interviews yielded highly variable results. Studies that used the Personality Disorder Examination (Loranger 1988) found both moderately high levels of diagnostic agreement ($r=0.76$; Pilkonis et al. 1991) and negligible agreement (median $\kappa=-0.01$; Riso et al. 1994). For the Structured Interview for DSM-III Personality Disorders (Pfohl et al. 1982), only a modest convergence was found between patient and collateral interviews for symptom ratings (median $r=0.29$), with essentially no agreement about diagnosis (median $\kappa=0.00$; Zimmerman et al. 1988). In light of these data, practitioners and researchers should not expect high levels of agreement, especially for prior episodes and prior occurrences.

The corroborative model should minimize its reliance on traditional interviews and other unstandardized methods. A pervasive problem with traditional interviews is the uncontrolled variability in 1) the wording of clinical inquiries, 2) the sequencing of clinical inquiries, and 3) the recording of the evaluatee's responses. This uncontrolled variability reduces unnecessarily the scientific rigor that is needed to validate retrospective evaluations.

An important caveat for the corroborative model is the avoidance of unnecessary method variance. *Method variance* refers to the variability in conceptualization and measurement of clinical constructs. For example, the Minnesota Multiphasic Personality Inventory—2 (MMPI-2) Psychopathic Deviance scale shares very little, besides its name, with psychopathy as measured by the PCL-R (Hare 1991). The use of dissimilar measures (e.g., multiscale inventories and structured interviews) introduces substantial method variance that likely confounds the results and their interpretation.

The best use of the corroborative model involves standardized measures, such as structured interviews (see Rogers 2001). The standardization provides a systematic method of studying the stability of the evaluatee's retrospective account. Likewise, it allows direct comparisons between the evaluatee's account and informants' reports based on the same clinical inquiries. In this same vein the standardization provides an objective method of recording clinical data from each source.

Time-Lapse Model

Description

The time-lapse model is an adaptation of test-retest reliability that is applied to the reproducibility of retrospective diagnosis and symptoms. In the classic test-retest paradigm patients are readministered identical measures after a predetermined period; both administrations focus on the present. In a time-lapse model the first administration is a *current* evaluation of an ongoing episode (e.g., June and July 1998). After a substantial interval the second administration is a *retrospective* evaluation of the same period covered by the first administration (i.e., June and July 1998).

Diagnostic studies with test-retest paradigms sometimes approximate the time-lapse model. For example, Loranger et al. (1994) examined Axis II symptomatology during the past 5 years on the Personality Disorder Examination (Loranger 1988). His readministration after a 6-month interval approximated the time-lapse model by covering nearly the same time period (i.e., 54 of 60 months). Likewise, Mazure and Gershon (1979) evaluated the stability of lifetime diagnosis on the SADS-C (Spitzer and Endicott 1978b) after a 6.7-month interval. These studies suggest the potential utility of time-lapse models but lack the following specification: the readministrations do not cover the identical time period as the first administration.

In evaluating prior occurrences, Fitchen et al. (1991) described the importance of systematic comparisons between current and retrospective accounts. They noted that a person's attributes about the event (see McFarland and Ross 1987) or his or her present circumstances (see Widom 1989) may substantially influence retrospective recall. Although their research does not correspond directly to the time-lapse model,[3] their results suggest that retrospective accounts may vary substantially from contemporaneous reports.

---

[3]Rather than readministrations to the same participants, they used two similar groups to compare current and retrospective accounts.

Examples in Forensic Research

The time-lapse model has direct relevance to prior episodes (e.g., insanity and personal injury evaluations) and prior occurrences (e.g., sexual harassment) that are often addressed in forensic evaluations. Despite its relevance, most forensic research has not used the time-lapse model.

McMillan et al. (1996) conducted a study with implications for forensic practice. They examined closed-head injuries and the length of posttraumatic amnesia based on patients' contemporaneous and retrospective accounts. They found that the two accounts were highly correlated ($r=0.87$). Unexpectedly, the retrospective estimates correlated more highly than did contemporaneous accounts with two external indices: 1) current emotional problems ($r=0.37$ and 0.24, respectively) and 2) ability to cope with work ($r=0.36$ and 0.29, respectively). The implications of this research for disability and personal injury evaluations have yet to be fully explored.

Critique

The time-lapse model is distinguished by both its experimental rigor and its clinical relevance. The capacity of persons with mental disorders to recall prior episodes can be assessed systematically via individual comparisons of symptoms and associated features. These systematic comparisons allow researchers and practitioners to examine the recall accuracy in clinical populations. In particular, symptoms and associated features may increase or decrease in salience. The time-lapse model provides a standard method of appraising these differences. When combined with structured interviews, the time-lapse model minimizes variations caused by the wording of clinical inquiries and the coding of responses (Rogers 2001).

The time-lapse model is conceptualized as a systematic method of assessing retrospective accuracy[4] in clinical and forensic populations. However, the model is not limited to persons with mental disorders or defendants. For example, the model can easily be adapted to the examination of informants and collateral sources (Bogler et al. 1998). Moreover, the retrospective accuracy of recalling prior occurrences could be systematically evaluated for different types (e.g., offenders, victims, and witnesses) of participants.

One limitation of the time-lapse model is that the *reasons* for discrep-

---

[4]As a point of clarification, *retrospective accuracy* does not suggest that a person's perspective is necessarily veridical; rather, it addresses whether the recall corresponds with contemporaneous accounts.

ancies between contemporaneous and retrospective accounts are not easily explained. Like the corroborative model, it focuses primarily on the potential for accuracy rather than on the reasons for inaccuracy. In forensic assessments evaluatees may have different motivations for distorting their retrospective accounts. In this regard, the analogue model has methodological advantages.

Analogue Model

Description

Analogue models are used in retrospective studies to address how specific factors may influence the recall or reporting of clinically relevant data. Within an experimental or quasi-experimental paradigm, participants are assigned to explicit experimental conditions to study the specific effects of those conditions. More specifically, research participants are exposed to a carefully controlled stimulus (e.g., a film of an automobile accident) under operationally defined experimental conditions (e.g., witnesses in a criminal investigation). After a predetermined interval, their accuracy at recall can be measured precisely. A primary advantage of analogue research is the ability to isolate and study how specific conditions affect patients' recall or reporting.

Examples in Forensic Research

A primary example of analogue research is the retrospective examination of eyewitness testimony. This extensive body of research focuses on memory accuracy and recall for salient prior occurrences, especially observations of criminal activity. Analogue design also has been extensively applied to response styles (e.g., malingering) in forensic populations. Although the predominant thrust of this research has focused on ongoing episodes, emerging research has addressed prior episodes and prior occurrences.

Eyewitness research. Research on eyewitness testimony (Cutler and Penrod 1995; Martin-Miller and Fremouw 1995; Penrod et al. 1995) provides a pellucid example of analogue research applied to prior occurrences. A common research design is for a particular crime to be staged under different witnessing conditions. Typically with the use of videotape, participants are randomly assigned to different experimental conditions. The time framework of "witnessing of the crime" is conceptualized as a prior occurrence. Participants' accuracy and confidence in their accuracy are tested against specific conditions. A sampling of the various conditions that have been extensively researched includes the following:

- Characteristics of the witness (e.g., age, race/ethnicity, and sex)
- Characteristics of the perpetrator (e.g., race/ethnicity, sex, attractiveness, and use of disguises)
- Characteristics of the crime (e.g., length of witnessing time, witnessing condition, and presence of a weapon)
- Potential confounds (e.g., elapsed time since witnessing and misleading questions)

Most research on eyewitness memories is limited to the investigation of several independent variables from one or two of these general categories. More complex analyses, including a large set of independent variables and their interactions, are frequently not practical, given the immense sample requirements for such analyses.

Malingering research.   Analogue studies on detection of malingering and other response styles constitute another major initiative in forensic research. The primary framework is ongoing episodes, although a few studies have focused on prior episodes. Because participants are asked to simulate a response style (e.g., a mental disorder for malingering), this type of analogue research is commonly known as a *simulation design*. The simulation design often augments the strict analogue design with one or more clinical comparison samples. These samples generally are designated as "comparison" groups because they often are not assigned randomly to experimental conditions but are typically samples of convenience used to test the generalizability of the results to mentally disordered populations.

The MMPI-2 and malingering provide a useful illustration of the analogue design applied to ongoing episodes. In a meta-analysis of the MMPI-2, Rogers et al. (1994) found that 13 of 14 studies were analogue-based research. Depending on the samples and the specific conditions, these studies yielded highly disparate findings. This study also showed the need for clinical comparison groups. When simulators were compared with only nonmalingering control subjects, the results appeared to be artificially inflated.[5]

Goodness (1999), in the context of feigned insanity, exemplified the potential utility of analogue studies specifically for the evaluation of prior episodes. For research purposes[6] she modified the Structured Interview of Reported Symptoms (SIRS; Rogers 1992; Rogers et al. 1992) so that ques-

---

[5]Beyond inflated results, the absence of clinical comparison samples is conceptually inelegant. If the purpose of malingering research is to distinguish feigned from genuine disorders, then both conditions need to be represented.

tions would be specifically framed for the time of the offense. Two observations are noteworthy: 1) prior episodes are likely to require different scoring to maximize classification, but 2) standard scoring produced moderately positive results.

Frederick et al. (1995) adapted an analogue-based method[7] for evaluating prior occurrences with defendants claiming amnesia to the alleged crime. Detailed information from the index crime is presented to the defendant in forced-choice paradigm. Persons feigning amnesia may not realize the level of performance expected from a person with no memory of the event and score unrealistically low (i.e., below chance probabilities) on the forced choices. As noted by Denney (1996), the forced-choice alternatives should be tested on a normative sample to ensure that items have a comparable likelihood of being selected.

Critique

A critical analysis of the analogue model relies heavily on constructs of internal and external validity (Kazdin 1992). The analogue model is distinguished by its attention to internal validity (e.g., careful operationalization of variables, precise experimental conditions, and rigorous methodology). These enhancements of internal validity are typically achieved at the expense of its external validity (Rogers and Cruise 1998). Simply put, the experimental rigor (internal validity) limits real-world applications (external validity). The following paragraphs examine the limitations of analogue research with examples from eyewitness research and malingering.

Critique of eyewitness. Yuille and Cutshall (1986), in collaboration with investigating officers, performed a naturalistic study of eyewitness accuracy and vulnerability to leading questions. Based on a robbery-homicide in Vancouver, British Columbia, with 21 witnesses, Yuille and Cutshall found that witnesses were moderately accurate at describing persons and comparatively more accurate at describing their actions and relevant objects during the crime. Follow-up data on 13 witnesses after a substantial interval (4–5 months) raised questions about the generalizability of analogue research to real-world applications. First, witnesses did not experi-

---

[6]Insufficient data are available for clinical use; no modifications of copyrighted materials are allowed without appropriate permission.

[7]This method is described as *symptom validity testing* (see Rogers 1997). Frederick et al. (1995) did not formally test symptom validity by analogue design but creatively applied this method to prior occurrences.

ence a substantial decrement in their delayed recalls of the crime, as suggested by analogue research. Second, unlike analogue-based studies, leading questions appeared to affect recall in only a minority of witnesses.

The Yuille and Cutshall article, as a single study with limited participants, does not disprove the vast body on analogue research (see also Yuille and Daylen 1998). However, it raises a key question yet unanswered by social scientists: "Is analogue-based eyewitness research relevant to the courtroom?" It also urges us to question leading experts in eyewitness research (Kassin et al. 1989) when they 1) achieve a consensus about the importance of their own analogue research and 2) advocate its direct application to courtrooms. A critical need exists for more naturalistic research to test further the real-world applications of eyewitness analogue research.

Critique of malingering.   Malingering research has clearly shown the potential drawbacks of analogue designs. An inherent problem is the simulation-malingering paradox (Rogers and Cavanaugh 1983). Simply put, research participants are asked to comply with directions to fake in order to study persons who fake when asked to comply. The generalizability across these dissimilar conditions cannot be assumed but must be tested empirically.

Rogers and Cruise (1998) examined how analogue research on malingering may not capture conditions faced by actual evaluatees. In a factorial study they evaluated the effects of experimental conditions on the malingered performances. Two issues, rarely considered in analogue research on malingering, appeared germane: 1) the presence of negative incentives (i.e., adverse consequences for being detected) and 2) a relevant scenario (i.e., a situation with which many participants could identify). Negative incentives for "caught" malingerers are especially salient in actual forensic evaluations. In criminal cases the adverse consequences are often lengthy incarcerations and possibly death. In civil matters the detrimental effects may include cessation of services or benefits, an unfavorable verdict, and even criminal charges of fraud.

Research on the M Test (Beaber et al. 1985) illustrates the dangers of relying solely on analogue designs for the validation of a malingering measure. Early analogue research (Beaber et al. 1985; Gillis et al. 1991) suggested that the M Test might be clinically useful with moderately high classification of malingerers (>75%). When a contrasted design[8] (i.e., suspected malingerers compared with genuine patients) was used, the classifi-

---

[8]In the malingering studies, the contrasted design is often referred to as *known-groups comparison*.

cation rates fell precipitously to 53.3% (i.e., the average of four studies; see Smith 1997) based on the original scoring.

The potential shrinkage in clinical utility from analogue to contrasted-groups design has been well established. Rogers et al. (1996) studied feigning on the Personality Assessment Inventory (PAI; Morey 1991) in a sophisticated analogue design. They used large samples for both the original ($n=204$) and the cross-validation ($n=199$) phases with clinical data drawn from multiple sites. Despite these efforts, the classification rate for the cross-validation phase (80.4%) was not sustained when applied to correctional-forensic cases in a contrasted-groups design (61.7%; see Rogers et al. 1998). The lesson from these studies is clear: analogue designs need to be supplemented with known-groups comparison. In this regard, the validation of the SIRS is instructive. Most studies relied on the analogue design, but their results were corroborated via known-groups comparisons.

Biological-Marker Model

Description

The biological-marker model is a useful but circumscribed paradigm for retrospective research. As its name describes, the evaluatee's retrospective account is confirmed by an established biological marker. The model is especially useful because its external validity (i.e., the physiological evidence) is often incontrovertible. The model is circumscribed in its clinical applications, based on its requirement of an established biological marker.

The basic paradigm uses physiological evidence of a prior episode to validate other measures of that same episode. For example, Rockwood et al. (1998) tested a semistructured retrospective interview for the evaluation of Alzheimer's disease. The results of retrospective interviews were verified by brain autopsies. Other examples include confirmation of neuroleptic malignant syndrome based on laboratory results (e.g., 5 of 15 cases; see Keck et al. 1989) and retrospective accounts of sleep disturbances as substantiated by 7 nights of polysomnographic monitoring (van Diest and Appels 1993).

A variation of the basic paradigm is the concurrent administration of a physiological procedure (e.g., Breathalyzer) at a specified time (e.g., arrest). In this variation, retrospective accounts of alcohol ingestion could be confirmed, at least partially, by laboratory results.[9] This variation of the bio-

---

[9]In this example, results are complicated by the variable rates of blood alcohol levels across individuals. However, additional testing could establish alcohol levels for a particular individual under conditions approximating the original testing.

logical-marker model has yet to be systematically implemented in clinical or forensic research.

Examples in Forensic Research

The use of hair analysis to confirm retrospective drug abuse represents the principal application of biological-marker research to forensic cases. Kelly and Rogers (1996) described the forensic applications of radioimmunoassay of hair; drug metabolites become embedded in hair shafts. Because scalp hair grows at a relatively consistent rate (approximately a half-inch per month), episodes of prior drug use can be evaluated for both the drug types and the relative usage. Positive radioimmunoassay of hair results, confirmed by gas chromatography/mass spectrometry, has a very high level of accuracy. As noted by Rogers and Kelly (1997), hair analysis provides a precise biological marker for researching the validity of clinical measures regarding prior substance abuse.

Critique

The biological-marker model has the potential to achieve a high level of both experimental rigor and clinical applicability. As in the case of substance abuse, self-report measures now can be validated against a stringent standard (i.e., radioimmunoassay of hair) for both ongoing and prior episodes. In addition, practitioners may use radioimmunoassay of hair directly in their assessments of prior episodes.

The biological-marker model faces one major challenge in its expanded application to clinical and forensic evaluations—namely, the identification of highly accurate markers that are not open to alternative explanations. For example, biological markers of suicide have yet to be achieved, despite sophisticated analysis of postmortem brain tissue (Bowden et al. 1997). At present the biological-marker model appears best suited for the retrospective evaluation of either substance abuse or syndromes with clear pathophysiological etiology (e.g., Alzheimer's disease).

Conclusions About Research Models

The bulk of forensic research has occurred in the last three decades, with major advances in both scientific rigor and clinical applicability. Regarding retrospective accounts, the recent emphasis has been placed on eyewitnesses rather than evaluatees. Different research favors different paradigms: eyewitness research focuses on the analogue model, whereas clinical and forensic research favors the corroborative model. Despite the reasons for these trends, investigators may wish to consider alternative models or the combination of models in their forensic research.

The following conclusions are provided for the four models of retrospective evaluations:

1. The corroborative model has the broadest clinical applicability and parallels forensic practice. However, care must be taken to use standardized measures that systematically assess the same clinical construct and minimize method variance.
2. The time-lapse model is especially useful for the retrospective measurement of symptoms and associated features, which are often the bedrock issues of forensic evaluations. For prior episodes or occurrences, time-lapse comparisons provide a rigorous methodology for studying the effects of time on recall. An elegant study would combine the time-lapse model for both evaluatees and informants; this model would allow a direct comparisons of time-lapse and corroborative designs. The time-lapse model is easily adapted to clinical research (e.g., first psychiatric hospitalizations) but is more challenging to implement in forensic cases (e.g., personal injury claims).[10]
3. The analogue model is noteworthy for its experimental rigor, which is often accomplished at the expense of its clinical applicability. For forensic practice its clinical applicability could be greatly improved by the use of persons with mental disorders. Despite obvious ethical concerns, the retrospective nature of personal injury evaluations might be better understood with the use of persons with mood or posttraumatic stress disorders and the simulation of a realistic accident or trauma.
4. The biological-marker model has exceptional experimental rigor and clinical applicability. With reference to forensic practice, its current application appears limited to the retrospective assessment of substance abuse. Within this circumscribed application, the biological-marker model has the remarkable potential to revolutionize the validation of retrospective self-report and psychometric methods.

Clinical Implications of Retrospective Research

Beyond understanding the methodological underpinnings of retrospective evaluations, forensic practitioners are highly invested in understanding the

---

[10]However, the time-lapse model can be approximated by successive forensic evaluations. For example, disability evaluations often span multiple years with direct comparisons of retrospective functioning possible across time periods.

clinical implications of this chapter. The main implications of this chapter for forensic practice are as follows:

- The present dichotomy of current versus retrospective evaluations is misinformed; it is likely to misdirect forensic practitioners.
- Within the tripartite typology (i.e., ongoing episodes, prior episodes, and prior occurrences), forensic practitioners are able to offer useful and empirically warranted conclusions about ongoing episodes, even though the episodes may extend weeks or possibly months into the past.
- The clinical implications of the corroborative model are readily apparent. Practitioners can apply standardized measures to the assessment of prior episodes with parallel clinical inquiries for evaluatees and informants. In addition the stability of both sources can be examined systematically via a repeat administration (i.e., test-retest reliability). For example, Rogers and Cunnien (1986) reported an insanity case in which identical portions of the SADS (Spitzer and Endicott 1978a) were administered for the time of the alleged offense to the male evaluatee with corroborative interviews with his mother and his girlfriend. When feasible, standardized measures should be used in forensic assessments for purposes of corroboration.
- Consistent with the corroborative model, forensic practitioners must exercise care in distinguishing informants' behavioral observations from speculative inferences and derivative reports.
- The retrospective assessment of personality disorders is complicated by largely untested assumptions about the stability of diagnoses and concomitant symptoms. In reality, evaluatees and their informants often show only modest agreement about Axis II symptoms. Therefore, forensic practitioners should not draw any unwarranted conclusions from discrepancies (e.g., the evaluatee reporting fewer symptoms than the informant) and their relevance to response styles (e.g., defensiveness or underreporting).
- One practical adaptation of the time-lapse model is successive evaluations for the same prior episode. In risk assessments, forensic practitioners often have an opportunity to reevaluate an individual for the same psycholegal issue (e.g., discharge an NGRI patient to a community placement). By focusing on a specified time period, a forensic practitioner may gain further understanding into the evaluatee's insight into prior episodes.
- From the section on analogue research, forensic practitioners must be satisfied that any measure of malingering successfully discriminates (i.e., cut scores or decision rules that are stable across studies) feigners from both persons without and persons with mental disorders. In addition,

malingering measures should not rely solely on analogue studies because of problems with clinical applicability.

- From the analogue model, practitioners may wish to consult the Frederick et al. (1995) article on how to evaluate purported amnesia for a prior occurrence. The likelihood of feigned amnesia sometimes can be established with substantial precision (see Rogers and Shuman 2000).

- An important contribution from the biological-marker model is the use of hair analysis (radioimmunoassay of hair) for the retrospective evaluation of substance abuse. Radioimmunoassay of hair has been successfully applied to both clinical evaluations and forensic cases (Kelly and Rogers 1996).

- Forensic practitioners should be aware that some measures of retrospective functioning do not use these four models and should be avoided. For example, the Retrospective Assessment of Traumatic Experiences (Gallagher et al. 1992) would appear to be relevant to many civil forensic cases. However, a careful review of the study indicated that traumatic events were simply assumed to be true and were not validated against external criteria.

References

an der Heiden W, Krumm B: The course of schizophrenia: some remarks on a yet unsolved problem of retrospective data collection. Eur Arch Psychiatry Clin Neurosci 240:303–306, 1991

Beaber RJ, Marston A, Michelli J, et al: A brief test for measuring malingering in schizophrenic individuals. Am J Psychiatry 142:1478–1481, 1985

Bogler JP, Strauss ME, Kennedy JS: Feasibility of retrospective assessments of behavioral symptoms in Alzheimer's disease: a preliminary study of postmortem caregiver reports. Int Psychogeriatr 10:61–69, 1998

Bowden C, Theodorou AE, Cheetham SC, et al: Dopamine D_1 and D_2 receptor binding sites in brain samples from depressed suicides and controls. Brain Res 752:227–233, 1997

Carnes M, Gunter-Hunt G, Rodgers E: The effect of an interdisciplinary geriatrics clinic visit on mental status. J Am Geriatr Soc 35:1035–1036, 1987

Cutler BL, Penrod SD: Mistaken Identification: The Eyewitness, Psychology and the Law. New York, Cambridge University Press, 1995

Denney RL: Symptom validity testing of remote memory in a criminal forensic setting. Archives of Clinical Neuropsychology 11:589–603, 1996

Fitchen CS, Libman E, Amsel R, et al: Evaluation of the sexual consequences of surgery: retrospective and prospective strategies. J Behav Med 14:267–285, 1991

Frederick RI, Carter M, Powel J: Adapting symptom validity testing to evaluate suspicious complaints of amnesia in medicolegal evaluations. Bulletin of the American Academy of Psychiatry and the Law 23:231–237, 1995

Gallagher RE, Flye BL, Hurt SW, et al: Retrospective assessment of traumatic experiences (RATE). J Personal Disord 6:99–108, 1992

Gillis JR, Rogers R, Bagby RM: Validity of the M test: simulation design and natural group approaches. J Pers Assess 57:130–140, 1991

Goodness K: Retrospective assessment of the malingering: R-SIRS and CT-SIRS. Unpublished doctoral dissertation, University of North Texas, Denton, TX, 1999

Grann M, Langstrom N, Tengstrom A, et al: Reliability of file-based retrospective ratings of psychopathy with the PCL-R. J Pers Assess 70:416–426, 1998

Hare RD: Comparison of procedures for the assessment of psychopathy. J Consult Clin Psychol 53:7–16, 1985

Hare RD: Manual for the Revised Psychopathy Checklist. Toronto, ON, Multi-Health Systems, 1991

Kassin SM, Ellsworth PC, Smith VL: The "general acceptance" of psychological research on eyewitness testimony: a survey of experts. Am Psychol 44:1089–1098, 1989

Kazdin AE: Research Design in Clinical Psychology, 2nd Edition. Boston, MA, Allyn & Bacon, 1992

Keck PE Jr, Sebastianelli J, Pope HG Jr, et al: Frequency and presentation of neuroleptic malignant syndrome in a state psychiatric hospital. J Clin Psychiatry 50:352–355, 1989

Kelly K, Rogers R: Detection of misreported drug use in forensic populations: an overview of hair analysis. Bulletin of the American Academy of Psychiatry and the Law 24:85–94, 1996

Loranger AW: Personality Disorder Examination (PDE) Manual. Yonkers, NY, DV Communications, 1988

Loranger AW, Sartorius N, Andreoli A, et al: The International Personality Disorder Examination: The World Health Organization and Alcohol, Drug Abuse and Mental Health Administration international pilot study of personality disorders. Arch Gen Psychiatry 51:215–224, 1994

Martin-Miller C, Fremouw WJ: Improving the accuracy of adult eyewitness testimony: implications for children. Clin Psychol Rev 15:631–645, 1995

Maurer K, Hafner H: Methodological aspects on onset assessment in schizophrenia. Schizophr Res 15:265–276, 1995

Mazure C, Gershon ES: Blindness and reliability in lifetime psychiatric diagnosis. Arch Gen Psychiatry 36:521–525, 1979

McFarland C, Ross M: The relation between current impressions and memories of self and dating partners. Personality and Social Psychology Bulletin 13:228–238, 1987

McMillan TM, Jongen EL, Greenwood RJ: Assessment of post-traumatic amnesia after severe closed head injury: retrospective or prospective? J Neurol Neurosurg Psychiatry 60:422–427, 1996

Morey LC: Personality Assessment Inventory: Professional Manual. Tampa, FL, Psychological Assessment Resources, 1991

Penrod SD, Fulero S, Cutler BL: Expert psychological testimony on eyewitness reliability before and after Daubert: the state of the law and the science. Behav Sci Law 13:229–259, 1995

Pfohl B, Stangl D, Zimmerman M: The Structured Interview for DSM-III Personality Disorders (SIDP). Iowa City, IA, University of Iowa, 1982

Pilkonis PA, Heape CL, Ruddy J, et al: Validity in the diagnosis of personality disorders: the use of the LEAD standard. J Consult Clin Psychol 3:46–54, 1991

Riso LP, Klein DN, Anderson RL, et al: Concordance between patients and informants on the Personality Disorder Examination. Am J Psychiatry 151:568–573, 1994

Rockwood K, Howard K, Thomas VS, et al: Retrospective diagnosis of dementia using an informant interview based on the Brief Cognitive Rating Scale. Int Psychogeriatr 10:53–60, 1998

Rogers R: Conducting Insanity Evaluations. New York, Van Nostrand Reinhold, 1986

Rogers R: Structured Interview of Reported Symptoms (SIRS). Odessa, FL, Psychological Assessment Resources, 1992

Rogers R (ed.): Clinical Assessment of Malingering and Deception, 2nd Edition. New York, Guilford, 1997

Rogers R: A Handbook of Diagnostic and Structured Interviewing. New York, Guilford, 2001

Rogers R, Cavanaugh JL: "Nothing but the truth."…a re-examination of malingering. Journal of Psychiatry and the Law 11:443–460, 1983

Rogers R, Cruise CR: Assessment of malingering with simulation designs: threats to external validity. Law Hum Behav 22:273–285, 1998

Rogers R, Cunnien AJ: Multiple SADS evaluation in the assessment of criminal defendants. J Forensic Sci 30:222–230, 1986

Rogers R, Kelly KS: Denial and misreporting of substance abuse, in Clinical Assessment of Malingering and Deception, 2nd Edition. Edited by Rogers R. New York, Guilford, 1997, pp 108–129

Rogers R, Shuman DW: Conducting Insanity Evaluations, 2nd Edition. New York, Guilford, 2000

Rogers R, Wettstein RE: Relapse in NGRI patients: an empirical study. International Journal of Offender Therapy and Comparative Criminology 29:227–236, 1985

Rogers R, Bagby RM, Dickens SE: Structured Interview of Reported Symptoms (SIRS) Professional Manual. Odessa, FL, Psychological Assessment Resources, 1992

Rogers R, Sewell KW, Salekin R: A meta-analysis of malingering on the MMPI-2. Assessment 1:227–237, 1994

Rogers R, Sewell KW, Morey LC, et al: Detection of feigned mental disorders on the Personality Assessment Inventory: a discriminant analysis. J Pers Assess 67:629–640, 1996

Rogers R, Sewell KW, Cruise KR, et al: The PAI and feigning: a cautionary note on its use in forensic-correctional settings. Assessment 5:399–405, 1998

Smith G: Self-report measures of malingering and deception, in Clinical Assessment of Malingering and Deception, 2nd Edition. Edited by Rogers R. New York, Guilford, 1997, pp 351–370

Spitzer RL: Psychiatric diagnosis: are clinicians still necessary? Compr Psychiatry 24:399–411, 1983

Spitzer RL, Endicott J: Schedule for Affective Disorders and Schizophrenia, 3rd Edition. New York, Biometrics Research, 1978a

Spitzer RL, Endicott J: Schedule for Affective Disorders and Schizophrenia— Change Version. New York, Biometrics Research, 1978b

van Diest R, Appels A: Vital exhaustion and perception of sleep. J Psychosom Res 36:449–458, 1993

von Zerssen D, Possl J, Hecht H, et al: The Biographical Personality Interview (BPI)—a new approach to the assessment of premorbid personality in psychiatric research, part I: development of the instrument. J Psychiatr Res 32:19–35, 1998

Ward MF, Wender PH, Reimherr FW: The Wender Utah Rating Scale: an aid in the retrospective diagnosis of childhood attention deficit hyperactivity disorder. Am J Psychiatry 150:885–890, 1993

Widom CS: Does violence beget violence? A critical examination of the literature. Psychol Bull 106:3–28, 1989

Wong S: Is Hare's Psychopathy Checklist reliable without the interview? Psychol Rep 62:931–934, 1988

Yuille JC, Cutshall JL: A case study of eyewitness memory of a crime. J Appl Psychol 71:291–301, 1986

Yuille JC, Daylen J: The impact of traumatic events of eyewitness memory, in Eyewitness Memory: Theoretical and Applied Perspectives. Edited by Thompson CP, Herrmann DJ, Read JR, et al. Mahwah, NJ, Lawrence Erlbaum, 1998, pp 155–177

Zimmerman M, Pfohl B, Coryell W, et al: Diagnosing personality disorder in depressed patients. Arch Gen Psychiatry 45:733–737, 1988

11

What Can Psychologists Contribute to the Examination of Memory and Past Mental States?

Amina Memon, Ph.D.
Sarah E. Henderson, B.Sc. (Hons)

Memory really has to be considered as a hypothetical construct because it is an intangible substance. It cannot be seen or felt or weighed. It cannot be fixed like a broken limb, it cannot be transplanted like other internal organs, and it cannot be saved for future generations to use. As such, the actual notion of having a memory has to be taken on some degree of trust. Of course we all know that we have a memory; without memory one would be unable to read these words—that is, unable to recognize the actual words, remember all the words to make up the sentence, or understand the meaning of them. Memory is one of the most important processes in the brain. It allows us to learn from the past and to some degree predict the future through the process of storing and recalling past experiences, events, and sensations.

The word *memory* itself is an umbrella term for the three main interrelated processes that allow individuals to convert episodes they have experienced into cognitive information that can be recalled at a later date. These processes are termed *encoding, storage,* and *retrieval.* Encoding is the process by which information is imputed to the brain to be remembered. Once this input has been encoded, it has to be retained (or placed in storage) until it is retrieved or remembered.

What are memories? Can they be likened to a videotape running in an individual's head and recording everything he or she looks at, to be played back at a later time? For those of us who feel they possess less than phenomenal memories, the answer is, in most cases, a reassuring "no." Rather our memories appear to summarize events (i.e., we remember the gist of the event), and then we can infer what else may have happened in order to fill in the missing information (Bransford and Franks 1971; Loftus 1979, 1993; Sachs 1967; Spanos 1996). Bartlett (1932) described memory as a reconstructive process and subsequently theorized that individuals construct memory from other information gathered from both past experiences and other related knowledge (or schemata). So if this is how a memory is formed, why do we forget?

Theories of Forgetting

The three main theories of forgetting are 1) the fading theory (Ebbinghaus 1885/1964), 2) the interference theory (Baddeley and Hitch 1977; McGeoch and McDonald 1931), and 3) the retrieval theory. The fading theory argues that the information has been converted into a memory trace; however, because it is not often used, it simply fades or decays away, rather like a poster exposed to sun and rain that gradually fades until it becomes quite illegible. Interference theory suggests that forgetting occurs because old and newly learned information compete, so memory traces are interrupted or written over by subsequently learned information. There seem to be two types of interference.

First, the replacing of old information with new information is known as *retroactive interference* (RI). Despite its name the process is not actually retroactive; rather the new information is superimposed on the old memory traces. As Sir Arthur Conan Doyle's most famous creation, the detective Sherlock Holmes, once remarked,

> I consider that a man's brain originally is like a little empty attic, and you have to stock it with such furniture as you choose. A fool takes in all the lumber of every sort that he comes across, so that the knowledge which might be useful to him gets crowded out, or at best is jumbled up with a

lot of other things, so that he has a difficulty in laying his hands upon it. Now the skillful workman is very careful indeed as to what he takes into his brain-attic. He will have nothing but the tools which may help him in doing his work, but of these he has a large assortment, and all in the most perfect order. It is a mistake to think that that little room has elastic walls and can distend to any extent. Depend upon it—there comes a time when for every addition of knowledge you forget something that you knew before. It is of the highest importance, therefore, not to have useless facts elbowing out the useful ones. (Doyle 1982, p. 21)

This is basically a fairly accurate summation of the notion of RI. As can be expected, RI frequently occurs as the individual's amount of learning increases and usually happens when the initial memory trace is relatively weak.

The second type of interference is termed *proactive interference* (PI). This is essentially the opposite idea of RI, whereby the old memory trace comes back into play and interferes with the newly learned memory (Kanak and Stevens 1992). An example of PI would be changing the password on your computer and then unthinkingly typing in an old password while logging on to your computer. The very fact that this can happen indicates that the original memory trace is not lost or destroyed forever; rather the problem appears to be one of accessibility.

The final theory of forgetting, the retrieval theory, states that the information has been poorly encoded and stored during the memory process, so the individual has problems finding and retrieving it.

Excluding the retrieval theory, which is basically just a breakdown of the memory process, can we know for sure which of the other two theories is more likely? If the original memory trace just fades away after a certain time, then the amount of time taken between the initial learning and the forgetting of the information should be examined. By this reasoning the longer the time that elapses, the greater the amount of information that is forgotten. If the interference theory is the more likely explanation, then the number and types of events that occurred in the intervening time should be examined.

Forgetting Curve

Hermann Ebbinghaus, a German psychologist, carried out exhaustive pioneering studies in learning and recall in which he was the subject. In one of his most well-known experiments, he arranged a series of nonsense syllables into 169 separate lists consisting of 13 nonsense syllables and learned and relearned each list over a period ranging from 21 minutes to 31 days. After this huge task he concluded that some forgetting had occurred and extrapolated the amount of time required to learn the list again as a measure of how much had been forgotten. He found that forgetting is rapid at first but then gradually slows down; thus people appear to forget 90% of what they learn in a class within 30 days. Ebbinghaus's study seems to suggest that the rate of forgetting is a more logarithmic than linear function. These findings have successfully been shown to apply across a very wide range of material and learning conditions.

The idea that forgetting starts rapidly, before slowing, also has been described in terms of Jost's Law (Jost 1894). Jost's Law states that if two equally strong memory traces are formed, then the older of the two will be more powerful and forgotten more slowly. This seems to suggest that memories do decay but also become more durable as they age, resisting further decay. These studies typically use nonsense words as the material to be learned and usually have only relatively short retention periods. But what happens when more ecologically valid, or everyday, events and material are used, and the retention period is much longer?

Warrington and Sanders (1971) conducted a study in which they selected several events that were considered to be important within the United Kingdom over the preceding 30 years. The idea was that these events were so singular that most people would know salient information about them. These people were then given a memory test for these events either by recall or by recognition tasks. Warrington and Sanders found a lot of forgetting of these public events, but, interestingly, younger people appeared to have better recall than did elderly people for both recent and older events. These studies adequately confirm the actions of forgetting curves; however, the material used usually is implicit (i.e., not expressly memorized).

Bahrick and colleagues (1975) asked American high school graduates to try and identify pictures and recall the names of other individuals in their class. They found that the ability to recognize a face or a name from a series of faces and names and then match these up remained at a fairly good degree of accuracy for more than 30 years. However, if asked to recall these names without prompting, evidence of extensive forgetting was seen. Interestingly, those tested after 50 years showed a significant deficiency in performance, which suggests that there could be an aging effect. However, Bahrick carried out a later study (Bahrick 1984) on the level of retention over many years. In this case he studied the individual's retention of a varied range of material, including tests of geography and foreign languages learned during college. In this study forgetting occurred only up to a certain point, beyond which memory traces appeared to be fixed, or frozen. Bahrick suggested an analogy with the frozen areas in the polar region, known as *permafrost*, and called this stable range of recall *permastore*.

Recently Schmidt et al. (2000) conducted a study of long-term retention of street names. Again the forgetting curve showed this permastore effect. Schmidt et al. hypothesized that this incidentally learned material underwent the same kind of processes of forgetting as those that affect intentionally learned material (e.g., Bahrick's tests of material learned in school). These results, although contradictory, suggest that different types of information are forgotten at different rates.[1]

Retrieval

Now that we have seen the basic theory behind the process of forgetting, some pertinent questions are raised about remembering. Can viable and accurate information be retrieved from the memory, and, if so, how? And perhaps most important, will it be reliable?

Retrieval Cues

Just because a memory trace has been disrupted does not necessarily mean that it cannot be accessed again. The phenomenon of knowing something but being unable to access it is a fairly common one. In most cases after concentrating on this "elusive" fact and recalling other related information, the original fact or event is soon remembered. This other related information, also known as *retrieval cues*, allows us to put several clues together until the memory trace is identified and recognized.

Context-Dependent Retrieval

As mentioned in the prior paragraph, retrieval cues help us to remember by allowing us to work back to the memory via a series of clues. A similar idea is that of context-dependent retrieval. The external environment in which an event occurred is reconstructed to help the individual remember it, so the individual replays the circumstances surrounding the event to be remembered and then works back from these. For example, if someone loses

---

[1] In 1961 an employee commenced an action for damages against his British employers based on alleged breach of duty to provide a reasonably safe means of access and on alleged breach of the shipbuilding Regulation 1931. The employers alleged that because of a lapse of time—2 years and 8 months—they were prejudiced and that the witness's memories had dimmed. It was held that there should be no trial by jury and that there should be an order for proof before answer (*Hunter v. John Brown and Co Ltd* 1961).

his or her car keys, then it is often helpful to go to the last place he or she remembers having them and then retrace the journey from this point.

The literature suggests that retrieval can be dependent on context. Godden and Baddeley (1975) carried out a series of experiments that examined the memory performance of divers on land and underwater. Free recall was better when the learning and test environments were the same, so divers who learned words underwater had a better level of recall underwater. Similarly, Smith (1986) carried out a study in which participants were given memory tests either in a room or in a flotation tank. Again a strong context-dependent effect was found. These studies indicate that each stage of learning is separated; for example, information learned in one context is kept apart from information learned in another context. So even if one feels as if he or she has forgotten a lot of information connected with one context, if he or she returns to that context, then the memories also should return. A good example of this is the Cognitive Interview (Fisher and Geiselman 1992; Memon and Higham 1999). The Cognitive Interview is a way of questioning a person so as to maximize the amount of information that can be obtained about a specific event. It draws on our knowledge of how memory works best and relies heavily on re-creating emotional, physical, and psychological contexts surrounding an event.

State-Dependent Memory

If context-dependent memory is concerned with the reinstatement of external cues to aid recall, then state-dependent memory involves the recreation of internal cues to aid recall. The few studies that have been conducted in this area involve changing the individual's internal state by way of a drug such as alcohol.

Goodwin et al. (1969) carried out a study in which individuals were given either a soft drink or a large amount of high-strength vodka and then were asked to perform several tasks. The next day the subjects were asked to perform these tasks again, either in the same state or in a different state. Goodwin et al. concluded that what is learned drunk is better recalled when drunk and vice versa. Researchers generally have concluded that state dependency seems to occur only with recall; as with context dependency it is not observed in recognition tests (Bower 1992; Eich 1980). This suggests that the internal or external cues are useful in accessing the elusive memory trace. However, if the individual does not have to initially find the memory trace because the item is already being presented for recognition, then these cues do not appear to be needed. This suggests that individuals first must identify the appropriate memory trace and then judge whether it is the correct one.

Mood-Congruent Memory Retrieval

If an individual's internal state can affect memory, then it also stands to reason that his or her emotional state can affect memory. Cognitive processes play a major role in the function and development of depression and anxiety (Beck et al. 1979, 1985), so they can play a significant role in the creation and perpetuation of mood-congruent memories. Beck theorized that depressed or anxious individuals process negative information (e.g., depressing or dangerous information) via a series of cognitive structures, and this negative information bias then perpetuates the individual's negative mood. So a type of self-fulfilling prophesy is created—the individual feels depressed but can think of only negative events and therefore feels more depressed.

Wagenaar (1986) conducted a series of experiments in which he recorded approximately 2,000 events over 6 years. Each of these events was then rated for pleasantness, saliency, and level of emotion. Additional pertinent information about who was involved, what actually happened, and when and where the event happened was recorded. Wagenaar then tested his memory for these events by using each of the information cues. The "what happened" information was the most effective cue, and events that evoked high levels of salience and emotionality and that were generally pleasant appeared to have a higher level of recall. Strangely the effects of highly emotional or more conspicuous events remained fairly constant over some considerable time (recall remained strong over intervals from 1 to 5 years); however, the effects of pleasantness declined after 5 years.

Similarly, Bower (1981) asked participants to keep a diary of the emotional aspects of their lives. After a short interval they underwent a mood-induction procedure: they were placed in a positive or negative mood via hypnotic suggestion. They were then asked to recall the events, and participants in a happy mood recalled more pleasant memories. This suggests a mood-congruency effect. Bower et al. (1981) conducted a follow-up study in which the participants again underwent mood induction to create a positive or negative mood. These participants were then told a story about a fictitious person who experienced a series of positive and negative events. Again a mood-congruency effect at recall was found. Quite apart from these studies, the memories of individuals who have mood disorders such as depression also may be influenced by mood. Lloyd and Lishman (1975) found that depressed patients took less time to recall negative events the more depressed they were. Likewise Clark and Teasdale (1981) found that when depressed patients were relatively happy, they recalled more pleasant than unpleasant memories, but when they were despondent, they recalled mostly negative memories.

Hypnosis

Hypnosis is a method of altering the individual's state of consciousness. The actual process of hypnosis has been used for centuries; researchers have examples of operations identifiable as hypnosis from more than 200 years ago. Hypnosis was originally associated with the occult, especially because it was believed to take away the individual's free will (Lynn et al. 1999). Today, however, after long processes of rigorous scientific investigation, hypnosis is being used as a tool in therapy. Lynn et al. (1999) defined clinical hypnosis as "the addition of hypnosis to accepted psychological or medical treatment…hypnosis is not a treatment in itself. Rather, hypnosis is a specialized technique that can be used as an adjunctive intervention integrated into a more encompassing treatment package" (p. 23).

There is a long association between hypnosis and the law. Hypnosis is an altered state of consciousness, usually performed by a hypnotist for the purpose of changing the subjects' conscious state (E. R. Hilgard 1975).

As stated earlier in this subsection, the common public perception of hypnosis is that it captures the individual's free will and places him or her under the hypnotist's complete power. However, research in this area has shown that a lot about hypnosis remains relatively unknown. For example, the literature on hypnosis suggests that everyone does not respond in a similar way to hypnotic suggestions. Two distinct schools of thought regarding hypnosis are apparent (Spanos 1986). First, the *state view* holds that different states can occur in the same person. However, all these states are not necessarily conscious at the same time, suggesting a certain degree of dissociation. Janet subscribed to this theory, believing that each of these states is isolated, with one being dominant at any given time; however, the others still have the chance to influence behavior or even replace the dominant state. J.R. Hilgard (1974) and E.R. Hilgard (1977) had a similar explanation, which they termed the *neo-dissociation theory of hypnosis*. J.R. Hilgard and E.R. Hilgard theorized that these various systems and states are controlled by an overriding main system, but the hypnotist takes control of this. This means that when people are hypnotized, they feel as if many of their actions are involuntary or distorted. The undetermined phenomenon of the *hidden observer* is often used to demonstrate the idea of dissociation across states (E.R. Hilgard 1977; J.R. Hilgard 1974). This was first observed in studies of hypnotic analgesia and consisted of seemingly independent responses from the same person at the same time.

Second, the *nonstate view* states that hypnosis does not cause involuntary actions but rather that the hypnotist and the hypnotized individual are playing specific roles (Sarbin and Coe 1972). In other words the "hypnotized" individual is playing a predetermined role and deliberately follows the instructions given by the hypnotist, no matter how strange they may sound (Wagstaff 1981).

Compliance is a powerful phenomenon, even in those who are not hypnotized; previous psychology experiments that examined examples of extreme compliance found that individuals will overstep the bounds of moral and ethical norms to comply. One of the most popular studies that caused ethical concern was Milgram's research on obedience (Milgram 1963). Milgram was testing the hypothesis that individuals would obey an authority figure no matter what. In this experiment a group of participants (who were not hypnotized) were asked to give an increasingly powerful electric shock to another individual, who was supposedly in another room. In reality no person was being shocked, but the participants were provided with audio feedback, which was supposed to be from the person being shocked. As far as these participants knew, they were inflicting severe pain on another person. The electrical generator was marked in such a way that the highest setting looked as if it would be possible to kill a person with that level of electricity. After prompting from the experimenter, 65% of the participants delivered this highest voltage, showing that compliance is a powerful factor.

This argument appears to suggest that hypnosis is a type of social encounter. Because the actions carried out by the hypnotized individual are often complex, they appear more likely to be an improvised act based on what he or she thinks the hypnotist wants him or her to do (Kihlstrom 1985; White 1941).

Despite this, there have often been claims that hypnosis can enhance memory, especially eyewitness memory (Parkin 1995). It does appear that hypnotized individuals can recall past events; however, can these memories really be called reliable? With this in mind, the American Medical Association (1985) cautioned against the systematic use of hypnosis for recollection purposes because of its potential to create vivid false memories with an artificially induced sense of certainty. Similarly, Erdelyi (1994) concluded that hypnosis is not a valid method to recover memories. Although hypnosis increases recall of meaningful stimuli, it also increases false recollections. Hypnosis does however seem to lower the threshold for reporting memories (both accurate and inaccurate) (Lynn et al. 1997). But as stated above, we cannot differentiate between real and false memories. Interestingly, the literature also shows that a positive relationship between hypnotizability and false memory reporting in both hypnotic and nonhypnotic contexts has been confirmed (Barnier and McConkey 1992; McConkey et al. 1990; Sheehan et al. 1991a, 1991b; Spanos et al. 1999). Murrey et al. (1992) conducted an experiment to determine whether the incident of false memory reports of highly hypnotizable participants would differ significantly from that of a control group. If response bias was controlled for, no significant difference in false memories was reported between the groups. Wagstaff et al. (1992) found that juries seem to give a greater level of credence to evidence elicited by hypnosis, which suggests that the public should be better educated about hypnosis and its effects on memory.[2] As Wagstaff (1993) pointed out, at the moment, practically either side of the argument—suggesting that hypnosis can be used as a tool for enhancing memory, or for robbing individuals of their free will—can be advanced. We still have a lot to learn about the process of hypnosis; thus, until hypnosis is studied in more depth, these claims should be examined carefully.

How Do Psychologists Study Memory?

Psychologists have developed several techniques to study memory. Unfortunately, it is not enough to merely ask individuals whether they think they have good memories, because these self-report techniques are mainly based on the processes of introspection and observation. Although the process of observation is often a particularly useful construct because it allows the researcher to note otherwise untestable phenomena (e.g., the effects of childhood experiences, which are usually impossible to examine under controlled experimental conditions because the participant's behavior is often constrained in some way), it is rarely ever unbiased. In an ideal world all scientific discoveries or theories would begin with simple unbiased observations; the researcher would simply carry out the experiment with no preconceptions or predetermined ideas. As Chalmers (1990, p. 49) argued, "Acceptable observation statements are those statements about observable states of affairs that are able to survive tests involving skilled use of the senses…objectivity is a practical achievement."

However, in reality this could never happen; observations can never be totally unbiased, and human observation is always directed toward something. After all, if it were not, we would not know when we had found what

---

[2]Recently it was held that evidence given under hypnosis is not inadmissible in law but is considered unreliable (*R. v. Mayes; R. v. McIntosh* 1995). It was decided that there also would be a danger of a miscarriage of justice if this evidence were ruled admissible. In a recent British court of appeals decision, it was held that precautions had to be taken to ensure that the subject could not be influenced in any way. In accordance with a Home Office circular (No. 66/1988), all such sessions should be carried out only by fully qualified practitioners and be videorecorded (*R. v. Browning [Edward]* 1995).

we were actually looking for (Medawar 1963; Popper 1972). One way in which researchers in the field of psychology have tried to combat the problem of subjectivity is through attention to reliability. An observation cannot be satisfactorily used as "evidence" (and therefore cannot be successfully incorporated into the larger body of scientific knowledge) unless its reliability is also known (Krietman 1961). This is why standardized tests and questionnaires are used (i.e., for the purposes of psychology, reliability can be conveniently measured in terms of interagreement between different observers examining the same subject).

Because of subjectivity, the participant's responses could significantly vary depending on his or her current state of mind, what he or she believes the "correct" response should be (i.e., what he or she believes most individuals would answer, or what he or she feels the researcher wants to hear), or even what kind of day he or she has had. Similarly experimenters scoring and analyzing these responses do so through their own personal perspectives. This could mean that the individual's views and reckoning could be inadvertently (or otherwise) changed, merely because the experimenter has different views from the participant. With this in mind it is more productive to give individuals a series of memory tasks and then score how well or badly they perform. This is important to remember because in the courtroom arena, even if witnesses believe they are telling "the whole truth and nothing but the truth," they are actually only recalling their perception of the events.

Amnesia

Before reviewing the processes involved in the assessment of past mental states and the problems that can occur in the remembering of information and events, a few terms such as *amnesia, repression,* and *dissociation* have to be defined. The distinction between *unconsciousness* and *insanity* also must be determined.

Amnesia is used to describe a severe loss of memory. However, the memory problems it refers to can result from a vast array of incidents and have various effects and symptoms. For example, *anterograde amnesia* describes an inability to recall events after whatever injury caused the memory loss, whereas *retrograde amnesia* describes an inability to recall events before the injury (Sternberg 1995). *Infantile amnesia* describes an inability to remember events that occurred during the first few years of life (Wetzler and Sweeney 1986). It is highly improbable that genuine episodic memories (a form of memory concerning autobiographical information; Parkin 1995) can be recalled from this period of life because regions of the brain, including the hippocampus (which plays a key role in the generation of memories), have not fully developed. Kolb and Whishaw (1996) suggested that infants and adults may use a different memory system, so the adult cannot access the infantile memories and therefore cannot remember those memories. Finally, *psychogenic amnesia* describes "a temporary loss of memory precipitated by a psychological trauma" (Schacter 1996).

Repression is another term that is commonly used in everyday language but has a specific meaning in psychology. Freud was the pioneering researcher in the area of repression, but he was inconsistent in his use of the term. In his early research he defined repression as the intentional rejection of distressing thoughts and memories from conscious awareness (although he also used the terms *suppression* and *repression proper* to explain this). However, over time he began to use the term to describe a type of unconscious defense mechanism designed to remove threatening material from the individual's conscious awareness (*primary repression*). Freud theorized that the unconscious is another part of the psyche. All memories, desires, and instincts that are considered too upsetting for the individual are exiled into the unconscious. Note that repression is seen as an involuntary process, unlike suppression, which is seen as voluntary (Memon and Young 1997).

Dissociation describes the "structured separation of mental processes (e.g., thoughts, emotions, connotation, memory and identity) that are ordinarily integrated" (Spiegal and Cardena 1991, p. 367).

Finally, there is a distinction between *unconsciousness* and *insanity*. The basic medicolegal argument is that mens rea (intent to harm) must be present in a criminal. This implies that the criminal acted out of a free choice of conduct. As a result, the basic law in most jurisdictions states that an individual cannot commit a crime if he or she is not conscious of it. In other words, since the individual has no memory of the event after it has occurred, it is likely that he or she was without consciousness during that period, even if he or she appeared to be acting normally. The problem then becomes one of the validity of the amnesia and its accompanying unconsciousness. The legal system has clearly separated the problems of "not guilty by reason of insanity" and not guilty by reason of "unconsciousness."

Effects of Emotion on Memory

Memories can be affected by emotional states, and it has been known for some time that humans are more alert and therefore more susceptible to learning and retaining information at certain times of the day. For instance, although individuals experience a wide-ranging level of alertness (or arousal) throughout the day, basically the optimum level of arousal occurs during the afternoon and early evening period. By this reasoning it would appear that this is the ideal time for memory formation (Baddeley 1999).

Baddeley's research is just one example from the literature that indicates that level of arousal can affect memory or at least the first stage of the memory process, encoding. In addition other stages in the memory process can be affected. When a person is experiencing extreme stress, he or she may have a reduced ability to perceive and recall the details of the event that caused the stress. The Yerkes-Dodson Law (Yerkes and Dodson 1908) states that, in general, cognitive abilities improve as arousal increases up to some peak, beyond which they deteriorate. Some clinical research has examined how trauma might influence memory. For instance, Chu and Dill (1990) reported that psychiatric patients with a history of childhood abuse reported higher levels of dissociative symptoms than did those without a history of childhood abuse. Similarly Carlson and Rosser-Hogan (1991), in a study of Cambodian refugees, reported a strong relation between the amount of trauma the refugees experienced and the severity of both traumatic stress response and dissociative reactions. Studies of adults with multiple personalities (Bliss 1986) and adolescents who went on to commit murder (Lewis et al. 1989) showed that these adults and adolescents very often were abused or traumatized in their own childhood. Chu and Dill (1990) suggested that this dissociative (or psychogenic) amnesia is particularly associated with chronicity of abuse, early age at onset, and severity of abuse.

The above studies suggested that there could be an association between traumatic life experience and a subsequent dissociative response. However, it should be remembered that this does not necessarily mean that trauma will always lead to dissociation. There have been a number of theories as to what these dissociative (for want of a better term) amnesias are and why they occur. Breuer and Freud (1895) first proposed that amnesia may result from a traumatic experience. Similarly, at the end of the nineteenth century, Janet (1889/1984) described dissociation as a key coping mechanism that allows the individual to function after an overwhelming trauma. Janet hypothesized a link between repressed memories that are stored apart from conscious awareness and the processes of dissociation and somatization in the form of hysteria. In other words, the individual cannot deal with the traumatic experience, so the associated memories are split off from the rest of consciousness. Ludwig (1983) proposed that dissociation may have evolutionary advantages. He maintained that dissociative processes bring about an experimental disengagement from overwhelming physical or psychological events because they have had species survival value and served many diverse adaptation-enhancing functions. He stated that, besides survival, dissociation may have other functions such as the cathartic discharge of feelings and the isolation of catastrophic experiences. In a connected vein, Parwatikar et al. (1985) suggested that certain individuals who commit a crime may undergo some form of dissociation because they do not want to consciously be reminded that they committed a "wrongful" act.

One fundamental aspect of the dissociative response to trauma concerns immediate dissociation at the time the traumatic event is unfolding. Victims of trauma often report alterations in their experience of time and place, which can confer a sense of unreality of the event as it is occurring. This suggests that these individuals may be experiencing a form of dissociation, which can take the form of altered time sense, with time being experienced as slowing down or rapidly accelerating. Profound feelings of unreality that the event is occurring or that the individual is the victim of the event; experiences of depersonalization; out-of-body experiences; bewilderment, confusion, and disorientation; altered pain perception; altered body image or feelings of disconnection from one's body; tunnel vision; and other experiences reflecting immediate dissociative responses to trauma also have been documented. This is succinctly illustrated in the phenomenon known as *event-specific amnesia*, in which memory loss is restricted to a particular time (Schacter 1996). Typically event-specific amnesia has been observed in individuals who have undergone extremely violent events (e.g., soldiers). Grinker and Spiegal (1945) studied many men who had developed amnesia following traumatic wartime episodes. Event-specific amnesia also has been claimed by violent criminals who assert that they cannot remember the crime they have been charged with (Kopelman 1987). Of course this may be a result of the influence of drugs. In fact alcoholism and inability to remember the actual commission of the assault are prominent factors in the history of many murder cases. As Markowitsch (1990) stated, "hysterical states, a labile personality, and criminal tendencies were common among patients with transient psychogenic amnesic states" (p. 182).

Despite these explanations the relation between emotion and memory is a complex one, and situational and individual factors may moderate the effects of emotion on memory.

Recovered Memories and False Memories

Recovered memories are, as the name suggests, memories that have been repressed for years and then spontaneously remembered and reported. For this process to occur, some facts have to be surmised. Individuals must have the ability to push certain emotions and experiences from their conscious awareness. These experiences must not be able to be actively recalled by the individual but often cause the manifestation of associated adverse reactions (e.g., depression). To address these associated reactions, these "forgotten" memories must be remembered via therapeutic intervention. Unfortunately, little evidence exists to support these claims; however, a few studies suggested that some individuals can have long-term amnesia for a traumatic event in childhood. For instance, Elliott (1997) conducted a study in which a random section of the general population was asked if they had undergone a traumatic experience, and 32% of those who responded in the affirmative reported some form of delayed memory for the event. Likewise, Feldman-Summers and Pope (1994) found that different forms of childhood abuse (both sexual and nonsexual) had been remembered after a delay. Interestingly, this reported forgetting appeared to be subject to the severity of the abuse.

Because memory is a reconstructive process rather than a continuous recording of information, we rely on information from multiple sources to re-create our memories. When an individual incorporates incorrect information into this reconstructive process, a false memory may be formed. *False memories* are typically defined as incorrect beliefs about past events that have been incorporated and experienced as genuine memories (Heaps and Nash 1999; Lampinen et al. 1998). What is in fact a memory illusion may appear to be the true picture of our past (Payne et al. 1997). These false memories may emerge during therapy and have sometimes been linked to the application of various therapeutic techniques, such as suggestion, social contagion, hypnosis (and the misuse of hypnosis), various types of dream analysis, and regression (Coons 1994). The therapists themselves also must understand their power over the patient. The literature indicates that a significant minority of practicing United States psychotherapists and United Kingdom psychologists use these types of therapeutic techniques to "help" their patients remember instances of childhood abuse. Thus much more research is needed into the area of memory-focused therapy (Poole et al. 1995).

Memory Implantation

As a direct result of concerns about the possibility that false memories can be created, several laboratories have developed paradigms to systematically study whether it is possible to implant an entire false memory in the mind of an adult. These studies go quite a way in describing how an entire false memory about a childhood event can be implanted in the mind of an adult.

Loftus and Pickrell (1995) described the typical procedure in the memory implantation studies. In the first part of their study, an older relative presented participants with four stories about their childhood. Three stories were true, and one was a false event (e.g., getting lost in a shopping mall). All participants were interviewed twice and asked to recall as much as they could. Loftus and Pickrell reported that 68% of the true events were remembered, whereas 25% of the false events were fully or partially recalled at the first and second interviews. These findings have been replicated. For example, Hyman et al. (1995; see experiment 2) implanted memories of an accident at a wedding reception that resulted in a punch bowl being overturned on the parents of the bride. Memory for true events was highly accurate over three separate interviews. For the false punch bowl event, no participants provided false recollections during the first interview, but 25.5% did so by the third interview. (The false recalls varied in clarity, with 6 of the 23 rated as "very clear.") Interestingly, subjects who incorporated general details that fit the event script into their first or second interview were more likely to have false recollections by the third interview.

Hyman and Pentland (1996), in an extension of the earlier studies of memory implantation, were interested in whether guided imagery–type procedures resembling those sometimes used in therapy would increase the recall of true and false memories and whether hypermnesia (or net increases in recall) would occur over repeated interviews. Students were interviewed three times about a series of true events based on information supplied by their parents and a false event (the accident with the punch bowl). They were given basic cues (age, nature of event, locations). When participants in the imagery condition failed to recall the event, they were asked for detailed descriptions (and asked questions about what happened). The control group was asked to sit quietly and think about the event for a minute. No significant differences were found between the imagery and the control condition in the percentage of true events recalled, but the tendency was for additional information to be reported following the first interview (this was most marked in the imagery condition), suggesting a form of hypermnesia. Not surprisingly, memories provided by subjects in the imagery condition were rated as higher in image clarity than were memories provided in the control condition. The false events were scored as clear false memory, partial memory, no memory, and no but trying (a memory recovered from the first to the third interview was referred to as a recovered memory). The number of clear false memories increased across interviews in both conditions (no clear differences were seen in partial memories, although some individuals went from partial to trying to clear). By the third interview 37.5% of the individuals in the imagery condition versus 12.4% in the control condition had created a false memory. Those who created a false memory tended to rate their image as clearer and were more confident. The data are compatible with source monitoring theory when an individual has to determine the original source of a memory.

Imagination Inflation

Garry and colleagues (1996) conducted a study that asked participants to imagine certain childhood events. They first gave some participants a copy of the Life Events Inventory (LEI) to complete. The LEI is a 40-item self-report questionnaire about a variety of events that may have occurred before age 10 years (e.g., broke a window with your hand). For each event the individual circled one of eight options (1 = definitely did not happen and 8 = definitely did happen) to indicate how certain he or she was that the event had actually happened to him or her. These pretest data were used to select eight target items (i.e., a significant number of individuals responded that these events probably did not occur). In the second session (2 weeks later), the participants were randomly split into two groups, one of which was given four of these target events and asked to imagine them (the other group acted as a control). Finally the experimenter told both groups that their original LEI had been misplaced and asked them to complete another copy. It was subsequently found that the imagined events were more likely to be believed as actual happenings than were the nonimagined events. Garry et al. termed this phenomenon *imagination inflation*. In much the same way in which imagination can be used to predict possible future events, it also seems to be able to affect an individual's subjective belief about whether a past event occurred (Sherman et al. 1985).

These findings would seem to suggest that caution should be exercised when imagination-based therapies are used in recovered memory situations. This effect is so strong that individuals even begin to believe that unlikely events were more likely to have occurred (Garry et al. 1996; Goff and Roediger 1998; Heaps and Nash 1999). Also when the participants initially reported a "know" judgment (i.e., the participants just knew that the event occurred, rather than specifically remembering its occurring), imagination could subsequently produce supporting, plausible, recollective experiences (Hyman and Pentland 1996; Hyman et al. 1998). This should not be surprising because imagination already has been found to be associated with suggestibility (Tousignant et al. 1986). Interestingly, Garry et al. also found a slight increase in estimation of certainty as the item was repeated; this supports the existing literature on rehearsal and hypermnesia effects (see below).

In a more recent study, Porter et al. (1999) attempted to obtain a false recovered memory for a highly stressful emotional event (the events were undergoing a serious medical procedure, getting lost, getting seriously harmed by another child, enduring a serious animal attack, having a serious indoor accident, and having a serious outdoor accident). The participants were then interviewed and asked about one real and one false event (from the preceding list). Two additional interviews asked specifically about the false event; guided imagery techniques were used in all these interviews. During the third session participants were asked to give a report of the incident; 26% of them recovered a full memory for the false event, and another 30% recalled various aspects of it.

However, it should be noted that despite all of, or maybe because of, the above arguments, a newly remembered memory may be either false or recovered, and it is virtually impossible to ascertain its genuineness. Recovered memories for events in one's past not only are relatively common but also seem to share certain characteristics with false memories. For instance, true and false memories initially appear to be very different (true memories are frequently rated as being better remembered and more emotional than are false memories) (Conway et al. 1996; Heaps and Nash 1999). However, these differences appear to be eliminated with use of rehearsal to try and recall the memory more clearly. This has led to some confusion as to the quality of false memories, recovered memories, and "true" memories of an event. Researchers maintain that without corroboration it is not possible to differentiate between genuine recovered memories and false memories (Ceci et al. 1994; Lindsay and Read 1994; Lynn et al. 1997). Although false memories appear to be less well defined than true memories, Loftus and Pickrell (1995) concluded that false memories are recounted with fewer words and are rated by the participants as being less clear. Schooler et al. (1986) found that when recalling false postevent information, individuals typically provided longer descriptions with more hesitations and fewer sensory details than when recalling objects that were actually present. Opposing research states that recollective experience in false memories often can be as full as that found with true memories (Kassin 1997; Loftus 1993; Reisberg 1997). Again this seems to be especially true in the interview and imagination procedures (Lindsay and Read 1994). In a related aside, Brainerd et al. (1995) and Poole (1995) stated that according to members of the legal profession, response consistency across interviews is one of the key methods the court uses to assess the credibility of evidence.

Other Causes of Amnesia

Amnesic states can be caused by several different circumstances, such as alcohol intoxication or head injuries. It is well known that even moderate drinking can impair cognitive, perceptual, verbal, and motor processes.[3] Chronic alcoholism may of course result in brain damage, but the alcohol-induced blackout is one of the better-known examples of amnesia (Whitty et al. 1977). A blackout can occur if the individual is intoxicated to the point of unconsciousness or impairment of consciousness. It also can affect a significant amount of time before the drinking and can cause amnesia for the time during which the alcohol was imbibed. Despite this, the individual's outward behavior may have appeared relatively normal; he or she may not even have appeared particularly intoxicated. The onset and conclusion of a blackout are abrupt; the blackout usually ends when a particular experience is remembered, which appears to trigger the recovery of other memories. The type of amnesia incurred would suggest that extreme drunkenness might prevent memory formation. Of course, total blanket amnesia is rare; isolated details may be recalled at a later time.

Some events may be recalled during subsequent periods of intoxication, which would suggest that the process of recall could be affected (Whitty et al. 1977). However, Wolf (1980) investigated this and found conflicting results. He studied several convicted murderers, all of whom had been extremely drunk at the time when they committed their crimes. Once the subjects became intoxicated again, no evidence indicated that they could now recall their crimes any better. It should be noted that most of the evidence of blackout is provided via subjective recall by the patients themselves, so it may be questionable. Chronic alcohol abusers can have more pronounced problems, including amnestic syndrome, exacerbated by several factors, including nutritional deficiency and lack of specific vitamins (namely, vitamin B_1), commonly known as Korsakoff's syndrome (Kolb and Whishaw 1996; Pinel 1993).

The legal system basically believes that intoxication cannot be used as an excuse to explain the committing of a crime; however, it will be taken into consideration if the individual is so intoxicated that it is unlikely that he or she would have had the necessary intent to commit the crime (Whitlock 1963).

Amnesia is most frequently associated with head injuries. A person who is knocked unconscious by a blow to the head may have a period of confusion on regaining consciousness, after which normal responses should return. However, it may subsequently be found that the individual

---

[3]The British courts appear to understand that there is a distinction between different amnesias. In *R. v. Hartridge* (1966) the accused shot and killed his wife while intoxicated and experiencing alcohol-induced amnesia. The court held that it would be a misdirection to direct the jury on the defense of automatism and amnesia, allowing the accused to be entitled to an acquittal; rather, the amnesia was relevant only to the degree of drunkenness and to whether the degree was such as to render the accused incapable of forming the necessary specific intent (*Attorney General [Northern Ireland] v. Gallagher* 1963; *DPP v. Beard* 1920).

has a posttraumatic amnesia (PTA), even after this period of confusion has apparently ended. During this PTA the individual's actions and behavior can appear normal. In addition, memory for a short period of time before the injury occurred can be lost; this is typically known as retrograde amnesia. Retrograde amnesias are typically much shorter than PTAs. In fact retrograde amnesias of more than a few minutes are unlikely if the PTA is less than 24 hours. Similarly if the retrograde amnesia is approximately 30 minutes, it is likely that the associated PTA is for several days or even weeks (Whitty and Zangwell 1977). Therefore it is usually best to assess memory after the patient's apparent recovery, in case the assessment falls into this PTA period. Also PTA can be used to assess the severity of the underlying brain injury. A PTA of less than 10 minutes indicates a very mild injury, 10–60 minutes indicates a mild injury, 1–24 hours indicates a moderate injury, 1–7 days indicates a severe injury, and more than 7 days indicates a very severe injury (Kolb and Whishaw 1996).

Malingering

Malingering also should be taken into consideration. If an individual who is accused of a crime claims some form of amnesia, he or she could be trying to fake memory loss as a way of gaining sympathy and reduction of sentence. *Malingering* is typically defined as the conscious production of, or embellishment of, physical or psychological disorders, usually for the purpose of gaining something that otherwise would not be given (Schwartz et al. 1998). In general, malingering should be considered if any combination of the following is noted (American Psychiatric Association 2000, p. 739):

1. Medicolegal context of presentation
2. Marked discrepancy between the person's claimed stress or disability and the objective findings
3. Lack of cooperation during the diagnostic evaluation and in complying with the prescribed treatment regimen
4. The presence of antisocial personality disorder

Because of the added problems of determining intentionality, the American Psychiatric Association's definition should be used only as a guideline rather than an assessment tool. Malingering may be determined through some psychological subtests (e.g., Structured Interview of Reported Symptoms, Minnesota Multiphasic Personality Inventory).

It should be remembered, however, that criminals also may have genuine memory problems; but, in order to make this assumption, both intoxication and malingering should be ruled out (Swihart et al. 1999).

It is generally agreed that the defendant may be highly motivated to malinger, and if no apparent organic basis exists for the amnesia (e.g., if no memory problems were present before the crime occurred), there is no way to know for certain whether the individual is simulating amnesia (*United States v. Sermon*, cited in Rubinsky and Brandt 1986).

Not only criminals may malinger. For instance, loss of memory is frequently associated with head injuries, so both exaggeration of symptoms and panic over their condition may prolong patients' own assessment of their loss of memory. Examiners must look for unusual or inconsistent performances as well as assess the patients' demeanor for evidence of deceit (Brooks 1999).

Caveat

This is but a cursory review of the psychological literature on memory. We have provided a basic introduction to the structure of memory and have shown that multiple processes may underlie remembering and forgetting. There is much research in this area, and those who keep abreast of the numerous developments in this field know that theories and interpretations are constantly being revised. For example, one of the most important recent developments is that we need to take into account individual differences. Just because one theory applies to one individual does not necessarily mean that it can be applied to all individuals per se.

Memory can function differently across individuals and situations. We cannot assume that all individuals will be affected by the same events or show the same set of memory biases. As Eysenck and Keene (1995, p. 185) stated, "It may well be that what we remember of our own lives is to some extent a reflection of our personalities." Our memory shapes us into the individuals we are, but conversely, that individuality also may to some extent affect our memories.

In a similar way our memory may operate differently depending on the context of remembering. This has been most clearly illustrated by the current debate on the reliability and validity of recovered memories, particularly those memories recovered in therapy. Although it is possible to retrieve accurate memories in the latter context, we know that memory distortions may readily occur under these conditions. Until we develop techniques that allow therapists to discriminate accurate from inaccurate memories, any memory for which the source cannot be identified must be subject to careful scrutiny by the courts.

References

American Medical Association Council on Scientific Affairs: Scientific status of refreshing recollection by the use of hypnosis. JAMA 253:1918–1923, 1985

American Psychiatric Association: Diagnostic and Statistical Manual of Mental Disorders, 4th Edition, Text Revision. Washington, DC, American Psychiatric Association, 2000

Attorney General (Northern Ireland) v Gallagher A.C. 349 applied (1963)

Baddeley A: Essentials of Human Memory. East Sussex, UK, Psychology Press, 1999

Baddeley AD, Hitch G: Working memory, in Recent Advances in Learning and Motivation. Edited by Bower GA. New York, Academic Press, 1974, pp 47–90

Bahrick HP, Bahrick PO, Wittlinger RP: Fifty years of memory for names and faces: a cross-sectional approach. J Exp Psychol Gen 104:54–75, 1975

Barnier AJ, McConkey KM: Reports of real and false memories: the relevance of hypnosis, hypnotizability, and context of memory test. J Abnorm Psychol 101:521–527, 1992

Bartlett FC: Remembering: A Study in Experimental and Social Psychology. Cambridge, UK, Cambridge University Press, 1932

Beck A, Rush AJ, Shaw BF, et al: Cognitive Therapy of Depression. New York, Guilford, 1979

Beck A, Emery G, Greenberg R: Anxiety Disorders and Phobias: A Cognitive Perspective. New York, HarperCollins, 1985

Bliss EL: Multiple Personality, Allied Disorders, and Hypnosis. New York, Oxford University Press, 1986

Bower G: Mood and memory. Am Psychol 36:129–148, 1981

Bower G: How might emotions affect learning?, in The Handbook of Emotion and Memory: Research and Theory. Edited by Christianson SA. Hillsdale, NJ, Lawrence Erlbaum, 1992, pp 3–31

Bower G, Gilligan SG, Monteiro KP: Selectivity of learning caused by affective states. J Exp Psychol Gen 110:451–473, 1981

Brainerd CJ, Reyna VF, Brandse E: Are children's false memories more persistent than their true memories? Psychological Science 6:359–364, 1995

Bransford JD, Franks JJ: The abstraction of linguistic ideas. Cognit Psychol 2:331–350, 1971

Breuer J, Freud S: Studies on hysteria (1893–1895), in Standard Edition of the Complete Psychological Works of Sigmund Freud, Vol 2. Translated and edited by Strachey J. London, Hogarth Press, 1955, pp 1–319

Brooks N: Compensation for brain injury, in Handbook of Psychology in Legal Contexts. Edited by Bull R, Carson D. Chichester, UK, Wiley, 1999, pp 411–426

Carlson EB, Rosser-Hogan R: Trauma experiences, posttraumatic stress, dissociation, and depression in Cambodian refugees. Am J Psychiatry 148:1548–1551, 1991

Ceci SJ, Huffman MCL, Smith E, et al: Repeatedly thinking about a non event—sources misattributions among preschoolers. Conscious Cogn 3(3–4):388–407, 1994

Chalmers AF: Science and Its Fabrication. Milton Keynes, UK, Open University Press, 1990

Chu JA, Dill DL: Dissociative symptoms in relation to childhood physical and sexual abuse. Am J Psychiatry 147:887–892, 1990

Clark DM, Teasdale JD: Diurnal variation in clinical depression and accessibility of positive and negative experiences. J Abnorm Psychol 91:87–95, 1981

Conway MA, Collins AF, Gathercole SE, et al: Recollections of true and false autobiographical memories. J Exp Psychol Gen 25:69–95, 1996

Coons PM: Reports of satanic ritual abuse: further implications about pseudomemories. Percept Mot Skills 78:1376–1378, 1994

Doyle AC: A Study in Scarlet, Reissue Edition. Harmondsworth, UK, Penguin Books, 1982

DPP v Beard A.C. 479 applied (1920)

Ebbinghaus H: Memory: A Contribution to Experimental Psychology (1885). Translated by Ruger HA, Bussenius CE. New York, Dover Publications, 1964

Eich E: The cue-dependent nature of state-dependent retrieval. Mem Cognit 8:157–173, 1980

Elliott DM: Traumatic events: prevalence and delayed recall in the general population. J Consult Clin Psychol 65:811–820, 1997

Erdelyi M: Hypnotic hypermnesia: the empty set of hypermnesia. Int J Clin Exp Hypn 42:379–390, 1994

Eysenck MW, Keane MT: Cognitive Psychology: A Student's Handbook, 3rd Edition. Hove, UK, Lawrence Erlbaum, 1995

Feldman-Summers S, Pope KS: The experience of forgetting childhood abuse: a national survey of psychologists. J Consult Clin Psychol 62:636–639, 1994

Fisher RP, Geiselman RE: Memory Enhancing Techniques for Investigative Interviewing: The Cognitive Interview. Springfield, IL, Charles C Thomas, 1992

Garry M, Manning CG, Loftus EF, et al: Imagination inflation: imagining a childhood event inflates confidence that it occurred. Psychonomic Bulletin and Review 3(2):208–214, 1996

Godden DR, Baddeley AD: Context-dependent memory in two natural environments: on land and under water. Br J Psychol 66:325–331, 1975

Goff LM, Roediger HL: Imagination inflation for action events: repeated imaginings lead to illusory recollections. Mem Cognit 26:20–33, 1998

Goodwin DW, Powell B, Bremer D, et al: Alcohol and recall: state-dependent effects in man. Science 163:135–1360, 1969

Grinker RR, Spiegal JP: Men Under Stress. New York, McGraw-Hill, 1945

Heaps C, Nash M: Individual differences in imagination inflation. Psychonomic Bulletin and Review 6:313–318, 1999

Hilgard ER: Hypnosis. Annu Rev Psychol 26:19–44, 1975

Hilgard ER: Divided Consciousness: Multiple Controls in Human Thought and Action. New York, Wiley Interscience, 1977

Hilgard JR: Sequelae to hypnosis. Int J Clin Exp Hypn 22:281–298, 1974

Hunter v John Brown and Co Ltd S.L.T. 302 (1961)

Hyman IE, Pentland J: The role of mental imagery in the creation of false childhood memories. Journal of Memory and Language 35:101–117, 1996

Hyman IE, Husband TH, Billings FJ: False memories of childhood experiences. Applied Cognitive Psychology 9:181–197, 1995

Hyman IE, Gilstrap LL, Decker K, et al: Manipulating remember and know judgements of autobiographical memories: an investigation of false memory creation. Applied Cognitive Psychology 12:371–386, 1998

Janet P: L'automatisme psychologique (1889), in Perry C, Laurence J-R: Mental processing outside of awareness: the contributions of Freud and Janet, in The Unconscious Reconsidered. Edited by Bowers KS, Meichenbaum D. New York, Wiley, pp 9–48

Kanak NJ, Stevens R: PI and RI in serial learning as a function of environmental context. Applied Cognitive Psychology 6:389–406, 1992

Kassin SM: The psychology of confession evidence. Am Psychol 52:221–233, 1997

Kihlstrom JF: Hypnosis. Annu Rev Psychol 36:385–418, 1985

Kolb B, Whishaw IQ: Fundamentals of Human Neuropsychology, 4th Edition. New York, WH Freeman, 1996

Kopelman MD: Crime and amnesia: a review. Behav Sci Law 5:323–342, 1987

Krietman N: The reliability of psychiatric diagnosis. Journal of Mental Science 10:876–886, 1961

Lampinen JM, Neuschatz JS, Payne DG: Memory illusions and consciousness: examining the phenomenology of true and false memories. Current Psychology 16:181–224, 1998

Lewis DO, Lovely R, Yeager C, et al: Toward a theory of the genesis of violence: a follow-up study of delinquents. J Am Acad Child Adolesc Psychiatry 28:431–436, 1989

Lindsay DS, Read JD: Psychotherapy and memories of childhood sexual abuse: a cognitive perspective. Applied Cognitive Psychology 8:281–338, 1994

Lloyd GC, Lishman WA: Effects of depression on the speed of recall of pleasant and unpleasant experiences. Psychol Med 5:173–180, 1975

Loftus EF: The malleability of human memory. American Scientist 67:312–320, 1979

Loftus EF: The reality of repressed memories. Am Psychol 48:518–537, 1993

Loftus EF, Pickrell J: The formation of false memories. Psychiatric Annals 25:720–725, 1995

Ludwig AM: The psychobiological functions of dissociation. Am J Clin Hypn 26:93–99, 1983

Lynn SJ, Lock TG, Myers B, et al: Recalling the unrecallable: should hypnosis be used to recover memories in psychotherapy? Current Directions in Psychological Science 6:79–83, 1997

Lynn SJ, Marmelstein L, Kirsch I, et al: The hypnotic Interview: conceptual and technical considerations, in Handbook of the Psychology of Interviewing. Edited by Memon A, Bull R. Chichester, UK, Wiley, 1999, pp 21–38

Markowitsch HJ (ed): Transient Global Amnesia and Related Disorders. Toronto, ON, Hogrefe & Huber, 1990

McConkey KM, Labelle L, Bibb BC, et al: Hypnosis and suggested pseudomemory: the relevance of test context. Australian Journal of Psychology 42:197–205, 1990

Medawar PB: The Art of the Soluble. Harmondsworth, UK, Penguin, 1963

Memon A, Higham P: A review of the Cognitive Interview. Psychology, Crime and Law 5 (special issue):177–196, 1999

Memon A, Young M: Desperately seeking evidence: the recovered memory debate. Legal and Criminological Psychology 2:131–154, 1997

Milgram S: Behavioral study of obedience. Journal of Abnormal and Social Psychology 67:371–378, 1963

Murrey GJ, Cross HJ, Whipple J: Hypnotically created pseudomemories: further investigation into the "memory distortion or response bias" question. J Abnorm Psychol 101:75–77, 1992

Parkin AJ: Memory: Phenomena, Experiment, and Theory, 3rd Edition. Oxford, UK, Blackwell, 1995

Parwatikar SD, Holcomb WR, Menninger KAD: The detection of malingered amnesia in accused murderers. Bulletin of the American Academy of Psychiatry and the Law 13:97–103, 1985

Payne DG, Neuschatz JS, Lampinen JM, et al: Compelling memory illusions: the qualitative characteristics of false memories. Current Directions in Psychological Sciences 6(3):56–60, 1997

Pinel JPJ: Biopsychology, 2nd Edition. Boston, MA, Allyn & Bacon, 1993

Poole DA: Strolling fuzzy-trace theory through eyewitness testimony (or vice versa). Learning and Individual Differences 7:87–94, 1995

Poole DA, Lindsay DS, Memon A, et al: Psychotherapy and the recovery of memories of childhood sexual abuse: US and British practitioners' opinions, practices, and experiences. J Consult Clin Psychol 63:426–437, 1995

Popper K: Objective Knowledge: An Evolutionary Approach. Oxford, UK, Oxford University Press, 1972

Porter S, Yuille JC, Lehman DR: The nature of real, implanted, and fabricated memories for emotional childhood events: implications for the recovered memory debate. Law Hum Behav 23:517–537, 1999

R. v Browning (Edward) Crim.L.R. 227 (1995)

R. v Hartridge 57 D.L.R. 2d 332 (1966)

R. v Mayes; R. v McIntosh C.L.Y. 930 (1995)

Reisberg D: Cognition: Exploring the Science of the Mind. New York, WW Norton, 1997

Rubinsky EW, Brandt J: Amnesia and criminal law: a clinical overview. Behav Sci Law 4:27–46, 1986

Sachs JS: Recognition memory for syntactic and semantic aspects of connected discourse. Percept Psychophys 2:437–442, 1967

Sarbin T, Coe W: Hypnosis. New York, Holt, 1972

Schacter DL: Searching for Memory: The Brain, the Mind and the Past. New York, Basic Books, 1996

Schmidt HG, Peeck VH, Paas F, et al: Remembering the street names of one's childhood neighbourhood: a study of very long-term retention. Memory 8:37–49, 2000

Schooler JW, Gerhard D, Loftus EF: Qualities of the unreal. J Exp Psychol Learn Mem Cogn 12:171–181, 1986

Schwartz SM, Gramling SE, Kerr KL, et al: Evaluation of intellect and deficit specific information on the ability to fake memory deficits. Int J Law Psychiatry 21:261–272, 1998

Sheehan PW, Statham D, Jamieson GA: Pseudomemory effects and their relationship to level of susceptibility to hypnosis and state instructions. J Pers Soc Psychol 60:130–137, 1991a

Sheehan PW, Statham D, Jamieson GA: Pseudomemory effects over time in the hypnotic setting. J Abnorm Psychol 100:39–44, 1991b

Sherman SJ, Cialdini RB, Schwartzman DF, et al: Imagining can heighten or lower the perceived likelihood of contracting a disease: the mediating effect of ease of imagery. Personality and Social Psychology Bulletin 11:118–127, 1985

Smith SM: Environmental context-dependent memory: recognition memory using a short-term memory task for input. Mem Cognit 14:347–354, 1986

Spanos NP: Hypnotic behaviour: a social psychological interpretation of amnesia, analgesia, and 'trance logic.' Behav Brain Sci 9:449–467, 1986

Spanos NP: Multiple Identities and False Memories: A Sociocognitive Perspective. Washington, DC, American Psychological Association, 1996

Spanos NP, Burgess CA, Burgess MF, et al: Creating false memories of infancy with hypnotic and non-hypnotic procedures. Applied Cognitive Psychology 13:201–218, 1999

Spiegal D, Cardena E: Disintegrated experience: the dissociative disorders revisited. J Abnorm Psychol 100:366–378, 1991

Sternberg RJ: In Search of the Human Mind. Orlando, FL, Harcourt Brace, 1995

Swihart G, Yuille J, Porter S: The role of state-dependent memory in "red-outs." Int J Law Psychiatry 22(3–4):199–212, 1999

Tousignant JP, Hall D, Loftus EF: Discrepancy detection and vulnerability to misleading postevent information. Mem Cognit 14:329–338, 1986

Wagenaar W: My memory: a study of autobiographical memory over six years. Cognit Psychol 18:225–252, 1986

Wagstaff GF: Hypnosis, Compliance and Belief. New York, St. Martin's Press, 1981

Wagstaff GF: What expert witnesses can tell courts about hypnosis: a review of the association between hypnosis and the law. Expert Evidence 2:60–70, 1993

Wagstaff GF, Vella M, Perfect TJ: The effect of hypnotically elicited testimony on jurors' judgements of guilt and innocence. J Soc Psychol 31:69–77, 1992

Warrington EK, Sanders HL: The fate of old memories. Q J Exp Psychol 23:432–442, 1971

Wetzler SE, Sweeney JA: Childhood amnesia: an empirical demonstration, in Autobiographical Memory. Edited by Rubin DC. Cambridge, MA, Cambridge University Press, 1986, pp 191–201

White RW: A preface to a theory of hypnotism. J Abnorm Soc Psychol 36:477–506, 1941

Whitlock FA: Criminal Responsibility and Mental Illness. London, Butterworths, 1963

Whitty CWM, Zangwell OL: Traumatic amnesia, in Amnesia: Clinical, Psychological and Medicolegal Aspects. Edited by Whitty CWM, Zangwell OL. London, Butterworths, 1977, pp 118–135

Whitty CWM, Stores G, Lishman WA: Amnesia in cerebral disease, in Amnesia: Clinical, Psychological and Medicolegal Aspects. Edited by Whitty CWM, Zangwell OL. London, Butterworths, 1977, pp 52–92

Wolf AS: Homicide and blackout in Alaskan natives: a report and reproduction of five cases. J Stud Alcohol 41:456–462, 1980

Yerkes RM, Dodson JD: The relation of strength of stimulus to rapidity of habit-formation. Journal of Comparative Neurology and Psychology 18:459–482, 1908

12

Psychiatric Diagnoses and the Retrospective Assessment of Mental States

Liza H. Gold, M.D.

Forensic psychiatrists and psychologists are frequently asked to make a determination of past mental status relative to a specific act or behavior in many types of litigation. Requests for such opinions can arise in cases involving criminal behavior, suicide, contractual agreements, wills, and other matters subject to adjudication that focus on the past rather than current or future mental status. The retrospective assessment of mental status often entails an attempt to formulate a diagnosis of past or present mental illness. However, the use of psychiatric diagnosis in the retrospective assessment of mental status raises some questions. Are such diagnoses legally required, relevant, or reliable? What does the use of psychiatric diagnosis add to the adjudication of the legal matter at issue?

The relevance of a current psychiatric diagnosis to past mental status is not straightforward. If the subject in question is available for an assessment of his or her current mental status, then the examination may indeed provide significant insight into past mental status and psychiatric diagnoses. However, in cases in which the subject is unavailable for direct examination, the evaluator may be asked to formulate an opinion regarding a diagnosis at some time in the past based on documentation and the observations of others and relate that diagnosis to questions about cognitive, behavioral, or psychological impairment. Under these circumstances the relation between diagnosis and past mental status is even more complex.

The diagnostic system of mental illness as described in DSM-IV-TR (American Psychiatric Association 2000) is the basis of all mental health diagnostic classification, clinical practice and research, and is the standard diagnostic nomenclature in use today. However, the use of psychiatric diagnoses in the legal process and their relationship to the retrospective assessment of mental states is frequently problematic in forensic evaluations. DSM-IV-TR diagnoses may create confusion rather than clarity as the finder of fact attempts to sort through complex and often conflicting levels of expert psychiatric and psychological testimony. Nevertheless, the legal system may require that such expert testimony be offered.

Diagnoses are often threshold requirements for meeting a specific legal sanction or determination. For example, in criminal law every legal test for criminal responsibility specifies that the legally relevant impairment must be due to "mental disease or defect," and many standards for incompetence to stand trial, including those of the Model Penal Code (American Law Institute 1962), require that the defendant's limitations be due to mental disorder. In civil law, the existence of a mental disorder may be necessary to establish that a party was incompetent to contract or unable to write a valid will (Halleck et al. 1992; Chapter 2, this volume).

Diagnoses serve these threshold functions because they are believed to be meaningfully associated with diminished abilities. However, they are also often used to validate critical legal contentions that certain relevant impairments were present at some time in the past. At times a diagnosis may be used as a substitute for an evaluation of specific impairments because the presence of a diagnosis implies the presence of impairments commonly associated with that specific diagnosis. Such uses can stretch the value of diagnosis beyond a reasonable limit.

Sorting through these complexities requires an examination of the relation between diagnosis and the retrospective assessment of mental states and the requirements of the legal process. Such an examination raises the following questions:

- *Is the DSM diagnostic classification system scientifically sound, and can it prove its scientific methodology under legal scrutiny?* This question is at the core of evidentiary issues surrounding the acceptability of expert testimony as defined by *Daubert* and the Federal Rules of Evidence. It is also at the core of parallel historical and philosophical issues, which address some of the questions posed by the legal system regarding expert testimony.

- *Does a present or past diagnosis of mental illness imply the presence of past mental impairment, and is that mental impairment relevant to the legal issue in question?* This issue is at the core of evidentiary issues regarding relevance and the specifics of forensic evaluation and is discussed in the section "Diagnoses and the Retrospective Assessment of Mental States."

Psychiatric Diagnostic Classification and DSM

DSM is the basis of the current diagnostic classification system and is widely used by mental health professionals and the legal system (Shuman 1989; M. Spitzer 1994). DSM-IV-TR diagnoses, when presented as expert testimony, typically are not challenged directly on their scientific credibility. The fact that such challenges do not occur on an appellate level indicates that attorneys and courts assume that DSM diagnoses meet the scientific reliability evidentiary criteria.

However, on occasion, the science behind a diagnosis can become a central point in court cases. In *United States v. Torniero* (1983), for example, the validity of the diagnosis of "pathological gambling," first described in DSM-III (American Psychiatric Association 1980), came into question. The judge ultimately ruled that the defendant could not introduce expert testimony regarding his diagnosis of pathological gambling on the grounds that it was only tangentially related to the charge of interstate transportation of stolen goods. However, the judge also took the position that the diagnosis of pathological gambling did not bear enough scientific validity to qualify as a threshold for the legal standard of insanity (Slovenko 1995). The judge reserved the right of the court, rather than the jury, "to consider whether the type of disease or defect alleged by the defendant is sufficient to constitute an allegation of insanity" (p. 721). The judge stated that he shared "the widespread and growing public concern that new mental disorders appear to be fabricated in unending succession...and that defendants increasingly seek to 'explain' their alleged criminal acts as somehow compelled by pathologies of vague description and scant relevance" (*United States v. Torniero* 1983, pp. 723–724).

History of DSM

Before the publication of DSM-III (American Psychiatric Association 1980), systems of classification for the diagnosis of mental illness were notably lacking in the methodology of modern scientific tradition. The absence of this methodology drew justifiable criticism of the reliability of psychiatric nomenclature, such as that of the judge in *United States v. Torniero* (1983). However, the publication and widespread acceptance of DSM-III and its revisions—DSM-III-R (American Psychiatric Association 1987), DSM-IV (American Psychiatric Association 1994), and DSM-IV-TR (American Psychiatric Association 2000)—marked a major change in the diagnostic classification of mental illness. Beginning with DSM-III, psychiatrists consciously attempted to use the scientific method in attempts to increase the accuracy and reliability of the diagnosis of mental illness. They devised a classification system, which as far as possible eliminated categories and concepts based on unproven (and unprovable) psychological theories. In doing so, they provided a standard diagnostic nomenclature, whose purpose was, as stated in DSM-III, "to provide clear descriptions of diagnostic categories in order to enable clinicians and investigators to diagnose, communicate about, study and treat various mental disorders" (DSM-III, p. 12) and to provide clinicians and researchers with "a common language with which to communicate" (DSM-III, p. 1).

Before the twentieth century, a number of systems of classification for mental illness had been devised. The first official psychiatric manual of mental disorders to focus on clinical rather than statistical utility was DSM-I (American Psychiatric Association 1952). This diagnostic nomenclature included brief descriptions of the symptoms and characteristics that typified each diagnostic category. DSM-I was widely used; it was reprinted 20 times through 1967 (Coolidge and Segal 1998). Its first revision, DSM-II (American Psychiatric Association 1968), incorporated some minor changes and added a few diagnostic categories, but it did not differ significantly from DSM-I in its fundamental approach toward classification or its underlying theoretical assumptions.

Some of the fundamental assumptions of the dominant professional philosophy of mid-twentieth-century psychiatry were reflected in the first DSMs, as any classificatory system incorporates the dominant theoretical influences of its time. During the 1950s and 1960s, these were the theories of Freud and of Adolf Meyer. Most psychiatrists used a broadly conceived psychosocial model that synthesized Freud's theories of personality and intrapsychic conflict and Meyer's psychodynamic and psychosocial theories (Grob 1991). The focus of psychiatric study based on these theories was the meaning of such symptoms, rather than the study of mental illnesses (Menninger 1963). Clinicians operating within this model often felt that careful, descriptive diagnosis obfuscated good clinical work by focusing attention on classificatory categories rather thanon the meaning of symptoms (Wilson 1993).

These models and their philosophy created weaknesses in the diagnostic classification system of DSM-I and DSM-II. Descriptions of disorders were brief and usually lacking in operational criteria for their application. For example, practitioners seeking guidance in differentiating schizophrenia from mania would find little to help them. Diagnosis was thus dependent on clinical supposition and was widely recognized to vary considerably from one clinician to another. Research demonstrated that measurements of diagnostic reliability failed to rise more than 50% for even the most severe mental illnesses (Scull 1989). "Through the 1950's and 1960's there were serious problems related to unreliability. We psychiatrists could not seem to agree with one another, particularly in courtrooms but more so in the consultation rooms and in research settings" (Klerman et al. 1984, p. 540).

However, in the 1970s the psychiatric profession's attitude toward diagnosis began to change. Internal and external pressures on the field of psychiatry arose, such as 1) the introduction of drug therapy and its implications for a biological basis of psychiatric illness and 2) the effect of the antipsychiatry movement of the 1960s and 1970s. These pressures resulted in a growing sense of need for diagnostic reliability, and a significant change in diagnostic classification became warranted (Wilson 1993). A group of psychiatrists began applying the methods of modern science to diagnostic classification in an attempt to address some of these problems of the existing diagnostic classification system.

These psychiatrists have been described as an invisible college of neo-Kraepelinians (Blashfield 1982; Klerman 1990; Rogler 1997). They believed, as did Kraepelin, that diagnostic categories needed to correspond to what were presumably natural disease entities. They felt that a diagnostic classification system could be based on a description of course and symptoms without necessarily proving etiological causes. They argued that the best method for arriving at these diagnostic classifications was to devise operational criteria based on research for determining exactly what symptoms must be present before a physician could make a given diagnosis. Such research-based operational criteria (Feighner et al. 1972; Spitzer et al. 1975), in conjunction with clinical expertise and judgment, would guide and standardize diagnosis from clinician to clinician, thereby increasing diagnostic reliability. Such a diagnostic system would enable clinicians to devise reliable differential diagnoses, to design appropriate treatment, and to promote research to expand the limits of knowledge regarding mental illness.

In 1974 a new APA task force, headed by Robert Spitzer, was formed to revise the DSM-II. The task force believed that the key to successful innovation in psychiatric classification was the application of scientific methodology. Using the neo-Kraepelinian principles to guide a reformulation of diagnostic classification, the task force set out to produce a science-driven document in which classification would not be based on etiology unless the etiology had been proved. The task force used and emulated the medical model of disease to attain a scientific ideal for the classification of mental illnesses. DSM-III, published in 1980, changed the focus of the diagnosis of mental illness from a clinically based biopsychosocial model to a science- and research-based medical model. It was a descriptive manual that empha- sized observable symptoms and etiological neutrality.

DSM-III thus represented a marked departure from the classification sys- tem of the earlier DSMs. The designers of DSM-III made explicit efforts to use research evidence in nosological constructions and to test for interrater re- liability the definitions developed. Between 1977 and 1979 the National Insti- tute of Mental Health sponsored a field trial in which approximately 550 clinicians from more than 200 facilities used successive drafts of DSM-III in evaluating 12,667 patients and compared diagnostic consistency (DSM-III, p. 5). The concerns with interrater reliability and with better-controlled clini- cal, laboratory, epidemiological, medical, and basic science studies with larger sample sizes showed that a classification system for psychiatric diagnosis could be based on the principles of modern science.

As a result of DSM-III's changes in the system of diagnostic classifica- tion, broad changes in both the utility and the popularity of the diagnostic classification of mental illness have occurred. DSM has become central to the vast system of mental health care and is the taxonomy of mental illness most widely used by all the professional mental health disciplines in teach- ing, research, and clinical practice. Directly or indirectly, it has influenced judicial deliberations, third-party payments, budgetary allocations by pri- vate and governmental bodies, and many other key institutional functions (Rogler 1997). A survey of psychiatrists reported that they considered DSM-III to be the most important psychiatric publication to appear be- tween 1970 and 1980 (Strauss et al. 1993).

DSM: Strengths and Limitations

With the publication of DSM-III, psychiatry adopted a research-oriented descriptive approach to the classification of mental illness based on the medical model of disease and accepted methods of scientific research to validate and improve diagnostic reliability. Some of the advantages of the DSM classification system are as follows:

- Provisions for the recognition of multiple disorders
- Inclusion of operational criteria with exclusion and inclusion criteria

- Demonstrable reliability based on field testing
- Multiaxial system of diagnosis, which allows accommodation of diverse aspects of patients' existence
- Recognition of and provisions for the implicit necessity for further change directed by research based on evidence rather than assertions of competing ideological camps (Klerman et al. 1984)

Taken together, these features of DSM-III's classification system affirmed that the treatment of mental illness is a branch of medicine that should focus on biological aspects of mental illness and attend explicitly to the codification, reliability, and validity of psychiatric classifications based on scientific research. As a result, the DSM nosologies have supplied much improved diagnostic criteria for many major categories of mental illness (Wallace 1994).

The DSM diagnostic classification of mental illness, however, has limitations as well as strengths and advantages. Critics of the current system often use these limitations to question its scientific basis, reliability, or utility. An examination of the strengths and limitations of the DSM classification system allows honest evaluation of both. Such an examination not only improves our understanding of the use of the classification system but also shows that these limitations do not invalidate the scientific basis of the system or its utility.

Classification is the foundation of any science. Thinking in terms of classification is part of human nature, and the construction of classifications for all sorts of phenomena, including mental disorders, is inevitable and unavoidable (Millon 1991). However, it is also a process that is inevitably subject to change, debate, and controversy, as the publication of DSM-III demonstrated. The classification system of DSM-III provoked significant controversy and criticism from inside and outside the profession of psychiatry and from philosophical, historical, cultural, social, political, and scientific perspectives. These critiques highlight some of the limitations of DSM that are unique to classifications of mental illness and some that are common to diagnostic systems in general.

All clinical diagnosticians confront certain fundamental problems in devising a classification of illness, one of which is the construction of the definitions of basic terms. For example, physicians treat *diseases* without being able to define the term *disease* precisely. The concept of *disorder* itself always involves a value judgment (R.L. Spitzer 1981). Similarly, DSM is a manual of *mental disorders*, but a precise and universally accepted definition of a *mental disorder* has yet to be devised (Follette and Houts 1996; R.L. Spitzer 1999; Wakefield 1992, 1999; Widiger et al. 1991). This failure of definition is not a reflection of the many individuals from medical, psychological, philosophical, and social disciplines who have attempted to define terms such as *mental disorder, disease,* and *illness.* Rather, it results from the essentially heterogeneous nature of the many elements that make up these terms.

DSM-IV-TR acknowledges the challenge presented by defining basic terms in devising a classification system. The introduction states that "although this manual provides a classification of mental disorders, it must be admitted that no definition adequately specifies precise boundaries for the concept of 'mental disorder'" (American Psychiatric Association 2000, p. xxx). "The concept of a mental disorder, like many other concepts in medicine and science, lacks a consistent operational definition that covers all situations" (American Psychiatric Association 2000, p. xxx).

DSM ultimately defined a *mental disorder* as a

> clinically significant behavioral or psychological syndrome or pattern that occurs in an individual and that is associated with present distress (e.g., a painful symptom) or disability (i.e., impairment in one or more important areas of functioning) or with a significantly increased risk of suffering death, pain, disability, or an important loss of freedom....Whatever its original cause, it must currently be considered a manifestation of a behavioral, psychological, or biological dysfunction in the individual. (American Psychiatric Association 2000, pp. xxxi)

However, it acknowledged the arbitrary nature of this definition. "The definition of *mental disorder* that was included in DSM-III and DSM-III-R is presented here because it is as useful as any other available definition and has helped to guide decisions regarding which conditions on the boundary between normality and pathology should be included in DSM-IV" (American Psychiatric Association 2000, p. xxxi).

Classification systems such as DSM-III are also subject to criticism for lacking objective measures that might serve to establish the presence or absence of a mental disorder (Widiger et al. 1991; Zarin and Earls 1993). Pathognomonic tests or imaging techniques are currently unavailable for most mental illnesses. These problems raise the question of what kind of evidence can be used to order a system of classification when "absolute" evidence is unavailable and how to ensure reliability of such diagnoses. Definitional criteria that guide inclusionary and exclusionary decisions for the manual have defied construction (Frances 1994)."The need for a classification of mental disorders has been clear throughout the history of medicine, but there has been little agreement on which disorders should be included and the optimal method for their organization" (American Psychiatric Association 2000, p. xxiv).

The lack of objective corroborative or diagnostic data becomes most acute when mental health professionals encounter difficult or controversial diagnostic issues that do not lend themselves to simple explanations or diagnostic labels. Medical diagnoses that lack such objective measures of validation are also often controversial and are criticized for susceptibility to external influences in much the same way as psychiatric diagnoses are. Consider, for example, the political and social complexities associated with the diagnoses of Gulf War syndrome and chronic fatigue syndrome, two medical syndromes described primarily by their clinical symptomatology. Even more straightforward medical diagnoses have been found to have significant problems with accuracy and reliability (R.L. Spitzer 1976).

Complex scientific, evaluative, and practical concerns are inextricably combined in medical diagnosis in general and in the classification of mental illness in particular. No system of categorization can completely embody the complexity of human emotion, behavior, and distress. Classifications of mental illness are rendered problematic by the fact that most mental illnesses consist of symptoms that, at the milder end of the spectrum, are clearly aspects of normal daily functioning. This raises sensitive issues of the use of judgment and value systems when drawing a line between a mental illness and a common or "normal" psychological function.

Nevertheless, although the boundary between mental health and mental disorder remains ill defined, without some system for classifying these experiences, investigators would be unable to communicate with one another, and knowledge would not advance. Individuals would have to develop their own personal systems that could not be applied beyond their subjective experience. When dealing with vegetation, insects, or rocks, these concepts are fundamental and rarely questioned. When the subject matter is human behavior in general, and psychological disorders in particular, controversy surrounds all aspects of the endeavor, including the very basic issues of whether classification even ought to be attempted (Millon 1991).

Other critiques of DSM-III questioned the "science" of devising a classification system by committee. Critics have argued that the process of consensus and compromise inherent in committees is unscientific and is a disadvantage in devising a diagnostic classification (Klerman et al. 1984). Work by consensus may have some limitations, and committee decisions may be influenced by factors other than pure science. Nevertheless, committee work serves a fundamental need in the development of a science. The dominance of any particular scientific theory over others arises from the joint efforts of individuals who use the same concrete models and are committed to the same rules and standards for scientific practice (Kuhn 1996). Such agreement can be reached only by consensus and compromise.

Thus the use of a process of compromise and consensus does not invalidate the classification system of DSM-III. Such consensus is a prerequisite for the development and practice of science (Kuhn 1996). What becomes accepted as science by any group results in part from successful social organizing (Cooksey and Brown 1998) and the negotiation of areas of controversy that exist in all scientific disciplines. In addressing arguments regarding the use of committees in DSM-III, Spitzer stated: "If you accept the proposition that classifications are man-made...then it follows that committees are all that we have....So I have no apologies for the fact that DSM-III was developed by committees" (Klerman et al. 1984, p. 546).

Criticism also has been directed toward the claims that DSM is atheoretical (Follette and Houts 1996; Rogler 1997; Sadler et al. 1994; Wakefield 1999; Wilson 1993). This criticism is largely justified; the dominance of the theories of the "invisible college of neo-Kraepelinians" is clear throughout the classification system. Although not explicitly stated, the underlying ontologies of the medical model of disease are easily deducible from the DSM's content (Follette and Houts 1996; Rogler 1997) and provide the theoretical model of the DSM classification system. The claims of an atheoretical position in DSM-III arose out of professional politics rather than the exigencies of diagnostic classification (Follette and Houts 1996). However, the incorporation of a theoretical bias does not of itself invalidate a classification system because it is not possible to have a classification system that is devoid of a theoretical basis (or bias). Every system of classification inevitably involves creating, defining, or confirming boundaries of theoretical concepts (Morey 1991). Theory provides a context and gives a classification system its scientific and clinical relevance (Carson 1991; Hempel 1994; Millon 1991; Wallace 1994).

Other criticisms of DSM-III related to theory and methodology have included DSM's emphasis on "transient surface phenomena," its lack of emphasis on clinical course and human development, and its emphasis on diagnostic reliability at the expense of diagnostic validity (Klerman et al. 1984). One of the most powerful of these criticisms includes concerns about the disadvantages of reductionism and its resulting increase in categories of illness (Klerman et al. 1984). These critics argue that the artificial quality of using methods based on observational phenomena to define mental illnesses is demonstrated by the increase in the number of diagnoses in each revision of DSM since DSM-I.

R.L. Spitzer and Williams (1994) stated that DSM should include all widely used diagnostic categories that clinicians find essential to their work, even if satisfactory reliability and validity data are lacking, to maximize clinical utility. Such an approach will inevitably result in the inclusion of less-well-validated diagnoses. DSM was expressly designed to highlight unknown areas and to mark them for future research. However, DSM does not distinguish between established and newer diagnoses in the main body of the classification system. Although they may have been included to stimulate research into their clinical validity and usefulness, some of the newer diagnoses, such as pathological gambling, can appear to carry the same degree of historical weight and diagnostic validity as more established diagnoses.

Classification is an inherently political process as well as a scientific endeavor. The importance and exclusiveness of a professional discipline are defined by the process of classification of its territory. The creation and widespread acceptance of DSM-III's classification system resulted in the remedicalization of psychiatry. "The decision of the American Psychiatric Association to develop the DSM-III and then to promulgate its use represents a significant reaffirmation on the part of American psychiatry of its medical identity and its commitment to scientific medicine" (Klerman et al. 1984, p. 539). However, this process of reestablishing a medical identity for mental illness also formed the basis for criticism of both the DSM and the psychiatric profession as an intentional attempt by psychiatrists to consolidate professional power and establish themselves as the preeminent authorities in mental illness (Cooksey and Brown 1998).

Critics also have argued that DSM embodies and codifies what are essentially value judgments about normality and deviance, based on the norms of a select group of predominantly white male professionals. This has resulted in giving the sex, culture, and racial biases of this group the appearance of scientific validity (Cooksey and Brown 1998). For example, feminist historians have drawn attention to psychiatry's negative and discriminatory stereotypes of women (Chesler 1972; Showalter 1985) and how these have influenced the definition of mental illness and certain diagnostic categories. Theories of a differential, sex-based etiology for mental disturbances correspond in some important respects to differential expectations and social roles for men and women. In addition, stereotypical images of mental illness and psychiatric explanations and treatments of mental disorders often contain overt and subliminal sexual references and assumptions. These historians point out the overrepresentation of women in certain stigmatized diagnostic categories such as histrionic and borderline personality disorder and the now abandoned category of self-defeating personality disorder (Caplan 1987; Kaplan 1983; Russell 1994; R.L. Spitzer et al. 1989).

Critics also point out that DSM-III reflects cultural parochialism as a result of the origins of the task force members, primarily on the East Coast of North America. Such critics observe that DSM-III does not reflect syndromes observed primarily in non-European cultures, uses distinctively American terminology and concepts, and ignores culture-specific disorders and the influence of cultural context on the specific presentations of disorders. Thus they have argued that DSM does not reflect the experiences, views, or histories of countries or cultures other than the United States (Fabrega 1992; Maser et al. 1991; Mezzich et al. 1999; Shorter 1997; Widiger et al. 1991).

Of all the criticism directed toward DSM's system of psychiatric diagnosis, some of the most powerful originated from the antipsychiatry movement and social historians. These groups focused on the political and social uses of the definition of mental illness and argued that by remedicalizing mental illness, psychiatrists enabled the repression of those labeled as different. Authors such as and Szasz (1960), Laing (1961), and Foucault (1965) approached the subject of mental illness with a strong antinosological bias. These authors doubted the very existence of mental illness and viewed the practice and institutions of psychiatry as reactionary enemies of civil liberties. They explained virtually all scientific, medical, and psychiatric developments as arising from external social forces and from psychiatrists' professional motives for prestige, power, and income. They considered assertions of internal determinants of mental illness at best as rationalizations of the true external social causes, value judgments, and hidden guild self-interests of the psychiatric profession.

Such critics pointed out the potential for political and social misuse of diagnostic categories (Wallace 1994). In support of these arguments against psychiatry and the DSM's diagnostic nosology, the history of homosexuality in DSM is often cited. In DSM-II, homosexuality was classified as a mental illness. After much controversy, acrimony, and public debate, homosexuality was declared not to be a "mental illness" and eliminated from DSM-III. Neither its original inclusion in nor its ultimate exclusion from DSM as a category of mental illness was related to evidence gleaned from scientific research but was clearly the result of social values and the application of political pressures. Other examples cited have included the political pressures from veterans groups that accompanied the introduction of the diagnosis of posttraumatic stress disorder in DSM-III and the inclusion and exclusion of self-defeating personality disorder as a result of feminist concerns. Debates regarding such value-laden diagnostic categories can never be purely scientific (Bayer and Spitzer 1982; Cooksey and Brown 1998; Rogler 1997; Spitzer 1981; Wallace 1994).

Validity of Psychiatric Diagnostic Classification

Some have considered the framers of DSM to be naive positivists because of their belief that an adequate and a comprehensive diagnostic system for mental illness could be devised. Clearly psychopathological states and processes may be classified from several perspectives (such as behavior, intrapsychic processes, or phenomenological data) or from a variety of attributes (interpersonal conduct, mood or affect, or self-image). The ideal classification would be clear, concise, and comprehensively inclusive of all the various scientific approaches in psychiatry and psychology (Sadler et al. 1994). Devising such a classification is as impossible as avoiding classification altogether.

When carried to an extreme, these critical perspectives distort an understanding of the value of the present diagnostic system (Wallace 1994). Following many of the arguments of the DSM's critics to their logical conclusions leads to nosological nihilism, in which the solution to avoiding the biases and limitations inherent in any classification system is to do without classification. Such a solution is not realistic. It is equally unrealistic to reduce the goals of formulating as complicated and intricate a diagnostic classification system as that of DSM-III to psychiatry's covert motivations to establish professional hegemony over mental illness or to provide the social and political establishment with a scientifically sanctioned tool with which to punish deviancy. The primary purpose of any classification of mental illness has been to make it easier for individuals with identifiable problems to receive care that may be helpful to them (R.L. Spitzer 1981).

Many of the criticisms of DSM have legitimately identified some of the inadequacies of the current classification system. Nevertheless, they do not invalidate its advantages and strengths. The concepts and categories that scientists construct are only tools to guide the observation and interpretation of the natural world. The nature of the task of developing such constructs is inevitably arbitrary at best, wholly political at worst, and subject to a variety of cultural, social, and political influences. Moreover, tacit assumptions are an unavoidable artifact of the human condition and thus are also present in such constructs. Because of the particular limitations these assumptions impose, all of our descriptive and explanatory tools in science, including classification systems, are limited in their scope and applicability (Sadler et al. 1994).

No scientific classification, particularly a classification of human behavior, can be constructed that is free of cultural, social, and political influences. "Classification systems are neither inherently self-evident nor given. On the contrary, they emerge from the crucible of human experience" (Grob 1991, p. 421). in addition, although science is practiced by individuals, scientific knowledge is intrinsically a group product. As such it is subject not only to scientific methodology but also to the values of the groups that produce it (Kuhn 1996). Nosological debates regarding mental disorders are inevitably influenced by the social origins and ideological, political, and moral commitments of psychiatrists; their desire for status and legitimacy; and the broader social and intellectual currents prevalent at a given time (Grob 1991).

The fact that science and its practitioners are influenced by values and assumptions held by members of that community does not invalidate the science of the group. However, this fact does imply that those who use any science or classification system need to have a conscious awareness of these influences and values. Certainly much can be learned from an examination of the external forces at work in any field of scientific endeavor, including psychiatry. Such factors have had profound and at times determinative effects on the fate of certain diagnoses, such as that of homosexuality, self-defeating personality disorder, and posttraumatic stress disorder. Nevertheless, the inevitable limitations caused by the presence of such influences do not invalidate the scientific basis of the DSM's nosological system.

The arguments posed by many of the critics of the DSM's classification system typify the conflicts found in the process of maturation in any scientific discipline. The sciences of psychiatry and psychology, despite recent advances, are still young. The influence of cultural, social, and political factors in the development of a science is greatest in its early years and lessens as the science becomes more theoretically and experimentally mature. This is partly because early developmental stages of most sciences are characterized by continual competition among several distinct views of nature. Each of these views is partially derived from and is approximately compatible with the dictates of scientific observation and method. The success of one view over another, an essential step in the development of a scientific discipline, is a multifactorial process. However, some of the factors deciding theoretical dominance are inevitably arbitrary and value laden (Kuhn 1996).

The scientific basis of DSM is the source of the strengths as well as many of the limitations of the DSM classification system. These limitations are not the result of the lack of scientific validity or methodology. Rather they arise from limitations due to the early stages of our knowledge regarding mental illness and to the forces that affect all scientific endeavors. The strengths of the DSM's system derive directly from its descriptive approach to the definition of mental disorders, the use of scientific methods in the classification of mental illness, and the benefits that have resulted from the application of this classification system to clinical practice, treatment, and research (R.L. Spitzer et al. 1980).

DSM: Science and *Daubert*

The DSM classification system was intended to be used for clinical and research purposes. The recognition that it might be used in other contexts resulted in the inclusion of certain caveats in its introduction. The advisory cautions regarding the use of DSM diagnoses for legal purposes occupy an entire page of text. In addition to this discussion, there is a separate "Cautionary Statement": "The clinical and scientific considerations involved in categorization of these conditions as mental disorders may not be wholly relevant to legal judgments, for example, that take into account such issues as individual responsibility, disability determination, and competency" (American Psychiatric Association 2000, p. xxxvii).

However, the legal issues regarding admissibility of expert testimony do not typically focus on the distinctions between clinical and forensic evaluations that worried the framers of DSM. Clinical evaluations and forensic evaluations have different goals and methodology, which are subject to different requirements and ethics (Greenberg and Shuman 1997; Strasburger et al. 1997). The caveats in DSM focus attention on these differences and the use of DSM in forensic evaluations. "When the DSM-IV categories, criteria, and textual descriptions are employed for forensic purposes, there are significant risks that diagnostic information will be misused or misunderstood" (American Psychiatric Association 2000, p. xxxiii). In contrast, legal concerns relating to the admissibility of expert psychiatric and psychological testimony are typically those addressed by *Daubert v. Merrell Dow Pharmaceuticals, Inc.* (1993) (Shuman, Chapter 2, this volume).

For the 70 years prior to the *Daubert* decision, the principle guiding the admission of expert testimony was that of general acceptance within the scientific community. This standard was delineated in the federal court case of *Frye v. United States* (1923). Although largely ignored until the 1960s, the *Frye* standard was binding in the federal courts. In *Daubert* the United States Supreme Court rejected the general acceptance test for scientific evidence and provided more flexible guidelines for admissibility of scientific evidence under the Federal Rules of Evidence, specifically Federal Rule 702. This rule states that when faced with a proffer of expert testimony, the court must consider whether the expert testimony being offered

1. Is beyond the scope of knowledge attributable to the fact-finder
2. Is relevant
3. Can be applied to the facts at issue
4. Can assist the fact-finder

In addition, such expert knowledge and testimony must be based on scientific, technical, or other specialized knowledge, which is subject to scrutiny for its reliability.

In *Daubert* the Supreme Court posed questions similar to those posed by historians and philosophers of science in regard to the nature and validity of the scientific method. The Supreme Court acknowledged that many factors would bear on such inquiries and specifically stated that they were not presuming to set out a definitive checklist. They indicated that they did not intend for a trial judge to automatically exclude relevant evidence if one of these conditions was not fully satisfied. However, the objective of *Daubert's* "gatekeeping" requirement was to ensure both the reliability and the relevancy of expert testimony.

A more recent Supreme Court decision, *Kumho Tire Co. v. Carmichael* (1999), held that Federal Rule 702 imposed a special obligation on a trial judge to ensure that all scientific testimony was both relevant and reliable (Shuman, Chapter 2, this volume). This decision expanded the *Daubert* gatekeeping obligations to proffers of all expert testimony involving scientific, technical, or other specialized knowledge in federal court and reemphasized the Court's determination to admit only reliable and valid expert testimony. Theoretically this ruling could affect the admissibility of expert psychiatric and psychological evidence.

Is the Psychiatric Classification System of DSM "Good Science"?

Because psychiatric diagnoses are often part of expert psychiatric testimony, the *Daubert* decision requires that psychiatric diagnoses be subject to examination regarding their scientific reliability. In considering the scientific reliability of expert testimony, *Daubert* instructed courts to focus solely on the principles and methodology used to generate knowledge, not on the conclusions generated. The justices of the Supreme Court recognized that scientific methodology is the key to distinguishing between genuine and specious knowledge.

The decision of the Court reflected our society's belief in the validity of modern scientific methodology. Methodology is concerned with establishing the legitimate bases for knowledge claims. Methodology addresses 1) the concepts and classifications that constitute the elements of these claims and 2) the larger theories, frameworks, and scientific attitudes into which such claims fit. Acceptable scientific methodology in our society is considered to be that which is consistent with the modern scientific tradition of empirical and deductive logic (Sadler et al. 1994).

The Court stated that the trial judge's assessment of the testimony's underlying reasoning or methodology should consider the following:

1. Whether the theory or technique in question can be and has been tested
2. Whether it has been subjected to peer review and publication
3. Its known or potential error rate
4. The existence and maintenance of standards controlling its operation

5. Whether it has attracted widespread acceptance within the relevant scientific community

The *Daubert* criteria for admissibility of expert testimony in the federal courts identified elements basic to modern scientific method as the main criteria for determining scientific reliability and validity. DSM-III and its subsequent editions have specifically and intentionally used these methods. Thus legal challenges regarding the scientific basis of the current diagnostic classification of mental illness can be addressed by the expert if they arise. As a general rule opinions about DSM psychiatric diagnoses tend to meet the *Daubert* criteria:

1. Current DSM diagnoses have been and continue to be tested and revised based on research evidence.
2. Current DSM diagnoses have been subjected to extensive peer review and have been widely published.
3. The known or potential error rate has been addressed, as far as possible, by investigating and quantifying interrater reliability.
4. The operational criteria of current DSM diagnoses and the continual review process create standards that control the appropriate use of DSM diagnoses.
5. DSM is the most widely accepted psychiatric classification system ever devised. All disciplines within the mental health community and mental health–related businesses and government policymakers outside the mental health community use this system.

Clinical experience is of course a crucial element in evaluating psychiatric illness and formulating diagnoses. By itself, however, it is not the basis of a scientific methodology of diagnostic classification, a fact that makes the use of idiosyncratic diagnoses in expert testimony problematic. Arguments that assignment of a diagnosis is a matter of clinical experience and that DSM diagnoses represent an idiosyncratic application of a vague and unreliable diagnostic system do not take into account the scientific methodology used to devise the current classification system and the training needed to apply it. The Task Force on DSM-III's attempts to resolve diagnostic disputes relied, as much as possible, on research evidence relevant to various kinds of diagnostic validity rather than on individual clinical experience. The science of the diagnostic classification of mental illness emphasizes shared knowledge, collected and tested on the basis of methods meant to overcome the inherent deficiencies of reliance on individual clinical experience alone.

In addition, diagnostic interrater reliability was assessed in the field trials for DSM-III and assigned an easily calculated and understood numerical value, referred to as *kappa* (κ) (American Psychiatric Association 1980). This value corrects for chance agreement between raters. Historically, κ solved a serious problem for diagnostic classification. By correcting diagnostic agreement data for the play of chance, the κ statistic provided an excellent measure of reproducibility. The initial numerical calculations of the DSM interrater reliability studies that used κ were published as an appendix to DSM-III. There have been criticisms of this methodology (Cooksey and Brown 1998), including debates over the difference between diagnostic reliability and validity and the difference between diagnostic accuracy and diagnostic reliability. Although reliability does not guarantee validity or accuracy, it is a necessary precursor of these desirable characteristics. As a result, κ is now the touchstone for assessing the quality of diagnostic procedures (Faraone and Tsuang 1994). Diagnostic classifications that have been assessed by its use meet the criteria for evaluation of the known or potential error rate of expert scientific testimony demanded by *Daubert*.

Acceptance by the scientific community, formerly the *Frye* standard, is another important aspect of any scientific endeavor. This standard remains one of the *Daubert* criteria for admissibility of expert testimony, in recognition of its importance in the determination of scientific validity. General acceptance by the community is, in fact, more important in a scientific discipline than are precise definitions of the subject under study (Kuhn 1977). DSM-III was widely accepted and used by all mental health professions within a few years of its publication, thus meeting another of the *Daubert* criteria.

The lack of consensus regarding important terms such as *mental illness* or *disorder* does not signify a lack of widespread acceptance of the classification system itself. Achieving consensus among a scientific community, an essential part of the process of "normal science," does not require that theoretical terms be precisely defined. Indeed, attempts to produce definitions of basic terms in the physical sciences such as *force* or *mass* often provoke pronounced disagreement. However, it does require agreement among the community on the standard methods used to solve selected problems in which such basic terms figure (Kuhn 1977). DSM attempts to use standard methodology for establishing diagnoses whenever possible and encourages research to validate or invalidate diagnostic criteria, even though certain terms still defy definition.

Psychiatric Diagnosis and Junk Science

In the context of litigation, psychiatric and psychological testimony is often accused of being "junk" science. *Junk science* is information presented as science that is not derived from a valid scientific methodology involving the development of hypotheses that can be tested through objective, quantifiable observation (Huber 1993; Parry 1998). Such critics point to the diversity of psychiatric or psychological theories on the same topics and cite conflicting studies and instances of conflicting diagnosis (often highly publicized, as in the Hinkley case [Stone 1984]) as evidence of their claims. They argue that the "soft" sciences, such as psychology or sociology, cannot achieve the same kind of scientific validity as the "hard" physical sciences, such as chemistry or physics.

Such accusations overlook the nature of science and the scientific method. Science investigates natural phenomena of every sort—from the physical to the biological to the social. Scientific method rests on the concept that ideas about the natural phenomena have consequences and that these consequences provide a basis for testing the idea itself. It is characterized by devising experimental conditions under which explanations for natural phenomena can be tested. Some areas of inquiry lend themselves easily to such methods, whereas others, for practical or ethical reasons, do not. *Daubert* does not state that only Western scientific methodology is valid. Other methods of inquiry into areas that do not lend themselves to scientific proposition and testing may have value, and *Daubert* suggests that these also should be considered if offered as the basis of expert testimony. However, the *Daubert* decision emphasizes that the essential question of scientific validity revolves around the process of the science.

Numerous characteristics of the methods used in generating knowledge mark the differences between genuine science and junk or pseudoscience and allow identification of each category. Genuine science tends to be self-correcting, whereas pseudoscience does not result in self-examination and correction. The findings of genuine science are always open to revision. Pseudoscientific claims rarely change much over time, and pseudoscientists take this aspect of their beliefs to be a scientific virtue. Genuine science embraces skepticism; pseudoscience tends to view skepticism as a sign of narrow-mindedness. Finally as a scientific discipline develops, it will gradually produce a maturing body of explanatory or theoretical findings. Pseudoscience produces very little theory.

in addition, the distinction between science and pseudoscience has nothing to do with the distinction between the hard sciences that investigate the physical world and the soft sciences, such as those that study human behavior. Despite their obvious differences, the hard and soft sciences are all proper science. All are attempts to explain phenomena of the natural world, whether those phenomena are the behavior of matter or of human beings. Genuine practitioners of both hard and soft sciences adhere to scientific methods in advancing and testing their theories. Although the soft sciences differ in several respects from the hard sciences, none of the differences are sufficient to support the accusation that the soft disciplines are pseudosciences. The social sciences may never produce the kinds of grand, unifying theories characteristic of the physical and biological sciences; the soft sciences may have to be satisfied with discrete bits of explanatory material, each suited to a limited aspect of human behavior. But insofar as research in the social and behavioral sciences conforms to the more general methods of good scientific research, it is capable of delivering genuine scientific results.

Finally, the distinction between science and pseudoscience cannot be drawn along lines of scientific discipline. Astronomy and psychology cannot be distinguished from astrology and psychic research as genuine scientific disciplines until the methodology behind the assertions of each field is explored. in addition, every discipline has examples of pseudoscientific theories and experiments that have ultimately been proven to be junk science. Both the justices of the Supreme Court and philosophers of science have recognized that genuine science, regardless of the area of inquiry, is distinguished from pseudoscience on the basis of its methodology rather than their conclusions.

Certainly the methods used by science can be abused, and even careful scientific investigation can result in errors. Critics of psychiatry and psychology may use such instances of errors, abuses, or even reevaluation of previously accepted theories as evidence of the pseudoscientific nature of psychiatry or of its lack of scientific rigor. They may embrace the difficulty in distinguishing science from pseudoscience and use it to imply that any science relating to the analysis of human thought and behavior is unreliable (Hagen 1997). For litigators it can be an advantage to maintain that science, especially soft sciences, can supply no reliable truth and that such scientific expertise can embrace any view, thereby invalidating the testimony of any mental health expert.

However, *Daubert* and scientific philosophy do not demand that all applications of scientific methodology must result in decisive explanations for every problem or exact answers to every question. For example, gravity is a force that can be described mathematically but whose nature still escapes precise definition. This does not render the use of gravitational physics in science problematic or unscientific. Similarly mental disorder itself, critical in the classification of mental illness, has not been precisely defined. Nevertheless, DSM has allowed psychiatry and psychology to abandon an essentially untestable taxonomy. in addition, it has emphasized some of the desirable features of any scientifically based classification system, including those specifically addressed in *Daubert*.

Honest practitioners of science do not attempt to defend the indefensible: they recognize that many questions cannot be settled by scientific inquiry and do not make claims that science is the only tool for investigating the natural world. Some of the critical pragmatic and moral considerations raised by philosophers of science show that empirical research might never resolve some important questions. Clearly issues relating to DSM's classification of mental illness exist that cannot be readily answered simply by gathering more empirical data (Wiggins and Schwartz 1994).

Honest assessment also compels recognition that science is never devoid of political, social, and cultural influences that can color its practice and its results. Nevertheless, despite its limitations, careful scientific investigation in the tradition of rational empiricism and experimental observation has proven to be a more accurate, reliable, stable, coherent, and evenhanded process in the pursuit of knowledge than other alternatives. These attributes, and the advances in knowledge that they have facilitated, account for the success of modern scientific tradition in our culture.

Although not often challenged, the scientific basis of DSM diagnoses may be questioned, as it was in *United States v. Torniero* (1983) in regard to the validity of the diagnosis of pathological gambling. Therefore the distinction between genuine science and pseudoscience, and hard and soft science, must be clear to those who base their expert testimony on knowledge derived from the conscientious application of scientific methodology in the empirical tradition. "Scientists may always be asked to explain their choices, to exhibit the bases for their judgments. Such judgments are eminently discussible, and the man who refuses to discuss his own cannot expect to be taken seriously" (Kuhn 1977, p. 337). Psychiatric testimony that can prove its underlying reliability based on the application of scientific methodology will be admissible if it can be related to the facts of the case before the court.

The *Daubert* and *Kumho* decisions underscore the need for psychiatrists and psychologists testifying as experts to understand the scientific methodology on which the DSM diagnostic system is based. They should be familiar with the empirical evidence that supports diagnosis as well as other testing or methodology that they rely on because they may have to defend it from challenges based on *Daubert* (Grudzinskas 1999). The use of DSM diagnoses serves as a check on poorly informed or biased experts who attempt to cloak their reasoning process by stating that their opinion is a clinical judgment. The methodology involved in the construction of DSM diagnoses and the requirement that symptom presentation must meet specific criteria to qualify for DSM diagnoses allows the expert's reasoning to be tested. This type of preparation will allow forensic experts to apply their clinical expertise with a surer understanding of the legitimate scientific basis on which that expertise rests.

Diagnoses and the Retrospective Assessment of Mental States

The *Daubert* and *Kumho* rulings also underscore the need to be aware of the limitations of DSM diagnoses when used in a forensic context. In addition to addressing the scientific validity of expert testimony, *Daubert* requires that such testimony have relevance to the legal matter at issue. Thus forensic assessment of the retrospective assessment of mental status must include consideration of whether a present or past diagnosis of any mental illness infers the presence of past mental impairment and whether that mental impairment is relevant to the legal issue in question. In other words, does any given DSM diagnosis impart information that is helpful or useful in a specific legal matter as determined by substantive law?

Legal concerns regarding mental illness address the relation between a person's psychological dysfunction and the legal criteria of eligibility at issue rather than between that dysfunction and the criteria for clinical diagnostic categories. The use of DSM diagnoses in the retrospective assessment of mental states is limited by the fact that testimony regarding the individual's diagnostic category may not be directly relevant. The legal requirements for the determination of a psychiatric diagnosis vary from standard to standard. Certain standards, such as civil commitment and insanity, may require or exclude certain disorders, whereas other legal standards, such as testamentary capacity and guardianship, are almost entirely functional and do not require the presence of a DSM diagnosis to adjudicate. Other legal standards may not mention disorders at all. Therefore although diagnostic considerations may not be relevant, expert testimony describing a person's impaired psychological capacities is directly relevant to the court's determination of legal mental illness.

Regardless of the legal standard, no diagnosis of mental illness establishes any legally significant findings about the past or present mental status of an individual. The presence (or absence) of a diagnosis does not provide specific information about an individual's mental status or functional capacity at a given time in the past or present. An individual may have any mental illness and still be legally responsible for his or her behavior or commitments. Conversely the lack of a diagnostic finding does not necessarily indicate that no significant functional impairment or psychological symptoms exist (or existed). The relation between the presence or absence of severe mental illness and issue-specific responsibility or competency does not provide any conclusive evidence about an individual's past mental state.

This apparent contradiction often generates confusion in the legal system about the value and meaning of diagnostic assessments and results in part from the "imperfect fit between the questions of ultimate concern to the law and the information contained in a clinical diagnosis" (American Psychiatric Association 2000, p. xxxiii). Legal mental illness is defined by statute or case law as psychological impairment that renders an individual ineligible for a specified legal status and thus for rights or liabilities associated with that status. Diagnostic nomenclatures, however, define categories of illness as identifiable patterns of impaired psychological processes for the clinical purposes of diagnosis and treatment. in addition, legal criteria contain terms such as *mental illness, mental disease or defect, insanity,* and *incompetence* that are not easily translated into related psychiatric terms. DSM explicitly states that, "In most situations, the clinical diagnosis of a DSM-IV mental disorder is not sufficient to establish the existence for legal purposes of a 'mental disorder,' 'mental disability,' 'mental disease,' or 'mental defect' (American Psychiatric Association 2000, p. xxxiii).

Individuals qualify for diagnostic categories if and only if they manifest psychological symptoms and impairments that meet the operational criteria for those categories. However, such individuals have legal mental illness for a particular purpose if and only if they manifest psychological impairment that renders them ineligible for the legal status at issue. Those who have impairments qualifying as legal mental illness for a particular purpose also might meet the diagnostic requirements of one or more clinical disorders. However, neither their specific diagnostic category nor the fact that they qualified for some recognized category would be directly relevant to their standing as legally mentally ill. In fact, in regard to legal considerations, DSM states the following:

> In determining whether an individual meets a specified legal standard (e.g., for competence, criminal responsibility, or disability), additional information is usually required beyond that contained in the DSM-IV diagnosis. This might include information about the individual's functional impairments and how these impairments affect the particular abilities in question. It is precisely because impairments, abilities, and disabilities vary widely within each diagnostic category that assignment of a particular diagnosis does not imply a specific level of impairment or disability. (American Psychiatric Association 2000, p. xxxiii)

Functional impairment, although typically a criterion of most DSM diagnoses, is not specifically assessed by Axis I diagnoses. More specific assessment of functioning is made through the use of various assessment scales, such as the Global Assessment of Functioning Scale, which is numerically quantified on Axis V. However, even the numerical score reflecting the degree of functional capacity or impairment in an individual does not give specific information about any particular functional capacity that may be at issue in a specific legal circumstance, such as perception, memory, comprehension, mood, or reasoning.

Diagnosis may create additional confusion when an individual meets the criteria for more than one diagnosis, as is often the case. Multiple diagnoses can result from overlapping criteria in several categories as well as definitional artifacts caused by the division of single complex syndromes into different DSM categories. This problem is derived in part from the change in DSM through its evolution from a monothetic to a polythetic model. The monothetic model used in DSM-I and DSM-II required that all formal descriptors must be present for a diagnosis to be made. The current polythetic model, first used in DSM-III, provides a list of descriptors (symptoms) and requires that only a certain number of these be present for a diagnosis to be made. The polythetic model allows much greater flexibility but also allows the same diagnoses to be applied to individuals who are arguably quite different. Conversely it also often allows multiple diagnoses to be made in reference to the same sets of symptoms in a single individual. As a result many patients have symptoms that meet criteria for more than one disorder (Widiger et al. 1991; Zarin and Earls 1993). In both clinical and forensic practice, this can and often does result in honest disagreement regarding assignment of diagnoses.

When such disagreement occurs in the adversarial arena of the courtroom, confusion and controversy can become magnified. The conceptual generality of nosology and the clinical specificity of any individual case will rarely be entirely congruent. Room for disagreement on diagnosis will always exist as a result of the use of a polythetic model and the individuality of each person's expression of symptoms or illness regardless of diagnosis. However, when experts come to different diagnostic conclusions in the forensic arena, diagnostic criteria often become overly emphasized, and endless debate may ensue about whether the individual meets all the criteria for a diagnostic category, whether the individual meets some of the criteria, or whether another category might be more appropriate. Each side will use such disagreement to its own advantage and attempt to discredit the expert, with the result that no psychiatric diagnosis appears valid. As a consequence the controversy over diagnosis may obscure the key factor in retrospective assessment of mental state: the specific functional impairment in question (Slovenko 1995).

Legal issues of responsibility or competence also may be confused by the use of the medical model of illness as a framework or basis for DSM diagnostic classification. In our society a person who is ill is typically not considered to be responsible for his or her symptoms. Similarly an individual with a mental illness is often assumed not to be responsible for his or her behavior. Thus the use of a medical model in the diagnosis of a mental illness often implies that the individual is not responsible for behavior that is the result of his or her illness. However, in forensic assessments, this implication may be quite misleading, and concern regarding such confusion warranted another caveat in DSM-IV-TR:

> The fact that an individual's presentation meets the criteria for a DSM-IV diagnosis does not carry any necessary implication regarding the individual's degree of control over the behaviors that may be associated with the disorder. Even when diminished control over one's behavior is a feature of the disorder, having the diagnosis in itself does not demonstrate that a particular individual is (or was) unable to control his or her behavior at a particular time. (American Psychiatric Association 2000, p. xxxiii)

The fact that each successive edition of DSM has included new diagnostic categories also has generated confusion in legal proceedings, as the judge in *United States v. Torniero* pointed out. Inclusion in the diagnostic taxonomy reflects a general consensus that some patients may be described meaningfully by the established criteria and that further study should occur, but it may not tell us much more. Although some new diagnostic categories are placed in the DSM section "Criteria Sets and Axes Provided for Further Study," new diagnostic categories in the main body of diagnostic classifications do not explicitly state their limitations. This can lead to the presumption that all DSM disorders carry equal weight and have achieved equal scientific stature unless otherwise specified, which is not the case. Considerable variability exists among diagnostic classifications on the basis of historical experience, knowledge about longitudinal course, and conviction about the validity of each disorder's place in the diagnostic taxonomy.

The application of a diagnostic classification also frequently results in the misconception that all individuals described as having the same mental disorder are alike in all important ways. The introduction to DSM states that no such assumption is made. Nevertheless this clinical distinction is often lost in forensic settings. Although all the individuals described as having the same mental disorder show at least the defining features of the disorder, they may well differ in other important ways that may affect clinical management and outcome (American Psychiatric Association 1980). The assignment of a diagnosis in the forensic setting may lead to the false assumption that disorders of a common name are consistently manifested in the same way, or that the disorders have a distinct symptomatology, or that a given disorder implies a certain state of mind at a time in the past.

Even the opportunity to personally evaluate an individual rather than simply review documents or interview witnesses is only one more piece of data in the retrospective assessment of mental state and does not make a DSM diagnosis more relevant to the legal issue in question. Clinical examination may find evidence of current or previous severe pathology. However, because of the episodic or cyclical nature of several mental illnesses, the absence of demonstrable pathology during examination does not mean that the person was not ill in the past. Evidence of the individual's mental state before or after the time in question is circumstantial as to mental state at that time. A description of the current mental state is relevant to the legal issue at hand only if it relates to the time in question.

The DSM diagnostic system was not intended to be used as a tool for legal purposes, as DSM makes clear. If DSM diagnoses create such confusion, then why use them in court at all? The Federal Rules of Criminal Procedure, which govern introduction of expert testimony relating to a defendant's mental condition, do not require the expert to specify or categorize the mental illness of the accused person (*United States v. Buchbinder* 1986). In fact it has been suggested that the use of diagnostic labels be eradicated in forensic settings (Schopp and Sturgis 1995).

However, the use of diagnoses in forensic mental health evaluations is unlikely to disappear. As noted earlier, formal mental disorders are threshold requirements in some legal statutes. These threshold requirements limit legally sanctioned excuses, entitlements, and curtailments of liberty to persons with mental illness. In general, mental disorders serve these threshold functions because they are believed to be meaningfully associated with diminished abilities or functional impairments. Additionally in some cases, the law makes the presence of a mental disorder an element of a party's prima facie case or defense (D.W. Shuman, "The Tyranny of Diagnostic Labels: Unmasking 'Forensic' Diagnosis," unpublished manuscript, 2001). Even when not specifically required by statute, both lawyers and forensic evaluators often think that they must have a diagnosis for credibility. Thus lawyers often will request a diagnostic assessment, and forensic evaluators frequently will offer a diagnosis, even if not specifically requested.

Moreover, despite all these limitations, diagnostic considerations can be quite relevant in the retrospective assessment of mental states. Although not dispositive, some degree of association clearly exists between DSM diagnoses, impaired mental capacity, and impaired functioning. Even though a diagnosis does not specify the nature of this association in regard to a specific functional capacity or a specific legal standard, the forensic evaluator's assessment of a relevant impairment may be informed or guided by a past or current psychiatric diagnosis. In making a diagnosis the forensic evaluator identifies a range of possible symptoms. Evaluators may be directed by their own diagnostic assessment or the earlier diagnostic impressions of others toward closer examination of those symptoms that are associated with the functional impairments and specific capacities that are legally relevant. Conversely, by identifying symptoms associated with a given illness, the use of diagnosis can serve as a restraint on ungrounded speculation regarding an individual's past mental states. The forensic evaluator, as result of his or her specialized knowledge, can draw reasonable connections or refute unreasonable claims between symptoms associated with a diagnosis and impaired functions associated with those symptoms for the trier of fact.

Diagnosis also may enhance an understanding of retrospective mental states by increasing an understanding of the nature and characteristics of the disorder. Use of diagnoses allows the forensic evaluator to make knowledgeable observations about the longitudinal course of a disorder, which can provide essential information about symptoms that may have affected relevant legal capacities. The identification of a chronic, episodic, or progressively deteriorating course of mental illness associated with various diagnostic categories provides the forensic evaluator with a framework for determining the course of a particular individual's illness and the likelihood of symptoms creating functional impairments at a certain point in time, past or future. Often it provides clues as to the possible duration of such impairment.

The use of an established diagnosis also can serve as a point of reference that enhances the value and reliability of psychiatric testimony, even though it may not be the determinative factor in the retrospective assessment of mental state. When a diagnosis is established, an extensive body of literature and research that can be of value in rendering legal determinations can be introduced to the court. The subject of the evaluation can be assessed in relation to others of the same diagnostic category aided by the cumulative experiences and research of the fields of psychiatry and psychology. Finally, when mental disorder is a threshold requirement for certain legal determinations, the diagnostic requirement is meant to serve as a validator of the main legal contention that certain relevant impairments are present (Halleck et al. 1992). Many diagnoses serve this function well.

Thus the use of diagnosis can enhance the reliability of testimony about mental disorders and retrospective assessments of mental states, particularly if the following guidelines are observed:

1. Identify the necessity for inclusion or exclusion of psychiatric diagnosis as per the relevant legal statute.
2. Identify the functional capacity directly relevant to the legal issue in question, and evaluate functional impairment, if any.
3. If required or requested, formulate a past or present diagnosis based on standard forensic and clinical methodology. Use DSM diagnostic categories. Be able to identify and substantiate the diagnostic criteria, the presence (or absence) of the specific DSM criteria in the evaluee, and the evidence supporting or refuting the diagnosis.

4. Explain the relation between the diagnosis and the relevant functional capacity. If an unreasonable or invalid inference of functional impairment is being made on the basis of any given diagnosis, explain the lack of correlation or incorrect reasoning between the diagnosis and the functional capacity in question.
5. Do not substitute the formulation of a DSM diagnosis for a careful forensic evaluation of the relevant functional capacity in question.

Conclusion

DSM is the most comprehensive and widely used diagnostic tool in the classification of mental disorders. However, DSM is a clinical guide whose function is to assist clinicians in making diagnoses and designing treatment interventions. Diagnostic classifications, despite their scientific basis, can create confusion in legal settings because of the imperfect fit between clinical and legal concepts. The caveats regarding the use of DSM in forensic settings have not arisen from concerns about its lack of scientific methodology or clinical reliability, as attorneys attempting to discredit diagnostic testimony may claim. Rather these caveats arise from concerns regarding the use and misuse of a diagnostic nomenclature for nonclinical purposes by individuals untrained in their application. The imperfect fit between psychiatric concepts and legal concepts underscores the importance of training and expertise in the accurate use of DSM, as stated in DSM-IV-TR: "The proper use of these criteria [in making diagnoses] requires specialized clinical training that provides both a body of knowledge and clinical skills" (American Psychiatric Association 2000, p. xxxvii).

In clinical practice a DSM diagnosis is the beginning, not the end, of understanding an individual's experience of mental functioning. A diagnostic assessment of recurrent major depression, for example, does not provide information about significant clinical and treatment issues, such as the presence of suicidality, response to past treatment, or the need for hospitalization. Once such a diagnosis is made, the clinician must go further and assess how that illness is affecting that particular individual and suggest treatment accordingly. The diagnostic category provides clinical guidance but cannot provide specific information about any individual.

Diagnosis in the retrospective assessment of mental states can serve the same useful purpose of providing guidance in a forensic evaluation. The forensic psychiatrist or psychologist's clinical training in diagnosing and treating mental illness, and the scientific methodology used to increase knowledge of and the ability to treat such illnesses, have resulted in the accumulation of experience that can be instrumental in clarifying forensic issues. However, the use of a DSM diagnosis to circumstantially support or refute a legal claim without an evaluation of the specific functional impairment related to the legal issue is misleading and potentially legally ineffective. Although it may meet the *Daubert* standard for scientific reliability, it may be successfully challenged on the basis of relevance.

Establishing a diagnosis in a forensic evaluation, although frequently necessary, is often a secondary issue in regard to informing the legal decision-maker about an individual's functional impairments relative to any legal standard. The assignment of a DSM diagnosis is not a substitute for a careful evaluation that considers the relations between DSM diagnoses, the retrospective assessment of mental state, and the evaluation of functional impairment relative to the legal capacities in question. DSM diagnoses can be instrumental in gaining access to clinical and research data defining the range of functional impairments associated with various symptoms. Nevertheless, in the evaluation of retrospective assessment of mental states, forensic evaluators must focus on the specific functional impairment relevant to the legal issue at hand, regardless of diagnosis.

References

American Law Institute: Model Penal Code, Proposed Official Draft. Philadelphia, PA, American Law Institute, 1962

American Psychiatric Association: Diagnostic and Statistical Manual: Mental Disorders. Washington, DC, American Psychiatric Association, 1952

American Psychiatric Association: Diagnostic and Statistical Manual of Mental Disorders, 2nd Edition. Washington, DC, American Psychiatric Association, 1968

American Psychiatric Association: Diagnostic and Statistical Manual of Mental Disorders, 3rd Edition. Washington, DC, American Psychiatric Association, 1980

American Psychiatric Association: Diagnostic and Statistical Manual of Mental Disorders, 3rd Edition, Revised. Washington, DC, American Psychiatric Association, 1987

American Psychiatric Association: Diagnostic and Statistical Manual of Mental Disorders, 4th Edition. Washington, DC, American Psychiatric Association, 1994

American Psychiatric Association: Diagnostic and Statistical Manual of Mental Disorders, 4th Edition, Text Revision. Washington, DC, American Psychiatric Association, 2000

Bayer R, Spitzer RL: Edited correspondence on the status of homosexuality in DSM-III. J Hist Behav Sci 18:32–52, 1982

Blashfield RK: Feighner et al., invisible colleges and the Matthew effect. Schizophr Bull 8:1–6, 1982

Caplan PJ: The psychiatric association's failure to meet its own standards: the dangers of self-defeating personality disorder as a category. J Personal Disord 1:178–182, 1987

Carson RC: Dilemmas in the pathway of the DSM-IV. J Abnorm Psychol 100:302–307, 1991

Chesler P: Women and Madness. Garden City, NY, Doubleday, 1972

Cooksey EC, Brown P: Spinning on its axes: DSM and the social construction of psychiatric diagnosis. Int J Health Serv 28:525–554, 1998

Coolidge FL, Segal DL: Evolution of personality disorder diagnosis in the Diagnostic and Statistical Manual of Mental Disorders. Clin Psychol Rev 18:585–599, 1998

Daubert v Merrell Dow Pharmaceuticals, Inc., 509 US 579, 113 SCt 2786 (1993)

Fabrega H: Diagnosis interminable: toward a culturally sensitive DSM-IV. J Nerv Ment Dis 180:5–7, 1992

Faraone SV, Tsuang MT: Measuring diagnostic accuracy in the absence of a "gold standard." Am J Psychiatry 151:650–657, 1994

Feighner J, Robins E, Guze S, et al: Diagnostic criteria for use in psychiatric research. Arch Gen Psychiatry 26:57–63, 1972

Follette WC, Houts AC: Models of scientific progress and the role of theory in taxonomy development: a case study of the DSM. J Consult Clin Psychol 64:1120–1132, 1996

Foucault M: Madness and Civilization: A History of Insanity in the Age of Reason. Translated by Howard R. New York, Pantheon, 1965

Frances AJ: Foreword, in Philosophical Perspectives on Psychiatric Diagnostic Classification. Edited by Sadler JZ, Wiggins OP, Schwartz MA. Baltimore, MD, Johns Hopkins University Press, 1994, pp vii–ix

Frye v United States, 293 F 1013 (DC Cir 1923)

Greenberg SA, Shuman DW: Irreconcilable conflict between therapeutic and forensic roles. Professional Psychology: Research and Practice 28:5–57, 1997

Grob GN: Origins of the DSM-I: a study in appearance and reality. Am J Psychiatry 148:421–431, 1991

Grudzinskas AJ: Kumho Tire Col, Ltd., v. Carmichael. J Am Acad Psychiatry Law 27:482–488, 1999

Hagen MA: Whores of the Court: The Fraud of Psychiatric Testimony and the Rape of American Justice. New York, ReganBooks, 1997

Halleck SL, Hoge SK, Miller RD, et al: The use of psychiatric diagnoses in the legal process: task force report of the American Psychiatric Association. Bulletin of the American Academy of Psychiatry and the Law 20:481–499, 1992

Hempel CG: Fundamentals of taxonomy, in Philosophical Perspectives on Psychiatric Diagnostic Classifications. Edited by Sadler JZ, Wiggins OP, Schwartz MA. Baltimore, MD, Johns Hopkins University Press, 1994, pp 315–331

Huber PW: Galileo's Revenge: Junk Science in the Courtroom. New York, Basic Books, 1993

Kaplan M: A woman's view of DSM-III. Am Psychol 38:786–792, 1983

Klerman GL: The contemporary American scene: diagnosis and classification of mental disorders, alcoholism and drug abuse, in Sources and Traditions of Classification in Psychiatry. Edited by Sartorius N. Toronto, ON, Hogrefe, 1990, pp 93–137

Klerman GL, Vaillant GE, Spitzer RS, et al: A debate on DSM-III. Am J Psychiatry 141:539–553, 1984

Kuhn TS: The Essential Tension: Selected Studies in Scientific Tradition and Change. Chicago, IL, University of Chicago Press, 1977

Kuhn TS: The Structure of Scientific Revolutions, 3rd Edition. Chicago, IL, University of Chicago Press, 1996

Kumho Tire Co. v Carmichael, 119 SCt 1167 (1999)

Laing RD: The Divided Self: A Study of Sanity and Madness. London, Tavistock, 1960

Maser JD, Kaelber C, Vies RE: International use and attitudes toward DSM-III and DSM-III-R: growing consensus in psychiatric classification. J Abnorm Psychol 100:271–279, 1991

Menninger K: The Vital Balance. New York, Viking Press, 1963

Mezzich JE, Kirmayer LJ, Kleinman A, et al: The place of culture in the DSM-IV. J Nerv Ment Dis 187:457–464, 1999

Millon T: Classification in psychopathology: rationale, alternatives, and standards. J Abnorm Psychol 100:245–262, 1991

Morey LC: Classification of mental disorder as a collection of hypothetical constructs. J Abnorm Psychol 100:289–293, 1991

Parry JW: National Benchbook on Psychiatric and Psychological Evidence and Testimony. Washington, DC, American Bar Association, 1998

Rogler LH: Making sense of historical changes in the Diagnostic and Statistical Manual of Mental Disorders: five propositions. J Health Soc Behav 38:9–20, 1997

Russell D: Psychiatric diagnosis and the interests of women, in Philosophical Perspectives on Psychiatric Diagnostic Classification. Edited by Sadler JZ, Wiggins OP, Schwartz MA. Baltimore, MD, Johns Hopkins University Press, 1994, pp 246–258

Sadler JZ, Wiggins OP, Schwartz MA: Introduction, in Philosophical Perspectives on Psychiatric Diagnostic Classifications. Edited by Sadler JZ, Wiggins OP, Schwartz MA. Baltimore, MD, Johns Hopkins University Press, 1994, pp 1–15

Schopp RG, Sturgis BJ: Sexual predators and legal mental illness for civil commitment. Behav Sci Law 13:437–458, 1995

Scull A: Social Order/Mental Disorder: Anglo-American Psychiatry in Historical Perspective. Berkeley, University of California Press, 1989

Shorter E: A History of Psychiatry: From the Era of the Asylum to the Age of Prozac. New York, Wiley, 1997

Showalter E: The Female Malady: Women, Madness, and English Culture, 1830-1980. New York, Pantheon Books, 1985

Shuman DW: The Diagnostic and Statistical Manual of Mental Disorders in the courts. Bulletin of the American Academy of Psychiatry and the Law 17:25–32, 1989

Slovenko R: Psychiatry and Criminal Culpability. New York, Wiley, 1995

Spitzer M: The basis of psychiatric diagnosis, in Philosophical Perspectives on Psychiatric Diagnostic Classification. Edited by Sadler JZ, Wiggins OP, Schwartz MA. Baltimore, MD, Johns Hopkins University Press, 1994, pp 163–177

Spitzer RL: More on pseudoscience in science and the case for psychiatric diagnosis: a critique of D.L. Rosenhan's "On being sane in insane places" and "The contextual nature of psychiatric diagnosis." Arch Gen Psychiatry 33:459–470, 1976

Spitzer RL: The diagnostic status of homosexuality in DSM-III: a reformulation of the issues. Am J Psychiatry 138:210–215, 1981

Spitzer RL: Harmful dysfunction and the DSM definition of mental disorder. J Abnorm Psychol 108:430–432, 1999

Spitzer RL, Williams JBW: Letter to the editor. Am J Psychiatry 151:459–460, 1994

Spitzer RL, Endicott J, Robins E: Research Diagnostic Criteria (RDC) for a Selected Group of Functional Disorders. New York, New York State Psychiatric Institute, Biometrics Branch, 1975

Spitzer RL, Williams JBW, Skodol AE: DSM-III: the major achievements and an overview. Am J Psychiatry 137:151–164, 1980

Spitzer RL, Williams JBW, Kass F, et al: National field trial of the DSM-III-R diagnostic criteria for self-defeating personality disorder. Am J Psychiatry 146:1561–1567, 1989

Stone AA: Law, Psychiatry, and Morality. Washington, DC, American Psychiatric Press, 1984

Strasburger LH, Gutheil TG, Brodsky A: On wearing two hats: role conflict in serving as both psychotherapist and expert witness. Am J Psychiatry 154:448–456, 1997

Strauss GD, Yager J, Strauss GE: The cutting edge in psychiatry. Am J Psychiatry 141:38–43, 1993

Szasz TS: The Myth of Mental Illness. New York, Harper & Row, 1960

United States v Buchbinder, 796 F2d 910 (7th Cir 1986)

United States v Torniero, 570 F Supp 721 (DC Conn 1983)

Wakefield JC: The concept of mental disorder: on the boundary between biological facts and social values. Am Psychol 47:373–388, 1992

Wakefield JC: The concept of disorder as a foundation for the DSM's theory-neutral nosology: response to Follette and Houts, part 2. Behav Res Ther 37:1001–1027, 1999

Wallace ER: Psychology and its nosology: a historico-philosophical overview, in Philosophical Perspectives on Psychiatric Diagnostic Classification. Edited by Sadler JZ, Wiggins OP, Schwartz MA. Baltimore, MD, Johns Hopkins University Press, 1994, pp 16–86

Widiger TA, Miele GM, Tilly SM, et al: An A to Z guide to DSM-IV conundrums. J Abnorm Psychol 100:407–412, 1991

Wiggins OP, Schwartz MA: The limits of psychiatric knowledge and the problem of classification, in Philosophical Perspectives on Psychiatric Diagnostic Classification. Edited by Sadler JZ, Wiggins OP, Schwartz MA. Baltimore, MD, Johns Hopkins University Press, 1994, pp 89–103

Wilson M: DSM-III and the transformation of American psychiatry: a history. Am J Psychiatry 150:399–410, 1993

Zarin DA, Earls F: Diagnostic decision making in psychiatry. Am J Psychiatry 150:197–206, 1993

13

Special Methodologies in Memory Retrieval

Chemical, Hypnotic, and Imagery Procedures

Alan W. Scheflin, J.D., LL.M., M.A.

Daniel Brown, Ph.D.

Edward J. Frischholz, Ph.D.

Jamie Caploe, Ed.M., J.D.

Introduction: Memory Recovery Techniques

In this chapter we address the relative usefulness, in clinical and forensic settings, of amobarbitol (Amytal) interviews, hypnosis, and guided imagery for the enhancement of memory, typically eyewitness memory and auto-biographical memory. Particular attention is paid to the issue of whether these methods of memory retrieval should pass a *Frye* or *Daubert* test for the admission of expert testimony into evidence.

The use of each of these procedures for memory retrieval has a long clinical and forensic history. Amytal interviews have been used extensively in clinical situations to explore past trauma (J.C. Perry and Jacobs 1982), as has hypnosis (Brown and Fromm 1986). Hypnosis also has been used frequently for clinical purposes and in forensic settings to refresh the memory of eyewitnesses and suspects of various crimes (Reiser 1980; Scheflin and Shapiro 1989). Many laboratory studies have been conducted on the effects of hypnosis on the completeness, accuracy, and confidence of memory for a target event. They are summarized in Brown et al. (1998).

Until the early 1980s the use of memory enhancement procedures in general was common in clinical settings where, for the most part, they were accepted uncritically. Hypnosis was approved for therapeutic purposes by the American Medical Association in 1958 (American Medical Association 1958) and by the American Psychiatric Association in 1961 (American Psychiatric Association 1961). Amytal interviews and guided imagery had been in clinical use for most of the century.

Courts generally have assumed that most memory recovery procedures were useful in establishing the kind of retrieval conditions that contributed to significant new and accurate information about the past event in question. This assumption, however, had not been subjected to adequate empirical testing. With regard to Amytal and hypnosis, however, courts made the opposite assumption, concluding that these memory retrieval techniques were not reliable; most courts rejected them as an appropriate means for the recovery of accurate memories, although empirical studies were lacking (Scheflin 2001). Studies of the efficacy of hypnosis as a means for accurate memory retrieval were virtually nonexistent until the late 1980s (McCann and Sheehan 1988). The ban on hypnosis was based on the judicial perception that linked hypnosis with truth serums and polygraphs, both of which were considered unreliable (Giannelli and Imwinkelried 1999; Moenssens et al. 1995).

Beginning in 1968, courts in the United States began to admit hypnotically refreshed recollection as testimony in civil and criminal trials. These courts rejected the old assumption that hypnosis was not a reliable means for inducing accurate memories. In response to this open admissibility policy, some serious questioning of the value of hypnosis as a technique of memory retrieval began based on the rapidly accumulating database of laboratory studies on hypnosis and memory in the late 1970s and early 1980s (Pettinati 1988). Previous claims that hypnosis was a reliable tool in retrieving accurate memories were soon challenged along two fronts: 1) that the alleged hypermnesic effect of hypnosis led to a mixture of both accurate and inaccurate information (the "hits and misses" viewpoint) and 2) that certain hypnotic expectancies and/or suggestive interviewing procedures inevitably led to "pseudomemories" and "confabulation" (Karlin and Orne 1996). These laboratory-based findings served as a serious scientific and political challenge to the previous uncritical acceptance by clinicians and by law enforcement of hypnosis as a memory enhancement procedure. In 1985 the American Medical Association issued a cautionary statement about the use of hypnosis, specifically for forensic purposes. The use of hypnosis in clinical settings was not the focus of the American Medical Association's position statement.

In the early 1990s a rapidly proliferating literature created a serious challenge to the use of any memory enhancement procedures, in either forensic or clinical settings. Professor Elizabeth Loftus's position paper in the *American Psychologist* in 1993 exemplified the then-emerging viewpoint (Loftus 1993). According to Loftus, memory in general is fallible and is vulnerable to postevent suggestive influences. Psychotherapy is not immune to distortion from memory's fallibility and responsiveness to suggestion. Loftus believed that certain therapists were implanting "false memories" (other writers called them "false beliefs") of childhood abuse in their adult patients through the practice of "recovered memory therapy." According to Ofshe and Watters (1994) "memory recovery therapy" is a new form of "quackery."

A definitional problem arose because the term *recovered memory therapy* is not a technical term found anywhere in the professional psychotherapy literature. For some writers the term may include "persistent encouragement to recall past events" (Frankel 1993, p. 25) or, simply, "memory work" (Ceci and Loftus 1994). Others have defined recovered memory therapy more specifically with respect to an extreme focus on recovering memories of abuse that previously had not been reported. Loftus and Ketcham (1994), for example, emphasized the "pressure to remember" (p. 25) and to "stockpile memory" (p. 27). Yapko (1994) wrote specifically of therapists who "pursue their memory work in a persistently suggestive manner."

As a result of this evolving literature, for the first time in legal history the actual practice of "talking cures" came under scientific attack and led to legal issues of whether certain testimony based on memory should be admissible in court. Substantial evidence has been marshaled to show that some therapists were not being sensitive to the ways in which memory may be deceptive. Other therapists often moved beyond their therapeutic role and became crusaders for the patients to bring lawsuits against others based on alleged false memories.

Litigators have claimed that therapists working with memory retrieval have fallen below an appropriate standard of care and are using dangerous and experimental techniques, such as hypnosis and Amytal, in the recovery of their patients' memories. These techniques, it has been argued, cause false memories to be created and believed of child abuse incidents that never actually occurred. The legal issue is raised by the leakage of the narrative truth of the therapy room into the historical truth of the courtroom. More recent developments indicate that litigators are also challenging the narrative truth of therapy sessions that never extend into courtroom confrontations. In these latter cases the argument has been that therapists have fallen below the standard of care because they did not strongly disbelieve their patients' memories (Scheflin 1998).

The recent controversies concerning the malleability of memory have left a cloud of legal and psychotherapeutic uncertainty. Should every therapy wherein the patient reports a memory be considered a form of recovered memory therapy inviting a malpractice suit? A focus on the past is characteristic of most therapies at one time or another and certainly of most psychodynamic therapy, as noted by Butler and Spiegel (1997):

> The very concept of psychotherapy is built on the reexamination of memory. Classic psychoanalytic and modern psychodynamic psychotherapy—not just so-called recovered memory therapy—assume that current problems may reflect memories of life experiences, such as traumatic events (incest, assault, accidents), family stresses, or warded-off fears and wishes, which may be only partially accessible to consciousness at a given time. In some cases, people simply may not connect an available memory with a symptom; in other cases they may not consciously remember the event. Consequently, many of the essential elements of psychotherapy—transference, working through, and restructuring—involve working with memories....Psychotherapy remains the primary treatment for trauma victims, with pharmacological agents playing only a secondary role. (pp. 13–14)

Some attorneys zealously involved in suing therapists have poured through medical records to find every reference to the past, and every reference to memory, and have labeled the therapy as "risky memory recovery treatments." Because a focus on the past is part of many dynamically oriented treatments, some plaintiff-oriented attorneys have attempted to characterize all such treatments as "experimental" because, in their view, such "memory work" has not been scientifically established as a reliable therapy. This strategy is used because it is easier to establish in a malpractice claim that an "experimental" treatment is below the standard of care. Furthermore if the treatment can be labeled as "experimental," any informed consent to it is objectionable unless the patient was told that the therapy was "dangerous," "not scientifically validated," and "experimental" (Scheflin 2000).

These arguments in some early cases resulted in large verdicts against therapists. The arguments, however, rest on two hidden premises. First, it is assumed that any technique that lacks full empirical scientific validation is necessarily below the standard of care and is also "experimental." Second, it is assumed that informed consent in therapy requires a written and signed detailed statement that chronicles the benefits and dangers of every treatment modality and expressly lists any differences held in the scientific community.

Opponents of these arguments claim that, with regard to the first assumption, the standard of care for psychotherapy has never been set by laboratory experimentalists or by long-term outcome studies, even though the field has recently moved in the direction of evidence-supported psychotherapy, as discussed in the special edition of the *Journal of Consulting and Clinical Psychology*, February 1998. The standard of care generally has been derived from the recognized practices taught in graduate schools and supported by professional organizations. Historically, they argue, the great strides in therapy have not come from laboratory experiments, nor could they have done so. Considerations of ecological validity and demand characteristics make it overwhelmingly clear that people behave differently in experiments than they do in their regular activities.

Opponents continue by noting that therapists treat real people in the real world, not laboratory subjects in experimental settings. Psychotherapy approaches seemingly supported by outcomes research are misleading in two respects. First, most psychotherapy outcomes research has been conducted on healthier college-based populations rather than the more disturbed clinic populations. Second, the use of exclusionary criteria in most outcomes research means that this research rarely addresses the issue of multiple comorbid psychiatric disorders in the same patient, a condition that most clinicians commonly treat. Thus the development of therapeutic insights in the clinical setting has been inductive, not deductive, as with experiments. Furthermore the crucial factor of rapport, so important in therapy because it may determine that the same technique used by one therapist succeeds, whereas the same technique used by another therapist fails, is untestable in the laboratory.

With regard to the second assumption, opponents claim that informed consent between patient and therapist is a relationship, not a document. Because the ebb and flow of therapy varies from patient to patient, the use of legalistic informed consent forms would freeze the necessary fluidity of the therapy. The rationale behind informed consent, that the patient is a knowing and consenting participant in the cure, is satisfied when the therapist explains the therapy and uses the patient's desire to be cured. By being actively and willingly involved in the treatment, the patient provides the necessary consent.

Resolution of these arguments and counterarguments must come from the courts, which are now hearing them. Therapy in the future will be shaped by what the courts decide.

In the debates concerning memory, certain specific methods for memory recovery have been targeted as being the main cause of alleged implanted false memories. Loftus (1993) attacked "memory recovery techniques" under which she included hypnosis, guided imagery, dream work, work with body memories, and journaling. Ofshe and Watters (1994) described "extensive use of memory recovery techniques [such as hypnosis, dream work, and guided imagery]…that encourage guesses, speculation, and confabulation" (p. 9). Lindsay and Read (1994) likewise addressed "extreme forms of memory recovery therapy" such as "hypnosis, dream interpretation, guided imagery, journaling, and body memories" (p. 326). Yapko (1994, p. 41) mentioned "suggestive therapy procedures." Ofshe and Watters added that these suggestive techniques encourage guessing and result in a confounding of fantasy and memory. Pezdek (1994), however, pointed out that these so-called memory recovery techniques were singled out because they were believed to lead to the creation of false memories in some patients. She emphasized, however, that "the phenomenon was never demonstrated [scientifically]" (p. 340).

Before the 1980s there was largely uncritical acceptance of most memory retrieval techniques. The professional attacks on memory enhancement procedures that began in the 1980s have resulted in the pendulum swinging entirely in the other direction—from uncritical acceptance of the efficacy of guided imagery and hypnosis for memory enhancement to uncritical acceptance of the view that these retrieval techniques inevitably contaminate memory and enhance the memory error rate.

The purpose of this chapter is to step back from the rhetoric of memory and instead critically review the available scientific data concerning memory retrieval. Although it has become common practice on both sides of this debate to cluster hypnosis, guided imagery, narcoanalysis, and other techniques together as memory enhancement procedures, no empirical justification exists for doing so. Conceptually, of course, these diverse procedures have common ground in their use as a means of recovering accurate memories. Because of the very modern development of scientific interest in the various techniques used to refresh recollection, so far there are no construct and discriminant validity studies on these procedures to establish scientifically that techniques as diverse as "truth drug" interviewing, hypnosis, and guided imagery are 1) significantly intercorrelated, 2) significantly discriminated from one another, or 3) significantly discriminated from the effects of other techniques. In short, studies comparing the various techniques do not exist. Given this lack of scientific data concerning the interrelation between truth drug interviewing, hypnosis, and guided imagery as memory enhancement procedures, we review each procedure separately in this chapter.

Although it recently has become fashionable to describe therapy as the realm of "narrative" truth, and courts of law as interested exclusively in "historical" truth, this viewpoint is now recognized as far too simplistic. Scheflin (1998) noted that therapists must be especially concerned with historical truth because of mandated reporting laws and required violations of confidentiality, and courts of law are social environments in which a form of narrative construction, which Scheflin calls "forensic" truth, is presented. Anyone who thinks the courtroom is the arena for historical truth has not spent much time there. It is important to recognize, however, that good psychotherapy need not be archaeological in terms of unearthing literally true memories. Good therapy is not the search for accurate memory; it is designed to make the patient functional, even if the memories themselves are not accurate.

The final third of the twentieth century witnessed an additional important expansion of psychology and psychiatry into the legal system. This time, however, the intervention was at the detection and preventive stage of criminal conduct rather than at the treatment end. Raymond Chandler (1959), the talented mystery writer, noticed the beginning of this trend in an extract from his novel *The Long Goodbye*:

> "You two characters been seeing any psychiatrists lately?"
>
> "Hell," Ohls said, "hadn't you heard? We got them in our hair all the time these days. We've got two of them on the staff. This ain't police business any more. It's getting to be a branch of the medical racket. They're in and out of jail, the courts, the interrogation rooms. They write reports fifteen pages long on why some punk of a juvenile held up a liquor store or raped a schoolgirl or peddled tea to the senior class. Ten years from now guys like Marty and me will be doing Rorschach tests and word associations instead of chin-ups and target practice. When we go out on a case we'll carry little black bags with portable lie detectors and bottles of truth serum."

Truth by Chemicals: The Use of Truth Drugs to Retrieve Memories

History

The extraction of drugs derived from plants and herbs, such as mandrake root, nightshade, belladonna, henbane, and Jimson weed, has an extensive history reaching as far back as our recorded history (Despres 1947; Mann 1992). Although these natural products were mostly used for the purpose of curing illnesses and psychological and social renewal, other users sought a deeper vision of life. Greek priestesses relied on drugs to summon their sought-after prophecies, and Native Americans used the hallucinogenic peyote, a form of mescaline, to create a "second sight" sensory-heightening effect in rituals. These users sought a "higher truth." Not until modern times have plants, herbs, and other natural products been used in an attempt to find literal, or historical, truth.

One of the first men to conduct a scientific study of mind-altering natural substances was the Austrian doctor Giovanni Antonio Scopoli. While working near the Idria mines of Carniola, Scopoli published his landmark *Flora Carniolica* in 1760. This labor of love resulted from his exhaustive collecting and cataloguing of more than 1,500 plants that he discovered in the Austrian mountains of the Carniola region. In his honor a foot-tall purple-blossomed shrub was dubbed *Scopolia carniolica* to commemorate his most significant discovery.

By the end of the nineteenth century, scientists were studying the medicinal effects of *S. carniolica* and other similar plants. Scopoli was again paid homage by German Professor Ernst A. Schmidt from the University of Marburg, who isolated and named scopolamine, the main substance derived from the dried rhizome of the shrub. Scopolamine, an odorless drug that is either colorless, white crystals, or white powder, was chemically matched with hyoscine, derived from *Hyoscyamus niger*, more commonly known as henbane. Henbane has a long history as a mind-altering weapon, as reported by Geis (1959):

> [Henbane]…figured in numerous stories about poisoning from remote times, being mentioned as early as 681 by Benedictus Crispus, the Archbishop of Milan. The dancing frenzy and the witches' madness of the Middle Ages was supposed to be traceable in part to the use of Black Henbane; the inhalation of fumes of hyoscyamus was alleged to have provided the stimulation for the processions of the flagellants, and, before these, the Scythians were reported to burn the seeds of Black Henbane in order to put themselves into a state of manic intoxication. More classically, in *Hamlet* there appears the murdered king, telling his son that he had been poisoned "with juice of cursed henbana in a vial", a "leperous distillment" which "holds such an enmity with blood of man." (p. 348)

Among the effects scopolamine produced were drowsiness, euphoria, amnesia, and dreamless sleep. The positive use of such effects led to scopolamine's role as an anesthetic for surgery. Its greatest fame, however, occurred in the early 1900s, as an aid in childbirth. The Germans called it *dammerschlaf*, a "twilight sleep," induced by a heady mix of scopolamine and morphine. Although women received substantial benefits from the procedure, which relieved pain during childbirth and provided amnesia for the entire process afterward, the potential dangers to both mother and child from such potent drugs resulted in an unresolved scientific conflict over its use.

Richard von Steinbuchel, J. Christian Gauss, and Bernard Kronig were in the forefront of the German research and implementation of twilight sleep (Geis 1959). Mothers-to-be, once labor had begun, were bedded in dark, quiet rooms with their eyes covered and ears stuffed with cotton. Efforts were made to remove all outside distractions, while uninterrupted supervision was used to ensure that the mother did not become agitated. A mixture of scopolamine and morphine was repeatedly injected throughout labor as needed according to the mother's mental state.

At its best twilight sleep allowed women to endure childbirth without pain and retain no memory of the event afterward. The difficulty for doctors was knowing what amount of the scopolamine and morphine mixture would best create that desired result. Too little medication could lead to free-floating fragments of memory; too much could prolong delivery or have a detrimental effect on the infant. To achieve the optimum dosage, Gauss devised what he termed *memory tests*, questioning the laboring mother at regularly timed half-hour intervals with a repeated series of inquiries. When she could no longer accurately answer the questions, proper dosage had been reached.

Dr. House's Crusade for Scopolamine

The most prominent champion of scopolamine in the United States was Dr. Robert Ernst House, a Texas obstetrician, whose true believer fervor fueled a lifetime of writings and experimentation with the drug. At the dawn of the twentieth century, Dr. House, newly degreed in medicine from Tulane University, opened his offices in the small town of Farris, Texas, just north of Dallas. Throughout his 30 years of practice, he extolled the virtues of scopolamine as an aid in medical procedures and, more important, as a forensic tool to establish guilt or innocence of suspects and defendants. Between 1921 and 1929 he authored 11 articles with ever-increasing praise for scopolamine's virtues (Freedman 1960; Geis 1959; Rolin 1956).

After observing the twilight sleep procedure in New York, he claimed to have used it himself in more than 300 births in Farris. His interest in drugs moved from the birthing bed to the prison cell in 1916 during a woman's labor; although she appeared deeply relaxed under the influence of scopolamine, she answered clearly and accurately a question the doctor asked of her husband about the whereabouts of the scales to weigh the newborn. From that initial incident, House proceeded to test the truthfulness of answers given by other women while sedated by scopolamine. This anecdotal evidence convinced House that individuals could answer only with the truth while under the drug's sway. According to House (1921), "under the influence of the drug, there is no imagination. They cannot create a lie because they have no power to think or reason."

While working at the Dallas County Jail, House conducted two experiments that emboldened his beliefs in scopolamine's truth-telling powers. One individual, sentenced to a 15-year term, offered information that enabled his attorney to go back to court and prove mistaken identity, releasing the unjustly convicted man from confinement. House's almost quaint enthusiasm overlooked the possibility that defendants and suspects might make self-serving exculpatory statements; he saw only truth and justice being served.

House never wavered in his evangelic support for the forensic use of scopolamine, even as newspapers of the day gave the drug lurid coverage, both for and against its use. The unfortunate side effect for House was that his opinions and writings became increasingly more strident when they were decreasingly met with approval. Although many professional institutions supported his work, such as the Texas Medical Society, he would not be satisfied unless the drug became a standard and essential element of crime detection. House traveled around the country advocating his position. In major American cities he gave demonstrations by interrogating local crime suspects who had been given the drug.

Equally enamored of early lie detector equipment, House thought the two in combination would eliminate a significant amount of legal errors and mistakes. In common with law enforcement officials, he had little tolerance for the privacy arguments being raised against the invasive quality presented by using drugs to elicit information from suspects. He did, however, recognize the need to regulate those who administered the potent drug to prevent improper, dangerous, or unprofessional conduct. House urged members of the legal and medical professions to work together to create appropriate safeguards for the use of his "truth" drug.

In House's later years he also directed his attention to the potential benefits of scopolamine in treating psychiatric patients, especially those whose behavior veered toward the criminal. Although he approached numerous mental hospitals, urging them to use narcoanalysis as a method of treatment, the response was minimal.

After House's death in 1930, scopolamine and other similar drugs continued to be used in forensic settings. The scientific effect across cases yielded varying results. In 1924 a slew of Birmingham, Alabama, ax murders terrorized that community (Geis 1959). Five individuals confessed to the hideous crimes while under the influence of scopolamine, and their inculpatory statements were later successfully corroborated. A 1928 Hawaii case cast a less positive light on narcoanalysis when a kidnap and murder suspect confessed while under the influence of hyoscine hydrobromide to writing the ransom note (Despres 1947). He also provided details of the events but then repudiated his confession after emerging from the haze of the drug. A second interrogation under the drug proved negative, although investigators stopped their pursuit of the man when the murderer—someone else—was caught. A 1931 Seattle, Washington, case involved the questioning of one Decasta Earl Mayer to find an alleged murder victim's body (Geis 1959). After an injunction successfully halted the use of any narcoanalysis, on the grounds that it violated the Fifth Amendment's privilege against self-incrimination and constituted an invasion of privacy, the legal climate around the United States supported these objections.

Scopolamine and its chemical cousins continued to be used for exculpatory purposes, as in a case in Kansas City, Missouri, in 1935 in which a local butcher willingly took the drug to help establish his innocence regarding a murder (Geis 1959). Because of the increasing legal objections to the involuntary drugging of criminal defendants, scopolamine proved more successful in clearing suspects than in capturing or convicting them.

Even this seemingly benign role for scopolamine came under judicial attack, however. The opinion on the use of truth serum drugs in criminal cases at the time, *State v. Hudson* (1926), was the only case of record for more than a decade. George Hudson of St. Louis, Missouri, was convicted of raping a 65-year-old woman. His defense attorneys wanted to introduce testimony that Hudson had denied his guilt while under the influence of scopolamine. The court unanimously rejected this proposition, as forcefully stated by Judge Robert Walker Franklin:

> Testimony of this character—barring the sufficient fact that it cannot be otherwise classified than as a self-serving declaration—is, in the present state of human knowledge, unworthy of serious consideration. We are not told from what well this serum is drawn or in what alembic its alleged truth compelling powers are distilled. Its origin is as nebulous as its effect is uncertain. A belief in its potency, if it has any existence, is confined to the modern Cagliostros, who still, as Balsamo did of old,[1] cozen the credulous for a quid pro quo, by inducing them to believe in the magic powers

---

[1] Guiseppe Balsame was the actual given name of Count Cagliostro, a well-known con man. His many exploits are written about in Bolitho W: *Cagliostro (& Seraphina), Twelve Against the Gods: The Story of Adventure*. New York, Simon & Schuster, 1929, p. 179.

of philters, potions, and cures by faith. The trial court, therefore, whether it assigned a reason for its action or not, ruled correctly in excluding this clap-trap from the consideration of the jury. (*State v. Hudson* 1926, court opinion, p. 921)

The fate of scopolamine in legal arenas has followed the opinion in *Hudson*. However, scopolamine generally has given way to more modern drugs, such as sodium Pentothal and sodium Amytal, which have proven safer and with fewer side effects (Freedman 1960). Scopolamine could create toxic effects, such as hallucinations, which clearly undermined its use as a truth serum for forensic purposes. Its use as an aid in the control of pain during childbirth continued successfully. With its antispasmodic element, it also has been useful for treating motion sickness and Parkinson's disease symptoms (Geis 1959; Rolin 1956).

The three general reasons for administering scopolamine, sodium Amytal, or sodium Pentothal for the purpose of lowering critical resistance are 1) to obtain material for clinical discussions, 2) to detect deception, and 3) to ascertain the truth.

Truth Serums in Clinical Settings

Humphry Davy used himself and his contemporaries Samuel Taylor Coleridge and Peter Roget (of thesaurus fame) as subjects to study the effects of nitrous oxide, commonly known as *laughing gas* (Freedman 1960). It was considered a delightful social activity to inhale the potent gas, but Davy took the fun a step further and recorded his and his friends' reactions as they fell under the sway of the drug. These gentlemen were particularly struck by the sensation of thoughts tumbling through their minds with lightning speed and vividness of detail, as if their mental faculties had been revved up beyond the normal pace. In mulling over this effect, Davy recognized that a soothing effect was reached whereby everyday worries simply fell away from consciousness.

William James, one of psychology's most gifted philosophers, also studied nitrous oxide, concluding that the altered state of consciousness it produced was actually another layer of the mind. Humans may spend most of their time confronting the world with their rational minds, but introducing a drug like nitrous oxide enabled one to tap into this coexisting state of mind, which, although ever present, blossomed to the foreground only when specifically accessed.

In 1916 Arthur S. Loevenhart at the University of Wisconsin stumbled into using the calming effects of mind-altering drugs to reach catatonic patients (Freedman 1960). He initially was investigating the drugs as an aid for stimulating patients' breathing. Catatonic patients were chosen for the study because their inert condition allowed researchers to observe their breathing quite easily and accurately and because researchers did not have to be concerned with obtaining informed consent. In the course of administering sodium cyanide, Loevenhart and his team were astonished when a comatose patient not only opened his eyes but also answered questions for the doctors. Other catatonic patients "awoke" in similar, albeit transitory, fashion while under the influence of the sodium cyanide.

This remarkable effect led to further experimentation in the 1930s with emotionally disturbed patients. Bleckwenn used sodium Amytal in the treatment of psychotic patients and also found that it was useful when interviewing nonpsychotic patients (J.C. Perry and Jacobs 1982). Some psychiatrists preferred large doses of medication that produced a deep sleep, after which catatonic patients returned to a normal waking state with alert mental functions for a while. Erich Lindemann at Massachusetts General Hospital took a different approach (Freedman 1960). He used much smaller doses and was able to revive catatonic patients into a relaxed, friendly, open frame of mind, allowing doctor and patient to communicate well, without having to first go through the deep sleep process. Lindemann experimented on the congenial effects of the drugs with emotionally stable people and found that they experienced both a sensation of euphoria and a noticeable increase in loquaciousness. Although they spoke far more, the drug did not produce any perceptual distortions or dreaminess; that is, the content of what they said remained the same, just more of it. This gabbiness was all the more remarkable given the unfortunate side effect of thickening of speech in the subjects. Lindemann concluded that the value of these drugs was their ability to suppress one's normal emotional reserve, resulting in freer communication with therapists. Khantzian (1975) described drugs such as these as "releasing agents" because they tend to release the individual from the normal inhibitory forces operating against the experience and expression of emotion.

The most commonly used drugs in the modern era for psychiatric purposes of inducing speech are sodium Amytal and sodium Pentothal, which produce the fewest side effects or toxic reactions and are the simplest to dispense (Freedman 1960). Therapists observe a tremendous relaxing effect in nervous patients, in both body language and verbal ease of expression. Some relax to the point of silliness, which generally subsides. Unlike the goal of reaching "truth" in terms of facts—dates, times, places, occurrences—many therapists find narcoanalysis useful in "loosening up" a patient so that he or she speaks more freely and also accesses emotions and thoughts that can lead to psychological insight and release. The effect of the drugs is that they speed up the therapeutic process by overcoming psychic inhibitions. Therapists and patients can deal with the substantive issues more readily, without having to tackle the superficial anxieties that block getting to those issues.

J.C. Perry and Jacobs (1982) studied Amytal interviews in the clinical setting and found that their greatest asset was in emergency situations, in which they quickly circumvent various difficulties in assessing psychiatric patients' conditions and required treatments. As already established, Amytal injections given to nonverbal patients manage to put them into a relaxed, awake, communicative state. These nonverbal states in which patients enter the emergency department include catatonia; hysterical stupor; unexplained muteness; and depressive, organic, and schizophrenic stupors (J.C. Perry and Jacobs 1982).

Amytal's effectiveness in rousing catatonic patients has been well established by Bleckwenn (1931) and Thorner (1935), who both used injections with excellent results. Although other medications are necessary to treat underlying psychiatric disorders, Amytal allows medical personnel to initiate lucid dialogue with patients to diagnose their condition on arrival in the emergency department.

Hysterical stupor is a condition found mainly in emergency circumstances. Individuals with this significant dissociation from customary consciousness generally cannot be roused, show no reaction to pain, oppose forcible opening of the eyelids, but have a modicum of voluntary muscle control. Even with all these symptoms, the electroencephalogram for individuals in such a stupor is consistent with someone who is awake. Often a person in a hysterical stupor will emerge from it unscathed within a relatively short time. However, in an emergency setting, the cause and treatment of the condition must be established. Amytal allows for this need, creating the necessary conscious state in which one can be interviewed and evaluated. One of the main benefits in this scenario is the avoidance of an unnecessary hospitalization.

A similar situation involves people who arrive in the emergency department fully conscious and attentive but mute. Indeed, although awake, these individuals make no effort to communicate by substituting hand gestures in place of their lost language skills. Hospitalization would be required until a diagnostic interview could be conducted; however, Amytal has been successful in lifting these patients out of their muteness.

In cases involving depressive, organic, and schizophrenic stupors, Amytal enables psychiatrists to gather information from the patient, which makes it possible to distinguish among these conditions. Often patients are elderly and in a stupor or a near-stupor. Depressed people are able to overcome their resistance to talking under the influence of Amytal. Schizophrenic patients can more easily relay their own delusional symptoms.

When an organic condition exists, patients, although communicative when injected with Amytal, are confused as to the role of the physician interviewing them, disoriented regarding where they are, or in denial about their medical condition.

In summarizing the therapeutic value of sodium Amytal in emergency room settings, J.C. Perry and Jacobs (1982) reached the following conclusion:

> the depressive patient given amytal will become more verbal, appear to brighten, perhaps, and have a normalization of mood. The schizophrenic patient will be less guarded and sometimes reveal additional symptoms. The patient with organic illness will become increasingly confused, however, and his or her performance on cognitive examination will deteriorate. Patients with one of these diagnoses will not appear more like patients with any of the other diagnoses. The ability to make this differentiation under amytal has been used as an aid to the Rorschach test in patients who are reticent. (p. 554)

In the clinical treatment setting, Amytal creates controversy as well as results. As in other situations it can make uncommunicative patients more talkative and move talking patients beyond their presenting resistant state to more substantive issues. Hoch (1946) noted that Amytal interviewing could lessen the time needed for psychotherapy because it could assist in establishing a transference more rapidly. Amytal's greatest strength as a clinical tool is its speed—by disinhibiting patients it allows them to progress more rapidly beyond their impeding symptoms.

In the more urgent case of posttraumatic stress disorders, Amytal has a history reaching back to World War I. For what was then termed *shell shock*, it again provided the relaxed state required to deal with repressed anxieties in response to combat horrors (Brown et al. 1998). The use of Amytal and sodium Pentothal with World War II soldiers facilitated recovery from stuporous conditions formed in reaction to experiencing and witnessing wartime atrocities. Noted film director John Huston, in his long-suppressed documentary *Let There Be Light*, recorded the remarkable achievements of narcoanalysis in the treatment of shell-shocked soldiers, some of whom had repressed memories of the war. Although the Pentagon kept the film unavailable for more than three decades as a threat to national security, it is now available on home video for a few dollars. As a result of medical developments during the Vietnam War, posttraumatic stress is now recognized as a common response to nonmilitary scenarios as well, such as rape, witnessing extreme catastrophes, and other stresses of modern life. In all these circumstances, J.C. Perry and Jacobs (1982) reported that "Amytal frees up a highly defended traumatic experience and aids in reintegration of dissociated ideas and affects. It provides a pharmacologic cushion that allows exploration and a lowering of defenses against the anxiety-provoking recollection of trauma" (p. 556).

For cases of dissociative amnesia (which entails lengthy memory loss for a distinct interval of time) and fugue states (which are characterized by a loss of identity), Amytal has proven to be more successful and swifter in treatment and recovery than has conventional therapy or hypnosis. For patients with a diagnosis of dissociative identity disorder, who characteristically disremember experiences, Amytal also has been useful specifically for exploring issues of dangerousness. For example, a patient with dissociative identity disorder may make a serious suicide attempt or series of attempts and claim no conscious knowledge of how the attempt happened. Amytal has been used to access consciously disremembered alter personality behavior associated with the suicide attempt.

Likewise, patients with conversion disorders and other somatoform disorders showed rapid and full improvement when treated with Amytal. Even suspected malingerers have been "cured" at the mere mention of the drug. One mute patient, on overhearing his doctor ordering the nurse to ready an Amytal injection to determine whether his symptoms were genuine or contrived, began to speak immediately.

In some situations the use of Amytal is not effective and therefore is not promoted. Patients with paranoia might react to the attempt to administer an injection as an attack or worry that they are being tranquilized against their will. Other medical conditions must be taken into consideration, such as liver or kidney conditions, respiratory tract infection or inflammation, hypotension, porphyria, and barbiturate addiction.

From the Clinical Setting to the Forensic Arena

Amytal is quite useful in clinical settings for a wide variety of purposes. For the most part, however, these purposes have not included establishing what has been called *historical truth* (Scheflin 1998). Therapists generally act without concern as to whether the patient is telling the truth. It is what the patient believes, not what actually happened, that serves as an important, although not exclusive, part of the therapy. Therapists have not been interested in investigating the factual accuracy of what their patients report. This conduct would move them beyond doing therapy and involve them in the construction of a carefully structured scientific test. Furthermore, experimenters have not been interested in establishing the historical truth of patient utterances in clinical settings. Thus in the clinical setting the Amytal literature does not address the issue of the veridicality of verbalizations induced by Amytal.

Two clinical cases that became widely publicized forensic cases show how a patient's utterance in therapy may become a relevant piece of evidence in a courtroom. The first case involves Richard Berendzen, a former president of American University, in Washington, D.C.

Berendzen fell from grace when the police arrested him for making obscene telephone calls to students. Berendzen resigned from the presidency and entered Johns Hopkins [University] Hospital for treatment. The treatment team used procedures such as guided imagery, age regression, writing imaginary letters to his mother, and focusing his attention on cases of child abuse that false memory advocates have labeled as unduly suggestive. in addition, sodium Amytal was administered. Berendzen began describing a series of sexual contacts with his parents that finally ended when he was 12 years old. These events had been eliminated from his mind. According to Berendzen (Berendzen and Palmer 1993) with regard to these sexual acts with his parents, "once it was over, it was erased" (p. xi). In later describing his story, Berendzen wrote "I now know I lived two childhoods, the one I remembered and the one I repressed. The one I remembered was the one that made it possible for me to survive. I was fifty-one years old before I remembered some of the repressed parts." (Berendzen and Palmer 1993, p. 7)

Paul McHugh, the chairman of the Department of Psychiatry at Johns Hopkins, monitored the treatment received by Berendzen. Based on the Amytal, guided imagery, regression, and other aspects of the treatment, McHugh concluded on a national television show that the events described by Berendzen really happened and that they shaped and caused his later conduct in making the obscene calls. McHugh further stated that the sexual contacts adversely affected Berendzen, who had a "kind of post-traumatic disorder, provoked by serious—the most serious kind of sexual abuse to him when he was a child" (ABC News 1990). McHugh further claimed that the calls were not obscene, although some of them involved strikingly graphic depictions of a 4-year-old girl kept as a sex slave who was locked up in a dog cage and fed only human waste. McHugh then filed a report with the court repeating his conclusions and further stating that Berendzen 1) made the telephone calls not because he had a prurient interest in sex but rather to resolve his own childhood sexual abuse, 2) was now fully cured, and 3) would never engage in making these telephone calls again (Pope 1995).

Another case attracted international press attention.

Gary Ramona was the vice president for marketing and sales and the chief executive officer of one of the satellite wineries of the Robert Mondavi Wineries. He had spent 20 years of hard work achieving those positions, which paid a salary of almost $500,000 a year. He was married to Stephanie and had three daughters—Holly, Kelli, Shawna.

Gary used the medical benefits from his job for his daughter Holly, who at the time was experiencing depression and an eating disorder (bulimia). Holly began seeing Marche Isabella, a marriage, family, and child counselor, in California. Therapy for the eating disorder began in late 1989. After 4 months of therapy, which did not involve any issues of sex or abuse, Holly, who was 19 years old, began having flashes of memory. These were not flashbacks because she did not feel that she was immediately immersed in the recollection. These flashes occurred outside of the therapy sessions. After several weeks these flashes of memory were discussed in the therapy sessions, but Holly did not recover any memories in an actual therapy session. Holly reported sexual abuse by her father, which began when she was approximately 5 years old and continued until she was about 10. Isabella decided to affiliate a psychiatrist, Richard Rose, on Holly's therapy to perform a psychiatric evaluation, including an Amytal interview.

On March 15, 1990, at Holly's insistence, Gary was invited to attend a meeting with Holly and her therapists. When Gary arrived, the day after the Amytal interview, Holly accused her father of multiple sexual assaults. Gary denied the accusations, but Holly's mother and sisters believed and supported her. Indeed, Holly's mother found confirmation from her own memories.

In March 1990, Holly filed a child abuse report against Gary for herself; Isabella, based on discussions with Holly and Shawna, filed a child abuse report on behalf of the younger daughters. In December 1990, Holly filed suit against her father for the abuse. In response Gary brought a lawsuit against his daughter's two therapists and the hospital for negligent treatment of his daughter and for intentional and negligent infliction of emotional distress on him.

Gary, in his verified second amended complaint (*Ramona v. Ramona* 1991), alleged that the therapists breached their duty of due care to him by negligently treating his daughter. In particular Gary alleged that the defendants failed in their duty, in part by

- Taking advantage of Holly's condition of extreme suggestibility caused by her major depression and bulimia, extreme anxiety, reduced self-esteem, and despair to subject her to the unwarranted and speculative suggestion that her condition must have been caused by childhood sexual abuse by her father
- Administering to Holly the sedative sodium Amytal, which has been shown to lead to disorientation, misidentification, and other errors and hallucinations
- Misrepresenting to Holly that the fantasies and hallucinations caused by suggestion and administration of sodium Amytal somehow corresponded to reality
- Failing to warn Holly and obtain her informed consent to the "therapy" embarked on by the defendants without advising her that there is no scientific evidence that the so-called therapy would reduce the major depression, reduce the bulimic behavior, or otherwise benefit the persons subjected to such "therapy"

Before the trial, Judge Snowden addressed the issue of whether Holly could testify after receiving a sodium Amytal treatment. He ruled that "a narcotized witness would be disqualified in a criminal proceeding just as a hypnotized witness is." The fact that the sodium Amytal was for treatment rather than for forensic purposes was irrelevant, especially because in this case the drugs were used to refresh memory. Judge Snowden (*Ramona v. Ramona* 1993) ruled that Holly's testimony was admissible because

> a central part of plaintiff's case is that the administration of sodium amytal was a cause of Holly's having false memories that he molested her. This makes this case quite different from one where narcosis is employed to supposedly enhance or recover a memory of some material fact; here, the very fact of the narcosis is a major element of plaintiff's lawsuit. Holly's testimony is in the nature of demonstrative evidence and it is evidence that the jury ought to be able to evaluate. Thus the court's ruling will be that the testimony of a narcotized witness should be admitted into evidence in a civil action where the plaintiff is suing over the narcosis itself and the memories allegedly engendered by it.

The case ended when the jury found in favor of Gary against the therapists but only awarded Gary $475,000 instead of the $8 million he had requested. Gary received no money for pain and suffering, only for past and future loss of earnings.

The *Ramona* case was not appealed because the verdict against the multiple defendants was so low that the costs of the appeal alone, not counting the new trial if the appeal were successful, would have been several times what the defendants had been found to owe. The appeal was not economically defensible. Some legal commentators argued that there was a strong likelihood that the case would have been reversed if it had been appealed.

Meanwhile Holly's own case against her father had not yet gone to trial. Because sodium Amytal had been used for memory retrieval, the original trial judge dismissed Holly's case against her father. Putting this initial judicial rejection aside, Holly and her attorney refiled the case in another court, this time relying on Holly's *pre*-Amytal memories. This second suit was dismissed on the grounds that the abuse issue had been decided against Holly in the *Ramona* case. In essence the judge ruled that Holly's personal case against her father was identical to her therapist's defense against her father, a defense that appeared to have been rejected by the jury verdict against the therapists. Holly successfully appealed this summary judgment dismissal. The path was now cleared for a jury trial on the merits of Holly's allegations that her recovered memories of her father molesting her years earlier were accurate. No trial was held, however, because the California Court of Appeals held that Holly's testimony was inadmissible because it had been influenced by the Amytal (*Ramona v. Superior Court* 1997).

Ironically, the commentators who predicted that the father's case would have been reversed on appeal were proven correct when the California Court of Appeals in *Trear v. Stills* (1999) ruled that nonpatients cannot sue therapists except in a few situations involving very special circumstances. As had occurred with Holly's father, the *Trear* case involved a father who had been sued by his adult daughter for alleged sexual abuse during her childhood. The father brought an action against the daughter's psychotherapist alleging that the psychotherapist had implanted false memories of childhood sexual abuse in the daughter and had encouraged her to take legal action against him. The court of appeals held that the psychotherapist owed no duty of due care to the father.

Thus Holly never got her own day in court to testify against her father. Her father, however, was permitted to collect the jury award he received despite the fact that the court of appeals subsequently refused to permit such legal actions to be brought. Even more interesting is the comparison between the *Ramona* case and the Berendzen incident. In *Ramona* the therapist's use of Amytal to confirm memories of childhood sexual abuse resulted in a successful lawsuit by the father against the therapist and also resulted in disqualifying the daughter, the alleged victim, from receiving compensation or even being heard. In the Berendzen incident, however, the therapist's use of Amytal to uncover memories of childhood abuse was applauded and served as the basis for the court to issue a suspended sentence after Berendzen pled guilty.

Thus an actual sex criminal received no sentence, an alleged perpetrator was permitted a financial recovery on a legal theory that existed for only that case alone, and an alleged victim was not permitted to testify on her own behalf against her alleged offender.

Current Legal Status of Narcoanalysis

Although the courts are aware of the power of scopolamine, sodium Amytal, sodium Pentothal, and other similar drugs to lower a person's inhibitions when administered by injection or intravenously, the reliability or veracity of statements made by suspects, defendants, and witnesses while under the influence of these drugs is not considered credible or trustworthy (Giannelli and Imwinkelried 1999; Moenssens et al. 1995). At best these drugs are viewed as a way to speed up the process (i.e., a person who is predisposed to confess may produce that confession more readily if narcoanalysis is used). However, the magic of confession is not attributed to the drugs themselves.

Most states regard the results of narcoanalysis interrogations as inadmissible and without scientific merit (Moenssens et al. 1995). A typical case in which narcoanalysis was rejected by the courts occurred in *State v. Pitts* (1989); the New Jersey Supreme Court declared the results of a drug-induced interrogation not scientifically reliable. The court refused to allow any expert testimony on the narcoanalysis at sentencing, relying instead on factual conclusions derived from the interview. Thus not only evidence both for and against defendants but also evidence from or about witnesses is inadmissible. However, if a suspect confesses following narcoanalysis, and that confession can be corroborated from other sources as well, the confession will be admissible. The courts are particularly attentive to the voluntariness of the narcoanalysis procedure and the protection of privacy rights.

A split of authority exists regarding whether experts can testify about what a defendant or witness said while under the influence of the drug. If the testimony is solely for the purpose of evaluating the expert's opinion of the subject's mental capacity or intent, then it usually will be admissible (Moenssens et al. 1995). Moenssens et al. (1995) noted that courts have rejected narcoanalysis test results in cases that involved the admissibility of the subject's statements under the influence of the drug, the admissibility of an expert's opinion based on factual conclusions derived from the drug interview, exculpatory statements made under the drug's influence, expert opinion that the drug tests proved that the subject was telling the truth, and the admission of a videotape of the drug test.

In two instances courts have not excluded evidence concerning truth drugs. In the first situation the drugs were used to refresh recollection, and the testimony admitted was the refreshed memory (*Sedgwick v. Kawasaki Cycleworks, Inc.* 1991; *United States v. Solomon* 1985). A pretrial hearing determined that the drug was administered according to stringent guidelines that offered a sufficient basis of belief that the memories were reliable.

The second situation involved the admissibility of postdrug memories or identifications. In the case of hypnotically refreshed recollections, states that follow the per se inadmissibility rule do not permit testimony about posthypnotic memories or identifications. In cases in which it could be shown that the drug was not the cause of a subsequent memory or confession, the memory or confession has been admitted into evidence (*People v. Heirens* 1954). When the confession or memory can be traced to the drug, it is inadmissible. Thus, a 15-hour gap between the administration of a drug and a confession rendered the confession inadmissible without a special hearing to determine whether the influence of the drug contaminated the confession (*Townsend v. Sain* 1963).

State legislatures have not enacted many statutes covering narcoanalysis. Currently three states have legislation on point. In Illinois both a criminal and a civil statute exist. For criminal trials the prohibition is that "in the course of any criminal trial the court shall not require, request, or suggest that the defendant submit...to questioning under the effect of thiopental sodium or to any other test or questioning by means of any mechanical device or chemical substance" (Illinois Statutes 1993a). This prohibition extends to sentencing hearings after trial (*People v. Ackerman* 1971). For civil cases that ban extends to pretrial and trial proceedings as well (Illinois Statutes 1993b).

Only two states have statutes permitting narcoanalysis in particular circumstances. Colorado sanctions narcoanalysis procedures when the defendant's sanity or eligibility for release from a civil commitment is being determined (Colorado Statutes 1993). Kentucky permits narcoanalysis when considering parole eligibility (Kentucky Statutes 1993).

Truth Drugs, Police Interrogations, and Intelligence Agencies

The search for historical truth through the use of chemical agents began a long time ago. As Loftus (1980) observed:

> An ancient Chinese test required a suspected wrongdoer to chew rice powder during an interrogation; the suspect then spit out the powder, and if it was dry, he was condemned. In Aztec Mexico, it was believed that peyote cactus (which contains mescaline) conferred the "power of second sight." This power could help in discovering the identity of a thief or in recovering stolen property. (p. 59)

Anecdotal incidents are sprinkled throughout the pages of history until the twentieth century, when the search for police drugs that were effective in interrogations (Rolin 1956) and that were useful for military and intelligence purposes (Lee and Shlain 1985; Scheflin and Opton 1978) became more systematic.

Rolin (1956) provided the fullest history, development, and use of truth drugs in print. He began with the following observation:

> This is an old story. It goes back to the times of Noah and his wine. The drunkenness of Noah is the first example of those states of self-abandonment in which, willy nilly, a man talks of things he would prefer to keep hidden, reveals things which are best not mentioned, gives away his secrets. Because it abolishes self-control and allows unchecked speech, alcohol is clearly the most ancient of those drugs now sometimes spoken of as "truth serums."
>
> The Romans coined an ironic proverb which expresses the meaning of this rather tragic collapse of the human mind: *in vino veritas*. (p. 11)

It is not surprising that Rolin reached the conclusion shared by others that "suggestibility and lucidity in interrogation are in some cases very marked, at other times the psychological defences remain unshaken. Sometimes the subject confesses, at other times he does not" (p. 29).

In a slightly later analysis, Gottschalk (1961) found "relatively few" studies of the use of drugs in interrogation settings. From these reports, and the literature in general, Gottschalk also concluded that "there is no 'truth serum' which can force every informant to report all the information he has" (p. 130). Some "criminal psychopaths" can lie under the influence of the drugs, and nonpsychopathic individuals may "disguise factual data." Fantasies may be reported as facts, and it would be very difficult for the interrogator to know whether fact or fantasy was being reported. Nevertheless, Gottschalk was not entirely dismissive of the use of truth serums because he urged further study and catalogued various uses and misuses of drug interrogations.

The development of viable truth drugs was one of the major goals of both the Office of Strategic Services and the Central Intelligence Agency, as well as several branches of military intelligence. Because the history of this search is still clouded in secrecy, no scientific tests have been declassified. From the reports that are available, however, it is clear that the truth drugs found several uses in covert operations. Clear evidence supports the fact that narcoanalysis was used in the Soviet bloc "show trials" of the 1940s, including the infamous trial of Cardinal Mindszenty. Truth serums were used by the Central Intelligence Agency, under the guise of a medical examination, to interrogate suspected enemy agents. After the questioning the drugs provided a mechanism to implant suggestions that the interrogation had been part of a dream or fantasy that never actually occurred beyond that nocturnal state (Scheflin and Opton 1978). Drugs also were used by hired prostitutes to secretly administer to their "lovers" while intelligence agents watched the sexual scenes from behind two-way mirrors (Farren 1999). The agents wanted to discover whether the power of the covertly administered drugs and the intimacy of the sexuality could loosen men's tongues into revealing secrets (Marks 1979). Indeed the Central Intelligence Agency hired a magician, John Mulholland, to write a manual on how the techniques of magic could be used by intelligence agents for purposes such as slipping drugs undetected into the drinks of unsuspecting individuals (Scheflin and Opton 1978). Massive experimentation was conducted with lysergic acid diethylamide for many purposes, including ascertaining truth (Lee and Shlain 1985).

One of the central figures in the intelligence agencies who was given the assignment of investigating the use of truth drugs for intelligence purposes reached the conclusion that no chemical substance reliably functioned as a truth serum (N. Hibler, personal communication with Alan W. Scheflin, February 2000). Truth drugs remain a subject of interest in, and are used by, many police departments (Danto 1979).

Is There "Truth" in Truth Serums?

Most commentators have concluded that sodium Amytal and sodium Pentathol are not very useful for interrogation purposes. For example, Freedman (1960) concluded that

> experimental and clinical findings indicate that only individuals who have conscious and unconscious reasons for doing so are inclined to confess and yield to interrogation under the influence of drugs. On the other hand, some are able to withhold information and some, especially character neurotics, are able to lie. Others are so suggestible or so impelled by unconscious guilt that they will describe, perhaps in response to suggestive questioning, behavior that never in fact occurred. The material produced is not "truth" in any sense of conforming with empirical fact. (p. 153)

In a paper motivated by political ideology more than by science, Piper (1994) joined the chorus of commentators who observed that narcoanalysis is no gateway to historical truth. It would be tempting to follow the weight of commentary and conclude that there is no "truth" in the truth serums. This conclusion would not be mistaken, but it would be misleading. Virtually all of the commentary on truth drugs fails to recognize three important variables. First, truth itself is an elusive concept, often depending on the eye of the beholder. Law Professor Geoffrey C. Hazard Jr. (1997) penned this crucial observation, which he then applied to the code of ethics for lawyers:

> In Lawrence Durrell's *Alexandria Quartet*, the author presents four narratives of a series of events about residents of Alexandria. The reader becomes aware, quickly or slowly, that the narratives address the same events. Yet Durrell never provides us with an external or objective viewpoint of these events. Hence, we can only surmise what "really" happened to the protagonists.
> Essentially, the same epistemological point is made in a Pirandello play ["Right You Are"].... [V]arious participants in a transaction view the events differently, interpret the events differently as they occur, remember them differently, and place different weights on the subsidiary incidents of the transaction....The same point is made in *Rashomon*, the Japanese play in which the same transaction is enacted serially from the respective viewpoints of the participants. (pp. 1041–1042)

The elusiveness of truth is sometimes captured in the way in which a person understands a communication. For example, a law enforcement official tells the story of interviewing a young boy who claimed to have been sexually molested. The boy's story was not believed because he said the molesting had occurred in a "rocket ship." The law enforcement official, quite by chance, was driving along a road and discovered an abandoned amusement park. He pulled his car into the park and found a rocket ship ride. In the rocket ship he found evidence confirming the boy's story.

Other truths hide behind screen memories or appear only in symbolic forms. On occasion a story that is very incomplete, or that contains several errors, may nevertheless be true concerning the gist of the events. Truth drugs may be highly useful for producing these elusive truths that may lead to important factual information.

Second, the criticisms of truth drugs are based on their failure to deliver pure, uncontaminated truth. But what procedure is capable of performing that function? Memory itself is not fully dependable, according to the currently popular reconstructionist model in effect since the writings of Munsterberg (1908) and Bartlett (1932). Should we therefore ban memory itself from the courtroom? Furthermore, because all memories are to some extent inaccurate, and because no memory carries with it any proof of its own truthfulness (no "Pinocchio" effect), every memory has a possibility or probability of accuracy. Whether a memory is sufficiently believable as reliable should be determined by the jury in assessing whether the burden of proof has been met in a particular case. Given the existence of the requirement that the burden of proof be met, there is little justification for excluding any memory, no matter how retrieved.

However, there is reason to believe that the inaccuracies of memory also have been exaggerated. Within memory research two schools of thought exist, although by careful analysis they can be synthesized (Brown et al. 1998). The "memory fallibility position," mostly argued by Loftus (1979), emphasized the inaccuracy of memory. This position, however, usually fails to specify the type of information for which memory may be more or less accurate. The "gist accuracy position" studies how frequently memory is accurate. This position emphasizes that under ordinary conditions memory for the gist of meaningful and emotionally salient personal experiences is generally quite accurate and reliable, whereas inaccuracies generally occur for peripheral, plot-irrelevant details (Christianson 1992). A detailed review of the scientific literature on laboratory studies for emotionally arousing events and on memory for real-life experiences showed that both positions have merit. It is clear that by focusing exclusively on how memory may go wrong, adherents of the memory fallibility position usually overstate their results. By adding the data from the gist accuracy position, it becomes clear that memory is remarkably accurate for the gist of crucial events but often inaccurate with regard to peripheral details.

A major forensic problem has been created because the memory fallibility position has been greatly overemphasized in the courts without the
necessary corrective of the other school of thought. Consequently, judges
have developed very negative impressions of memory in general and have
failed to make the crucial distinction between gist and peripheral details.
Furthermore, adherents of the memory fallibility position have overgener-
alized the belief that emotional stress hampers memory. In fact, emotionality or stress in many circumstances improves memory. The crucial
question is not "*is* memory involved?" (as the memory fallibility position
insists) but rather "*what* memory is involved?" (as the memory literature in
toto requires).

Because no studies have compared memory retrieval techniques with
each other, we cannot scientifically assess the value of truth serums in retrieving reliable (truthful) memories.

Third, Piper (1994) and others have argued that truth drugs are fail-
ures because they retrieve false as well as true memories. This criticism ignores the fact that memory itself delivers a concoction of truth, falsity, and
incompleteness. More important, however, is that the criticism does note
that some truth is delivered, although it is intertwined with error or lies. At
least under certain conditions, free from extreme interviewing, it can be expected that the gist of what is recovered by truth drugs is accurate, although
not all the details are likely to be fully accurate. No finder of fact can easily
distinguish which parts of a memory are true and which are false. To criti-
cize all memories refreshed by truth drugs on this ground is poor reasoning. If it could be confirmed that truth drugs produce substantially more
error in recollection than do other techniques of memory retrieval, a valid
objection could be lodged against them. But Piper does not make this
point. Furthermore, with any memory no matter how retrieved, police investigators may need only one small piece of truth to solve a crime. The fact
that 50 false leads are followed before one truthful tip cracks the case may
be insignificant with respect to the new information.

Rather than universally condemn truth serums on the grounds that
equally apply to memory itself, it seems wiser to experiment with them to
determine the exact conditions under which they are and are not useful.
This chapter shows that truth serum drugs have a variety of important clinical uses, apart from the issue of narrative memory. For example, they are
valuable in helping to overcome inhibitions, reduce anxiety, access emotional states, and explore disremembered behaviors. In this sense these
drugs serve an important clinical function as "releasing agents" (Khantzian
1975). With respect to the exploration of narrative memory, it is also clear
that such drugs are not a reliable type of truth serum. Nevertheless, even
in a forensic setting the new information that drug interviews may yield

may be useful both for enhancing memory for the gist of what happened and for identifying additional details, even if these details represent a mixture of accurate and inaccurate information. McHugh (ABC News 1990) listed an Amytal interview as one of the tests "which could validate our opinions or invalidate them" (p. 7) concerning his conclusion that his patient had been sexually molested as a child.

In our opinion, the problem with the use of truth serums in the forensic setting has less to do with the drug effects per se and more to do with the nature of the interview. Interviews characterized by 1) unrealistic expectancies (e.g., that the drug will reveal all the details of the truth or that everything reported will be accurate) and by 2) a systematic pattern of misinformation introduced or suggested by the interviewer are likely to yield highly unreliable recollections. However, interviews characterized by realistic expectancies, appropriate warnings about inaccuracies, and relatively nonsuggestive interviewing, at least under certain circumstances, may yield quite useful new information about both the gist and the details of an event.

Furthermore, the usefulness of truth serum drugs may in part depend on the type of individual for whom we use them. Little research has been done on what personality types respond better to them and what personality types easily resist them. Overall, the usefulness of truth serum drugs represents a complex interaction of drug effects, personality characteristics, and the nature and purpose of the interviewing. Among these variables the relative "truth" of the recollections reported through drug interviewing probably has much less to do with the effects of the drug per se and much more to do with 1) whether the interviewing is unduly suggestive, 2) whether the individual being interviewed has personality characteristics associated with proneness to distort memory, and 3) the potential consequences to the individual of disclosing or concealing the truth.

Truth by Relaxation: The Use of Hypnosis to Retrieve Memories

The use of hypnosis significantly and uniquely to influence each of the three "human response systems" (physiological, behavioral, and psychological) has been acknowledged by the scientific community from the time of Mesmer (about 1780–1790) (Hilgard 1965). In fact, since the eighteenth century, the increasing accumulation of empirical observations that human physiological functions (standardized measures of biological processes such as heart rate, blood pressure, respiratory rate, and body temperature), behavioral responses (descriptions of external, objective actions such as the tendency to sway back and forth while standing at attention with eyes closed, the distance of moving in a particular direction, and the number of button presses), and psychological experiences (communications about internal, subjective perceptions such as verbal reports about the intensity of loudness or deafness; the degree that something tastes sweet or sour; the inability to detect a noxious odor; the sense of involuntariness over one's own motor movements; and the ability or inability to recall past events) can be specifically influenced by hypnosis has been used as compelling evidence for its existence as a real, but directly unobservable, theoretical construct (Frischholz 1985; Hilgard 1965; Orne 1977; Spiegel and Spiegel 1978/1987). However, although there appears to be a growing consensus that such effects constitute the domain of "hypnosis" (Hilgard 1977; Orne 1977; Spanos 1986; Spanos and Barber 1974; Spiegel and Spiegel 1978/1987), there is little theoretical agreement about how to explain the underlying mechanisms by which hypnosis uniquely influences these various human response systems (Hilgard 1965; Kihlstrom 1985; Lynn and Rhue 1991).

Two Operational Definitions of Hypnosis

The lack of consensus about the unique mechanisms underlying hypnotic influences does not mean that there is a lack of agreement about how to operationally define *hypnosis*. Rather, two distinguishable (and not necessarily mutually exclusive) operational methods have evolved over the last 200 years and have been used in more than 90% of the published clinical and experimental literature on hypnotic effects. The first method is basically an attempt to define hypnosis by its *antecedent* conditions, such as whether subjects were or were not initially exposed to a *situation/context* characterized as a "hypnotic induction ceremony" *before* their response systems were subsequently assessed. Thus reports and studies that use this type of operational definition typically contrast subjects who have received some kind of commonly acknowledged hypnotic induction ceremony with subjects who have not received any hypnotic induction ceremony (either a no-hypnosis or a waking-baseline control condition; see Hilgard 1965; Hull 1933; Sheehan and Perry 1976; Weitzenhoffer 1953) or have instead received a recognized set of nonhypnotic instructions: nonhypnotic *comparison* conditions such as "relaxation" instructions (Edmonston 1972; Hilgard 1965), "imagination" instructions (Hilgard 1965; Katz 1979), "task-motivation" instructions (Barber 1969), and "simulation" instructions (Orne 1959, 1979). Obviously this type of operational definition is somewhat circular and speciously universal. According to the definition, all subjects exposed to a hypnotic induction ceremony should therefore be "hypnotized." From this perspective they should all manifest unique "hypnotic" effects on each of the three human response systems, which can be differentiated from the same measurements taken on subjects who had been exposed to either a nonhypnotic control or a nonhypnotic comparison condition.

In contrast, the second method for operationally defining hypnosis conceptualizes it as an identifiable human *trait/characteristic*. A range of individual differences on each or all of the three human response systems are a *consequence* of being exposed to a recognized hypnotic induction ceremony. Thus this method focuses on variations among subjects on the same measures that are seen *after* exposure to a hypnotic induction ceremony relative to such variation after exposure to either a nonhypnotic control condition (waking baseline) or a nonhypnotic comparison condition (relaxation instructions, imagination instructions, task-motivation instructions, and/or simulation instructions). This type of operational definition postulates that subjects should differ in terms of the degree to which they will manifest "unique" hypnotic effects. This means that some persons should not be expected to show any significant differences on each or all of the three human response systems after the administration of a hypnotic induction ceremony relative to responses on the same measures after exposure to either a nonhypnotic control or a nonhypnotic comparison condition (low hypnotizable subjects). Likewise other persons should show profound differences (high or medium hypnotizable subjects) on such variables that are considered to be distinct after exposure to a hypnotic induction ceremony relative to such responses following exposure to nonhypnotic situations/ contexts. In other words, unique hypnotic effects are probably *not* universally observed or found in all subjects. Rather, some persons show remarkable responsivity after exposure to a hypnotic induction ceremony, whereas others manifest few or no effects.

Empirical observations and investigations that have been published in the scientific literature on hypnosis for more than a century have repeatedly confirmed the validity of this second method that operationalizes hypnosis as a *trait* (Hilgard 1965; Tellegen 1979). A variety of scales and methods have been developed for measuring these individual differences (Barber 1969; Hilgard 1965; Spiegel and Spiegel 1978/1987). For example, empirical data collected on the standardization sample for the Stanford Hypnotic Susceptibility Scale, Form C (Weitzenhoffer and Hilgard 1962), show that approximately 11% of the sample earned a score of 10 or higher (i.e., were found to be highly hypnotizable) on this 0- to 12-point scale. In contrast, 26% of the sample earned scores of 2 or lower (i.e., low hypnotizable subjects). Thus the data clearly indicate that responsivity to hypnosis is not universal. Approximately 10% of the population should show the unique effects of being exposed to a hypnotic induction ceremony on each of the three human response systems, whereas approximately 25% of the population should not show any such effects despite such exposure. Therefore the only way to determine whether a subject would be likely to manifest a unique hypnotic effect on one or more of the three human response systems would be to measure his or her responsivity with one of the various hypnotizability scales. Based on such hypnotic responsivity scores, one could estimate which subjects would be expected to manifest unique hypnotic effects and which would not.

During the last 30 years numerous studies have reported that scores on these various hypnotizability measures are internally consistent, are temporally stable (even after a period of 10–25 years), and show high levels of interrater agreement (e.g., Frischholz et al. 1992).

In summary, two specific, but related, methods have become accepted by the scientific community for operationalizing the construct of hypnosis: 1) determining whether subjects were administered a hypnotic induction ceremony and 2) empirically demonstrating that subjects are hypnotizable or not hypnotizable by virtue of their score(s) on one or more of the various standardized hypnotic responsivity scales. Interestingly the scientific community has almost universally accepted the second method for operationally defining hypnosis based on the accumulated empirical data, whereas the courts still operationally define hypnosis based on the first method. The consequences of using these two distinct operational methods for defining hypnosis when evaluating how it can affect human memory are drastic and have led to different, and sometimes opposite, conclusions about such influences.

Another important point about the difference between the science of hypnosis and the conception of hypnosis is held by the courts. Almost every published experimental study that sought to detect a unique hypnotic effect on one or more of the three human response systems has used a methodology that included measuring a subject's hypnotizability and comparing subjects who have been administered some type of hypnotic induction ceremony with subjects who were exposed to a nonhypnotic control or comparison condition. By contrast, courts have rarely addressed the issue of the hypnotizability of the litigant. Perhaps even more interesting is the fact that most states have adopted a per se exclusion rule prohibiting the introduction into evidence of any memory occurring during or after hypnosis is used (Scheflin and Frischholz 1999). These states claim that hypnosis inevitably contaminates memory. Yet in dozens of court cases in which hypnosis was used, the subject had no additional recall and no loss of the prehypnotic memories. No court or commentator has explained how the claim that hypnosis must always harm memory can be squared with the large number of case reports of no memory alterations with hypnosis.

Criticisms of the Use of Hypnosis to Influence Memory

Since the publication of Dr. Orne's 1979 paper on forensic hypnosis, various new criticisms were made of the use of hypnosis to influence memory. Essentially they revolve around three central issues: suggestibility, reliability, and believability. Each of these criticisms is identified and evaluated briefly in the following subsections.

Suggestibility

Criticism 1. The subject becomes "suggestible" and may try to please the hypnotist with answers he or she thinks will be met with approval.

Evaluation. This criticism is not specific to "hypnotic" influences on memory alone, but it is of equal application in any social interaction that involves communication between an individual and an authority figure. Is it true that a person will be more likely to want to please the hypnotist than to please the police officer asking questions? Or the family members who want the crime to be solved?

in addition, no empirical study shows a significant and unique increase in a person's memory suggestibility (Brown et al. 1998) relative to the same types of significant memory suggestibility effects that have been found in a nonhypnotic context. The many cases in which subjects have no additional recall also would be evidence against the criticism that subjects will overly try to please the hypnotist. If the criticism were true, then the subjects would generate confabulated or inaccurate memories.

Thus this criticism is misdirected at hypnosis, and it lacks empirical and scientific support.

Criticism 2. The hypnotized subject experiences a loss of critical judgment.

Evaluation. This criticism is based on one of the many myths about hypnosis, which never was true (but still is thought to be). There has never been empirical documentation that hypnotized subjects exposed to a hypnotic induction ceremony, or highly hypnotizable subjects with or without a hypnotic induction ceremony, experience any loss of judgment as a unique effect of hypnosis. Instead some investigators, most notably Orne (1959, 1979), have reported that highly hypnotizable subjects exposed to a hypnotic induction ceremony appear to have a tolerance for logical incongruities in certain types of experimental situations. For example, Orne (1959, 1979) reported that highly hypnotizable subjects who were hypnotized and able to experience a suggested hallucination that a particular person was actually sitting in an empty chair to their left did not seem to be upset when they turned their heads and saw the actual person sitting in a chair to their right. In other words, they appeared able to accept the logical impossibility that the same person could be in two different places at the same time. Orne called this phenomena "trance logic." However, when asked if they could detect which person might be a hypnotic hallucination from the real person, most hypnotizable subjects correctly distinguished the real person from the hallucinated person. This suggests that their critical judgment was still intact despite the fact that they were temporarily able to accept an illogical perception. Indeed Spiegel (1974) proposed that some people are immediately critical of new information, whereas others will first accept this information and critically judge it at a later time. Furthermore, examples of "trance logic" have typically been found in some highly hypnotizable subjects exposed to a hypnotic induction ceremony, which means that this phenomenon, if assumed to be real, occurs in less than 10% of the population. It is not a universal or a specific "hypnotic" effect.

Criticism 3.   The subject is highly responsive to the creation of pseudo-memories.

Evaluation.   This criticism appears to be based on the work of Orne (1979, cited in Laurence and Perry 1983 and Scheflin and Frischholz 1999). This criticism also appears to be a faulty overgeneralization from the experimental data. For example, in the Laurence and Perry (1983) study, only one-half of the highly hypnotizable subjects had a pseudomemory, and about a quarter of the subjects thought that the memory was "real" and were certain that the event had occurred. This means that the pseudomemory phenomena did not even universally occur among a highly selected sample of subjects who represent 10% of the overall population (one-half of highly hypnotizable subjects is about 4.3% of the general population). Furthermore, because the experiment entailed suggestion of a minor detail (hearing a loud sound), it is likely that pseudomemory acceptance rates for suggested false complex events would be even lower. Furthermore, among the half that did report a pseudomemory, 50% were still able to distinguish between true memories and pseudomemories. Again this further proves that there is little empirical support for this criticism.

Other evaluations of this criticism have highlighted additional methodological problems (Brown et al. 1998). Loftus (1979) reported that she could create pseudomemories for the presence of a barn that did not really exist in the original stimulus event in more than 17% of nonhypnotized subjects (who were unscreened for their level of hypnotizability) with a single leading question. This finding suggests that the creation of pseudomemories for both peripheral and central details is not a unique "hypnotic" effect, and no significant increase in their likelihood of occurrence was found relative to nonhypnotized subjects.

Additional studies have attempted to show that hypnotic pseudomemories can be created not only by directly suggested misinformation but also indirectly, through the pattern of expectancies inherent in the hypnotic context. Thus certain motivational patterns (Murray et al. 1992) and expectancies about memory recall (Barnier and McConkey 1992; Lynn et al. 1992) significantly influence the production of hypnotic pseudomemories, especially when combined with suggested misinformation.

Several carefully designed studies have reported that pseudomemories occur in hypnotic experiments irrespective of whether a formal hypnotic induction ceremony or a waking control condition is used (see Brown et al. 1998). It is now clear that "hypnotic" pseudomemories are primarily a function of suggestive interviewing (wherein the interviewer directly suggests misinformation) and somewhat a function of unrealistic expectancies in the hypnotic context, combined with a personality trait of high hypnotizability. Thus hypnosis—as an induction ceremony or as a procedure—contributes very little to pseudomemory creation (Brown et al. 1998).

The conclusion of Lynn and Kirsch (1996), shared by most hypnosis experts, represents the current state of the scientific opinion: "False memories can be created with or without hypnosis, and the role of hypnosis in their creation is likely to be quite small....Hypnosis does not reliably produce more false memories than are produced in a variety of nonhypnotic situations in which misleading information is conveyed to participants" (p. 151).

Reliability

Criticism 1. The subject experiences "memory hardening," which gives him or her great confidence in both true and false memories, making effective cross-examination more difficult.

Evaluation. This criticism is specious for several reasons. First, no empirical study has yet found a significant increase in difficulty related to cross-examining a hypnotized witness's recollection compared with a non-hypnotized witness's recollection. Second, if a subject's prehypnotic recollections are available, then one can evaluate any differences between these and his or her later posthypnotic recollections in a variety of ways. For example, Spanos and McLean (1985–1986) and McCann and Sheehan (1987) reported different ways to help subjects distinguish between their original nonhypnotic recollections and pseudomemories created by hypnosis in their posthypnotic recollections. Likewise the findings reported by Laurence and Perry (1983) discussed earlier also suggest that at least one-half of the highly hypnotizable subjects who manifest a "hypnotic" pseudomemory are later able to distinguish between their original memory and the pseudomemory during a simple posthypnotic interview.

Other evaluations of this criticism can be found in other sources (Brown et al. 1998).

Criticism 2. The subject is likely to "confabulate," that is, to fill in details from the imagination, to make an answer more coherent and complete. According to this viewpoint the expectancies inherent in the hypnotic context cause some hypnotized individuals to shift their response criteria so that the boundary distinguishing fantasy and memory becomes blurred, and thus their report is likely to represent a mixture of fantasy and memory (Orne 1979).

Evaluation. This criticism is not unique to hypnotic recollections and is typically present in almost any type of memory report about a specific stimulus event (Bartlett 1932). Mixing fantasy and memory in response to memory instructions is more a function of contextual and expectancy variables than of any hypnotic procedure per se. in addition, no empirical studies to date have reported a significant increase in confabulation among hypnotized subjects, relative to nonhypnotized subjects, when the instructions and context for memory recall were *exactly the same* for both groups of subjects.

Criticism 3. The subject has source amnesia, which prevents properly identifying whether a memory occurred before or during hypnosis or whether the memory is real or suggested.

Evaluation. The phenomenon of hypnotic source amnesia is very rare and is typically observed only among a small number of subjects preselected for high hypnotizability (i.e.,<10% of the population). Furthermore, the studies reported by Spanos and McLean (1985–1986) and McCann and Sheehan (1987) clearly indicate that more than half of the subjects who do experience a hypnotic pseudomemory are later able to distinguish the source of the pseudomemory. In other words, approximately 2% of the population may manifest an unbreachable source amnesia, making it an unlikely event.

Believability

Criticism 1. Juries will disproportionately believe testimony that is the product of hypnosis.

Evaluation. This criticism has no empirical basis. In fact studies have shown that mock juries rated the testimony of a witness that was labeled as "hypnotically" influenced as being significantly less credible than the same testimony that was not labeled as hypnotic. Furthermore, warnings regarding the differential credibility of specific kinds of testimony have been used by the courts and attorneys when there is reason to believe that some types of evidence are more reliable than others.

Criticism 2. The subject can easily feign hypnosis and can be deceptive in trance.

Evaluation. No empirical study has shown that lies reported by subjects who are feigning hypnosis are significantly more difficult to detect than are lies from subjects who have never been hypnotized. Furthermore, one court case showed that an expert could detect a subject who was both feigning hypnosis and lying while under its alleged influence (*State v. Bianchi* 1979; see also Scheflin and Frischholz 1999 for a more detailed discussion of this issue).

Other Recent Criticisms

C. Perry (1995) proposed that many procedures routinely used in psychotherapy, such as relaxation, visualization, and guided imagery, are in fact "disguised" hypnosis. Hence these procedures have the same contaminating influence on memory as do those alleged above (i.e., issues regarding suggestibility, reliability, and believability). Perry's view in effect indicts most forms of psychotherapy as a contaminating influence on a person's memory. This contention, however, would be too extreme if, as discussed above, little or no empirical evidence supports the various criticisms that have been made against hypnosis as a contaminating influence on memory. Thus it also must be acknowledged that no evidence indicates that these other procedures are equivalent to hypnosis or that they always cause memory contaminations.

Another recent criticism alleges that even low hypnotizable subjects are negatively influenced by the use of hypnosis with memory (Orne et al. 1996a, 1996b). This argument is entirely unsupported by empirical data and illogical. Low hypnotizable subjects, by definition, are individuals who are unlikely to manifest any type of hypnotic effect based on their demonstrated lack of responsivity to test suggestions following a hypnotic induction ceremony.

Finally, Kebbell and Wagstaff (1998) have argued that the Cognitive Interview, a memory enhancement technique, is superior to hypnosis because it stimulates additional, accurate recollection while minimizing confabulations and errors. Unfortunately, empirical studies comparing the Cognitive Interview with hypnosis have not shown any significant increases in accurate recollection or consistent decreases in memory contamination or errors. In fact the major thrust of the Kebbell and Wagstaff argument

can be shown to be based on faulty assumptions about the scientific literature about hypnosis and memory. Once again, the few available comparative studies failed to control for contextual and expectancy effects.
Therefore it has not been shown that, under equivalent or comparable con-
textual/expectancy conditions, the Cognitive Interview is superior to hypnosis for memory enhancement, and the few available data imply that the
seeming superiority of the Cognitive Interview is an artifact of a more realistic set of expectancies about memory enhancement inherent in the Cognitive Interview than has been true for hypnosis.

Based on a careful review of the extensive research on hypnosis and
memory, Brown et al. (1998) concluded that "hypnotic techniques do not
appear to contribute anything unique to producing pseudomemory reports" (p. 340). McConkey (1992), likewise, concluded that "there may not
be anything particularly hypnotic about hypnotic pseudomemory" (p. 423).
A recent task force convened by the American Society of Clinical Hypnosis, representing the input of about 100 professionals in the field of hypnosis, drew a similar conclusion: "Based on the scientific evidence from
numerous studies, this panel concludes that contaminating effects on memory are no more likely to occur from the use of hypnosis than from many
nonhypnotic interviewing and interrogative procedures. Therefore, legal
rules that single out hypnosis for restrictive treatment are unwarranted"
(Hammond et al. 1994, pp. 22–23).

This statement represents a careful update of the science since the
1985 report on hypnosis issued by the American Medical Association, and
thus some of the conclusions of the American Medical Association report
are outdated and in need of modification. Overall, it has become clear that
hypnotic pseudomemories are the result of a complex interaction among
personality variables (hypnotizability, fantasy-proneness), suggested misinformation in an interview, and contextual/expectancy variables and that
hypnosis (defined in terms of a formal hypnotic induction ceremony or
specific procedures used after the induction of hypnosis) per se contributes
very little to pseudomemory production. Pseudomemory production is
more likely to occur in a context of unrealistic expectancies about memory
recovery combined with systematic misinformation suggested by the interviewer and rarely occurs when realistic expectancies are created and the interviewing is based on nonsuggestive free recall.

Truth by Imagination: Guided Imagery

The claim has been made that guided imagery creates false memories, although no empirical support has been offered to support this hypothesis.
Furthermore, there is no single definition as to what constitutes guided im-

agery specifically with respect to memory enhancement. The literature on the use of guided imagery in the clinical setting can be classified into two broad categories: 1) the use of imagery spontaneously emerging from the patient and 2) the use of structured scenes introduced by the therapist, such as a meadow, a safe place, and a house with many rooms to explore (Brown and Fromm 1986). The use of the latter approach, which is more accurately viewed as *guided* imagery for memory enhancement, has not been studied in the laboratory. Thus virtually no empirical evidence exists either to support or to refute the claim that guided imagery per se is a "risky memory recovery technique."

However, a good deal of laboratory research exists on at least one type of imagery used for memory enhancement—imagery in association with the Cognitive Interview. The Cognitive Interview was developed as an interview procedure to be used in forensic psychology. It is based on scientific research on conditions that improve accurate memory retrieval and was designed to maximize new information without increasing the memory error rate (Geiselman et al. 1984). The original Cognitive Interview contained four memory retrieval strategies (context reinstatement, report everything, varied order, and varied perspective), the most important element being context reinstatement (Geiselman et al. 1984). In essence the subject is instructed to reconstruct the time, physical surroundings, and self-experience at the time of the target event, followed by free recall of any and all details about the event, and subsequently followed by successive free recall attempts and specific questioning about the event.

The Cognitive Interview also contains explicit imagery instructions (Fisher and McCauley 1995). The interviewer is told "to encourage and assist the witness to generate focused concentration" (Fisher et al. 1989, p. 723). During the context reinstatement phase of the interview, the subject is encouraged to generate mental images of the event (George 1991). Memon (1998), for example, stated that

> the interviewer can help witnesses by asking them to form an image or impression of the environmental aspects of the original scene (e.g., the location of objects in a room), to comment on their emotional reactions and feelings at the time (surprise, anger, etc.) and to describe any sounds, smells and physical conditions at the time (hot, humid, smoky, etc.). Geiselman and his colleagues...have suggested that it may be helpful for child witnesses to verbalize out loud when mentally reinstating context. For example, to describe the room as the image comes to mind, to describe smells, sounds and other features of context. (p. 172)

Memon goes on to give the details of the imagery instructions that she used in much of her research:

> First of all I'd like you to think back to that day. Picture the room in your head as if you were back there....Can you see it? (pause for reply). Think about who was there (pause). How were you feeling? (pause) What could you see? (pause). What could you hear? (pause) Could you smell anything? (pause) (Memon 1998, p. 172)

Elsewhere Memon adds, "The CI interviews used a combination of context reinstatement and imagery instructions in the questioning phase. The interviewers actively encouraged the children to generate images of the event and to describe them" (Memon et al. 1997a, p. 192). In this sense the Cognitive Interview could be considered an imagery-type of "memory recovery technique." The revised Cognitive Interview consists of the same context reinstatement and varied retrieval strategies combined with more careful attention to interviewing methods that allow the subject to have more control over the interview and its pace and that use more open-ended questions (Fisher et al. 1987).

To date we have located a total of 42 laboratory studies that have used imagery, the great majority using either the original or the revised Cognitive Interview. Of these studies only five (Malpass and Devine 1981; Ceci et al. 1994a, 1994b; Poole and Lindsay 1995; Yuille and McEwan 1985) used imagery per se, not combined with the Cognitive Interview. In most of the 42 studies, college research subjects were shown some stimulus event, typically a brief film of a complex event such as a bank robbery or a car accident, or sometimes they witnessed a live staged theft. A few studies were conducted on eyewitnesses to actual crimes and accidents (e.g., Fisher et al. 1989). After viewing the stimulus event, the subjects were asked to recall the event. The imagery-based Cognitive Interview (original or revised version) was administered to the experimental group, and a standard or structured interview was administered to a control group. Results were formulated in terms of the percentage of new, accurate information retrieved about the stimulus event in the imagery-based Cognitive Interview relative to the control interview procedure. However, the interview style used in the Cognitive Interview and in the control interview also was not the same, so that comparisons made across the experimental and control conditions are partly limited by the nonequivalence of the conditions (Bekerian and Dennett 1993). This observation is similar to the situation regarding research on hypnotically refreshed recollection, in which the experimental hypnotic condition differs from the control or comparison condition on factors other than the presence or absence of a hypnotic induction ceremony. Nevertheless, the research design does permit conclusions about the relative efficacy of the Cognitive Interview over conventional interviewing.

The memory error rate is determined in one of several ways: 1) the total number of errors occurring after the experimental or control procedure, 2) the total number of errors adjusted to the total amount of information (the memory error rate), and 3) the total number of inaccurately reported details that were not part of the original stimulus event (the confabulation rate). Of these three measures, the memory error rate is given particular emphasis in this chapter.

As can be seen in Table 13–1, there are 42 laboratory studies (2 using guided imagery per se and 40 using guided imagery as part of the Cognitive Interview) in which the imagery procedure was combined with a free recall memory retrieval strategy. Specific open-ended questions were asked in addition to encouraging free recall. A few studies also included warnings not to guess. The total amount of new information from the imagery-based procedure relative to the control interview varied considerably across studies (Bekerian and Dennett 1993). Table 13–1 shows that between 4% and 105% new information occurred following the imagery-based Cognitive Interview. However, several critical reviews of these studies concurred that the original imagery-based Cognitive Interview typically yields an impressive 20%–35% significant new information relative to a control procedure (Bekerian and Dennett 1993; Fisher et al. 1987, 1989; Geiselman et al. 1984; Koehnken et al. 1994), and the revised Cognitive Interview yields about 45% new information (Fisher and McCauley 1995).

A meta-analysis of more than 30 experiments that used the Cognitive Interview with more than 1,000 subjects showed that the Cognitive Interview resulted in significantly more correct information about the target event (36%) relative to control interview conditions, although there was a smaller but significant increase in the amount of incorrect information (Koehnken et al. 1994).

According to our analysis in Table 13–1, despite variability across studies, a statistically significant amount of new information was retrieved in the Cognitive Interview as compared with the control procedure in 37 of the 42 studies (the 5 studies with insignificant results all were from the same research group). Overall, these findings are remarkably consistent across many independent replication studies from different research groups, most of which support the conclusion that the imagery-based Cognitive Interview yields a significant amount of new information relative to an ordinary control interview about a target event. This conclusion is consistently true when the imagery is used to reinstate the context of the target event, following which free recall is encouraged.

Several of these laboratory studies also found that the amount of incorrect information sometimes significantly increased along with the amount of new, correct information. A total of 8 of the 42 studies reported a significant increase in the number of memory errors, whereas 24 studies did not

Table 13–1. Imagery and memory enhancement: completeness and accuracy data

Study	Target	# Int	% new information	Error rate	Style	Strategy
Yuille and McEwan 1985	Bank robbery videotape	1		#NS		FR, specific questions
Malpass and Devine 1981	Staged vandalism	1	20	#NS	GI	Photo lineup vs. guided imagery
Geiselman et al. 1984	Staged theft	1	29		CI	CI vs. H
Geiselman et al. 1985	Violent police training film	1	40		CI	
Geiselman et al. 1986	Bank robbery videotape		29		CI	
Fisher et al. 1987		1	45	#NS c NS	CI R	CI vs. R
Scrivner and Safer 1988	Burglary videotape	4	23	#NS		FR replay of videotape
Fisher et al. 1989	Field study; witnessed crimes	5–7	47	#NS	R	R used in field trial
MacKinnon et al. 1990	Slides of number plates		23			
George and Clifford 1991	Staged argument	1	35	#NS	R	United Kingdom study
Aschermann et al. 1991	Videotape of amusement arcade	1	40	#NS	CI	German study
Koehnken et al. 1991	Film of blood donation		35	#NS r NS c*		German study

Table 13–1. Imagery and memory enhancement: completeness and accuracy data *(continued)*

Study	Target	# Int	% new information	Error rate	Style	Strategy
George and Clifford 1992	Field study of crimes and accidents		14			
Mantwill et al. 1992	Blood donation		25	#NS c NS	R	
Koehnken et al. 1992			52	#NS c NS	R	
Koehnken et al. 1994	Blood donation	1	52	#NS c NS	R	Control Q matched to CI
Turtle and Yuille 1994	Robbery	4	11	#* r NS		Repeated FR, review previous statements
Memon et al. 1994	Staged robbery	1	4 NS	#NS *Person		
Fisher and McCauley 1995	Videotape of car accident	1	65	#* r NS	R	
McCauley and Fisher, in press			84		R	
Dasgupta et al. 1995	4 types of stimuli		16 13.5	c NS	CI H	Comparison of CI and hypnosis
Mantwill et al. 1995	Blood donation		25	#* r NS c NS	R	Retrieval aids rarely applied
Koehnken et al. 1995	Blood donation	1	35	#NS r NS c*	R	CI's effect on statement analysis

Table 13–1. Imagery and memory enhancement: completeness and accuracy data *(continued)*

Study	Target	# Int	% new information	Error rate	Style	Strategy
Memon et al. 1996	Videotape of magic show	1	24	#NS	CI	Resistance to misinformation
Memon et al. 1997a	Staged magic show	1	41	#* r NS c NS	R	
Memon et al. 1997b	Videotape of shooting	1	11 NS	#* r* c*	R	
Clifford and George 1996	Actual crime witnesses	1	19	#NS	R	Field setting
Hernandez-Fernaud and Alonso-Querty 1997	Videotape of theft	1	105	#NS c*		Signifcant errors only for people and descriptions
Child studies						
Geiselman and Padilla 1988	Film of robbery	1	21	#NS	CI	CI plus warnings
Geiselman et al. 1990	Simon Says	1	26	#NS	CI	
McCauley and Fisher 1992	Simon Says	1	65	#NS	R	
Koehnken et al. 1992	Short film	1	93	c*	R	
Saywitz et al. 1992 #1	Staged event	1	26	#NS	CI	CI plus warning
Saywitz et al. 1992 #2	Staged event	1	18	#NS	CI	CI plus practice with CI
Memon et al. 1992		2	45 NS			

Table 13–1. Imagery and memory enhancement: completeness and accuracy data *(continued)*

Study	Target	# Int	% new information	Error rate	Style	Strategy
Memon et al. 1992	Vision test		NS	#NS		
Memon et al. 1993			NS	#* / r NS	CI	
McCauley and Fisher 1995	Simon Says		64 / 46	#* / r NS	R	
Poole and Lindsay 1995	Mr. Science staged event	1	56–68	NS		5 open-ended questions
Hayes and Delamothe 1997	Videotape of store adventure	1	78	#* / *c		
Chapman and Perry 1995	Videotape of road accident			#NS		
Dietze and Thompson 1993				#NS		
Misinformation						
Poole and Lindsay 1995	Mr. Science staged event	1		**24%		FR+9 misleading Q+coaching
Ceci et al. 1994a	Mousetrap study	10		20%		As if event happened+warning
Ceci et al. 1994b	Mousetrap study	10		NS		Warnings

Note. #Int=number of interviews; #=number of errors; GI=guided imagery; r=error rate; CI=cognitive interview; c=confabulation rate; R=revised cognitive interview; *=significant effect; H=hypnosis; NS=no significant effect; Q=questioning; FR=free recall.

find any significant increase in the total number of errors when the imagery-based Cognitive Interview was used. Some studies found that the greater portion of the variance of memory errors occurred in the later questioning phase of the Cognitive Interview relative to the earlier imagery/context reinstatement and free recall phase (Aschermann et al. 1991).

A more recent methodological improvement is the use of an adjusted memory error rate as another important dependent variable instead of just using a measure of the total number of errors. The memory error rate assesses the number of errors adjusted to the total amount of new information. Thus if a memory retrieval procedure yields a lot of new information, this information may contain some errors, but the memory error rate may not necessarily increase relative to ordinary recall. A total of 10 of the 42 studies reported memory rate as an outcome measure. Only 1 of these studies (Memon et al. 1997b) found that the Cognitive Interview procedure significantly increased the memory error rate. The other 9 studies that specifically addressed whether the memory error rate significantly increased reported that the use of the Cognitive Interview to enhance memory did not result in any significant increase in the memory error rate. Once again the data are remarkably robust across studies in showing that the imagery-based Cognitive Interview does not generally lead to a significant increase in the memory error rate.

Another methodological refinement is the inclusion of a confabulation rate as a measure of memory error. A response is scored as a confabulation when the subject recalls a detail that was not part of the original stimulus event (Memon et al. 1997a). A total of 13 of the 42 studies assessed confabulation. These results were equivocal; 7 studies did not and 6 did find a significant increase in the confabulation rate when the Cognitive Interview was used relative to the control procedure.

Clifford and George (1996) investigated the relative contribution of imagery to the overall efficacy of the Cognitive Interview as a memory enhancement procedure. They found that context reinstatement and imagery each made an independent contribution to overall effect. Significantly more information was reported about the target event when subjects were explicitly instructed to use imagery across all types of interview questions as compared with when no imagery instructions were given. Imagery may serve as an aid to context reinstatement (Bekerian and Dennett 1993) but is perhaps less useful during the open-ended questioning component of the revised Cognitive Interview (Clifford and George 1996).

The obvious finding across nearly all of these 42 data-based studies is that under ordinary interviewing conditions (free recall and careful non-suggestive questioning), imagery used as a focusing and context reinstatement device is not a "risky" memory recovery procedure at all but just the opposite—it is a very useful procedure. The consistent finding is that the imagery-based Cognitive Interview leads to significant new information about a target event relative to control interview procedures without significantly increasing the memory error rate. This is not to say that the information retrieved through the imagery-based Cognitive Interview is entirely free from error, because all memory is a mixture of accurate and inaccurate information. The use of a memory enhancement technique such as the Cognitive Interview does not pose any unique risk, in that the significant new information typically retrieved generally is not accompanied by a significant increase in the memory error rate. Overall, these data across studies support the conclusion that the imagery-based Cognitive Interview is a very useful memory enhancement technique, provided that the free recall is encouraged after imagery is used to reinstate the context of the target event. In other words, the conclusion from this large body of data-based laboratory studies is exactly the opposite of the claim that guided imagery per se is an allegedly "risky memory recovery technique" (Lindsay and Read 1994; Loftus 1993).

However, when guided imagery is combined with systematic misinformation characteristic of highly suggestive interviewing, a very different picture emerges. Numerous studies have reported that information supplied after an event can significantly alter a memory report. This is known as the *postevent misinformation suggestion effect* (for a review, see Brown et al. 1998). Table 13–1 contains 3 laboratory studies with children in which imagery was combined with a systematic pattern of suggested misinformation (Ceci et al. 1994a, 1994b; Poole and Lindsay 1995). In 2 of these studies the memory commission error rates increased remarkably to 20% or higher. These three studies are not exactly comparable to the other 42 studies because none of the 3 studies used the Cognitive Interview; nevertheless, these data clearly show that systematically suggestive interviewing substantially increases the memory error rate when an imagery procedure is being used to enhance memory.

What kind of overall conclusions are fair to these data? In our opinion, the conclusion best supported by the data is that imagery per se is a useful memory recovery procedure, provided that it is combined with a context reinstatement and free recall interviewing style. However, when imagery is combined with a systematically suggestive interview style (wherein the interviewer is supplying content), there is risk of both significantly increasing the memory error rate and producing false memories. Those who believe that false memories exist and that guided imagery is a risky memory recovery technique (e.g., Lindsay and Read 1994; Loftus 1993) have committed a logical error: misplaced emphasis. They have misattributed a significant memory error to the technique (the use of imagery per se), even though virtually no scientific studies support this speculation, and they have failed to see that the real problem is that of unduly suggestive interviewing, in which the interviewer is systematically supplying misinformation. The effectiveness of imagery as a memory enhancement procedure is largely a function of the quality of the interview procedure. Modest expectancies, appropriate warnings that not all memory information reported is accurate, and above all a free recall style of interviewing generally lead to significant new information without a significant increase in the memory error rate when an imagery-based interview procedure is used. Unrealistic expectancies, like those given in many studies on hypnotically refreshed recollection (e.g., "memory is like a tape recorder, and you will be able to remember absolutely everything about the event") without accompanying cautions, combined with a systematically suggestive style of interviewing in which the interviewer supplies misinformation, generally lead to a mixture of accurate and inaccurate information, to a significant increase in the memory error rate, and sometimes to false memory reports.

One interesting recent study explored the effects of guided imagery on reported confidence about childhood events (Clancy et al. 1999). The study used two samples of women—one group who had reported recovered memories of childhood sexual abuse and a control group of women who had not reported such memories but who had reported other childhood events. Both groups were pretested on the degree of confidence they had about whether certain childhood events had or had not actually happened to them. The experimental group received guided imagery instructions to "picture the event…given more details to imagine….Try to picture each event as clearly and completely as you can. It may help you to form a more complete mental picture if you include familiar places, people, and things in the imagined event" (p. 563). Control subjects did not use the imagery instructions. After the procedure, confidence was reassessed for both groups. Contrary to the anti-imagery hypothesis, "guided imagery did not significantly inflate confidence that early childhood events had occurred," and the effect size for inflated confidence was "twice as large in the control group as in the group with recovered memory" (p. 559). They added, "women who report recovered memories of sexual abuse are able, at least in the laboratory, to resist the potentially memory-distorting effects of guided imagery" (p. 567).

What conclusions can be drawn from the laboratory studies on guided imagery and memory enhancement?

First, imagery per se appears to be a useful memory enhancement procedure when associated with skilled, nonsuggestive interviewing, as exemplified by the Cognitive Interview method. Classification of guided imagery, at least the kind of imagery associated with the Cognitive Interview, as a "risky memory recovery procedure" has virtually no support across the large database of current laboratory studies. Nevertheless, it is important to remember that the use of imagery as a memory enhancement procedure must be associated with nonsuggestive interviewing.

Second, imagery, when combined with unduly suggestive interviewing, results in a significant increase in the memory error rate. False memories and memory distortion are apparently more a function of suggestive interviewing and have little to do with imagery as a technique per se.

Third, no evidence indicates that imagery unrealistically inflates confidence about memories.

Fourth, the conclusions drawn about the effects of guided imagery on memory enhancement are limited to certain types of imagery procedures, and the question remains open as to whether other types of guided imagery procedures might prove to be risky memory recovery procedures. However, based on the scientific evidence now available, the hypothesis that guided imagery is a "risky memory recovery technique" has virtually no empirical support.

Overall Conclusions

Our review of the literature on drug interviews, hypnosis, and guided imagery leads to consistent findings across all three of these memory enhancement procedures. First drug interviews, hypnosis, and guided imagery have a variety of important clinical uses, apart from the specific issue of exploring or enhancing narrative memory. These uses have not tended to attract legal controversy.

Second, as techniques, drug interviews, hypnosis, and guided imagery per se are not "risky memory recovery techniques" and may be useful under certain conditions with select subjects. Their usefulness is enhanced in a context of realistic expectancies about memory recall combined with a relatively nonsuggestive, free-recall interview style. On the other hand, these techniques may contribute to significant memory distortion, confabulation, or false memory creation *if* they are used in a high-demand context to remember "everything" accurately, combined with a pattern of systematically suggested misinformation by the interviewer. Thus the problem of memory distortion has much less to do with the use of the technique (drug interview, hypnotic induction, or guided imagery) per se and much more to do with the context, the pattern of expectancies, the quality of the interviewing, and the personality characteristics of the subject.

Third, blanket condemnation of these techniques represents a logical problem of misplaced emphasis; it is not the technique per se that causes memory distortion but rather how the interviewing is conducted, what sort of expectancies are created, and what type of individual is being interviewed. In short, one does not universally condemn a knife because it can cut a throat as easily as it cuts bread. Although it is certainly easier to attack a technique wholesale and claim that its every use is harmful, experts who so testify are violating their ethical responsibilities to report the scientific literature with accuracy.

Reasonably prudent clinicians who use these procedures, even in ways that have little to do with memory recovery, must be very mindful of the type of expectancies they create and the type of interview they conduct if they wish to minimize memory and other distortion. Triers of fact must relinquish the easier, but misleading, task of deeming testimony unreliable simply because a technique such as a drug interview, hypnosis, or guided imagery had been used. Experts must stop condemning techniques and instead look more carefully and closely at how those techniques were actually used in the particular case. Judges must, in their instructions and rulings, squarely address the factual issues concerning what type of expectancies might or might not have been created, whether the interviewing style was unduly suggestive, and whether the interviewee's personality characteristics posed a reasonable risk for significant memory distortion. Once this is done, the modern tests for the admissibility of expert testimony, which emphasize flexibility and the judge's role as the gatekeeper of admissibility, will have been satisfied, a better brand of justice will be administered, and patients will not lose the services of techniques that have proven therapeutic value.

References

ABC News, Nightline, May 23, 1990 (no 2348 in program series)

American Medical Association: Council on Mental Health, "Medical use of hypnosis." JAMA 168:186–189, 1958

American Medical Association: Council on Scientific Affairs: Scientific status of refreshing recollection by the use of hypnosis. JAMA 253:1918–1923, 1985

American Psychiatric Association: Regarding hypnosis: a statement of position by the American Psychiatric Association. February 15, 1961

Aschermann E, Mantwill M, Koehnken G: An independent replication of the Cognitive Interview. Applied Cognitive Psychology 5:489–495, 1991

Barber TX: Hypnosis: A Scientific Approach. New York, Psychological Dimensions, 1969

Barnier AJ, McConkey KM: Reports of real and false memories: the relevance of hypnosis, hypnotizability, and context of memory test. J Abnorm Psychol 101:521–527, 1992

Bartlett FC: Remembering: A Study in Experimental and Social Psychology. New York, Cambridge University Press, 1932

Bekerian DA, Dennett JL: The Cognitive Interview technique: reviving the issues. Applied Cognitive Psychology 7:275–297, 1993

Berendzen R, Palmer L: Come Here: A Man Overcomes the Tragic Aftermath of Childhood Sexual Abuse. New York, Villard Books, 1993

Bleckwenn WJ: The use of sodium amytal in catatonia. Res Pub Assoc Ner Ment Dis 10:224–229, 1931

Brown D, Fromm EF: Hypnotherapy and Hypnoanalysis. Hillsdale, NJ, Lawrence Erlbaum, 1986

Brown D, Scheflin AW, Hammond DC: Memory, Trauma Treatment, and the Law. New York, WW Norton, 1998

Butler LD, Spiegel D: Trauma and memory, in American Psychiatric Press Review of Psychiatry, Vol 16. Edited by Dickstein LJ, Riba MB, Oldham JM. Washington, DC, American Psychiatric Press, 1997, pp II-13–II-53

Ceci SJ, Loftus EF: Memory work: a royal road to false memories? Applied Cognitive Psychology 8:351–364, 1994

Ceci SJ, Loftus EF, Leichtman MD, et al: The possible role of source misattributions in the creation of false beliefs among preschoolers. International Journal of Clinical and Experimental Hypnosis 42:304–320, 1994a

Ceci SJ, Crotteau-Huffman MLC, Smith E, et al: Repeatedly thinking about a nonevent: source misattributions among preschoolers. Conscious Cogn 3:388–407, 1994b

Chandler R: The Long Goodbye (1953). New York, Vintage Books, 1988

Chapman AJ, Perry DJ: Applying the cognitive interview procedure to child and adult eyewitnesses of road accidents. Applied Psychology: An International Review 44:283–294, 1995

Christianson S-A: The Handbook of Emotion and Memory: Research and Theory. Hillsdale, NJ, Erlbaum, 1992

Clancy SA, McNally RJ, Schacter DL: Effects of guided imagery on memory distortion in women reporting recovered memories of childhood sexual abuse. J Trauma Stress 12:559–569, 1999

Clifford BR, George R: A field evaluation of training in three methods of witness/victim investigative interviewing. Psychology, Crime, and Law 2:231–248, 1996

Colo Rev Stat Annotated § 16-8-106 (1993)

Danto B: The use of brevital sodium in police investigation. The Police Chief, May 1979, pp 53–55

Dasgupta AM, Juza DM, White GM, et al: Memory and hypnosis: a comparative analysis of guided memory, cognitive interview, and hypnotic hypermnesia. Imagination, Cognition, and Personality 14(2):117–230, 1995

Dietze PM, Thompson DM: Mental reinstatement of context: a technique for interviewing child witnesses. Applied Cognitive Psychology 7:97–108, 1993

Edmonston WE Jr: Relaxation as an appropriate experimental control in hypnosis studies. Am J Clin Hypn 14:218–229, 1972

Farren M: The CIA Files: Secrets of "The Company." New York, Quadrillion Publishing Limited, 1999

Fisher RP, McCauley MR: Improving eyewitness testimony with the cognitive interview, in Memory and Testimony in the Child Witness. Edited by Zaragoza MS, Graham JR, Hall GCN, et al. Thousand Oaks, CA, Sage Publications, 1995, pp 141–159

Fisher RP, Geiselman RE, Raymond DS, et al: Enhancing eyewitness memory: refining the Cognitive Interview. Journal of Police Science and Administration 15:291–297, 1987

Fisher RP, Geiselman RE, Amador M: Field tests of the cognitive interview: enhancing the recollection of actual victims and witnesses of crime. J Appl Psychol 74:722–727, 1989

Frankel FH: Adult reconstruction of childhood events in the multiple personality literature. Am J Psychiatry 150:954–958, 1993

Freedman LZ: "Truth" drugs. Scientific American 202, March 1960, pp 145–154

Frischholz EJ: The relationship among dissociation, hypnosis, and child abuse in the development of multiple personality disorder, in Childhood Antecedents of Multiple Personality. Edited by Kluft RP. Washington, DC, American Psychiatric Press, 1985, pp 99–126

Frischholz EJ, Lipman LS, Braun BG, et al: Psychopathology, hypnotizability, and dissociation. Am J Psychiatry 149:1521–1525, 1992

Geis G: In Scopolamine Veritas: the early history of drug-induced statements. Journal of Criminal Law, Criminology and Police Science 50:347–357, 1959

Geiselman RE, Padilla J: Interviewing child witnesses with the Cognitive Interview. Journal of Police Science and Administration 16:236–242, 1988

Geiselman RE, Fisher RP, Firstenberg I, et al: Enhancement of eyewitness memory: an empirical evaluation of the Cognitive Interview. Journal of Police Science and Administration 12:74–80, 1984

Geiselman RE, Fisher RP, MacKinnon DP, et al: Eyewitness memory enhancement in the Cognitive Interview. Am J Psychol 99:386–401, 1985

Geiselman RE, Fisher RP, Cohen G, et al: Eyewitnesses responses to leading and misleading questions under the Cognitive Interview. Journal of Police Science and Administration 14:31–39, 1986

Geiselman RE, Saywitz KJ, Bornstein GK: Cognitive interviewing techniques for child witness and witnesses of crime. Report to the State Justice Institute, 1990

George R: A field and experimental evaluation of three methods of interviewing witnesses and victims of crime. Unpublished master's thesis. Polytechnic of East London, 1991

George R, Clifford B: A field comparison of the Cognitive Interview and conversation management. Paper presented at the British Psychological Society Annual Conference, Bournemouth, UK, 1991

George R, Clifford B: A field comparison of the cognitive interview and conversation management. Paper presented at the British Psychological Society Annual Conference, Bournemouth, UK, September 1992

Giannelli PC, Imwinkelried EJ: Scientific Evidence, 3rd Edition. Charlottesville, VA, Lexis Law Publishing, 1999

Gottschalk LA: The use of drugs in interrogation, in The Manipulation of Human Behavior. Edited by Biderman AD, Zimmer H. New York, Wiley, 1961, pp 96–141

Hammond DC, Garver RB, Mutter CB, et al: Clinical Hypnosis and Memory: Guidelines for Clinicians and for Forensic Hypnosis. Des Plaines, IL, American Society of Clinical Hypnosis Press, 1994

Hayes BK, Delamothe K: Cognitive interviewing procedures and suggestibility in children's recall. J Appl Psychol 82:562–577, 1997

Hazard GC Jr: The client fraud problem as a Justinian quartet: an extended analysis. Hofstra Law Review 25:1041–1061, 1997

Hernandez-Fernaud E, Alonso M: The Cognitive Interview and lie detection: a new magnifying glass for Sherlock Holmes? Applied Cognitive Psychology 11:55–68, 1997

Hilgard ER: Hypnotic Susceptibility. New York, Harcourt, Brace & World, 1965

Hilgard ER: Divided Consciousness: Multiple Controls in Human Thought and Action. New York, Wiley, 1977

Hoch PH: The present status of narco-diagnosis and therapy. J Nerv Ment Dis 103:248–259, 1946

House RE: The Physiological Effects of Scopolamine—The Revised Method of 'Twilight Sleep,' Medical Insurance and Health Conservation. 30:391–394, 1921

Hull CL: Hypnosis and Suggestibility: An Experimental Approach. New York, Appleton-Century Crofts, 1933

Ill Stat S.H.A. 725 ILCS 125/8b (1993a)

Ill Stat 735 ILCS 5/2–1104 (Smith-Hurd) (1993b)

Karlin RA, Orne MT: Commentary on Borawick v. Shay: hypnosis, social influence, incestuous child abuse, and satanic ritual abuse: the iatrogenic creation of horrific memories for the remote past. Cultic Studies Journal 13:42–94, 1996

Katz N: Comparative efficacy of behavioral training, training plus relaxation, and a sleep/trance hypnotic induction in increasing hypnotic susceptibility. J Consult Clin Psychol 47:119–127, 1979

Kebbell MR, Wagstaff GF: Hypnotic interviewing: the best way to interview eyewitness? Behav Sci Law 16:115–129, 1998

Khantzian E: Self selection and progression in drug dependence, Psychiatric Digest 36:19–22, 1975

Kihlstrom JF: Hypnosis. Annu Rev Psychol 36:385–418, 1985

Koehnken G, Thuerer C, Zoberier D: The cognitive interview. Unpublished manuscript, University of Kiel, Kiel, Germany, 1991

Koehnken G, Finger M, Nitschke N, et al: Does the Cognitive Interview interfere with a subsequent statement validity analysis? Paper presented at the conference of the American Psychology-Law Society, San Diego, CA, March 1992

Koehnken G, Milne R, Memon A, et al: A meta-analysis on the effects of the Cognitive Interview. Paper presented at the meeting of the American Psychology and Law Society, Santa Fe, NM, March 1994

Koehnken G, Schimossek E, Aschermann E, et al: The Cognitive Interview and the assessment of the credibility of adult's statements. J Appl Psychol 80:671–684, 1995

Ky Rev Stat Annotated §439.335 (Michie/Bobbs-Merrill) (1993)

Laurence JR, Perry C: Hypnosis, Will and Memory: A Psycho-Legal History. New York, Guilford, 1983

Lee MA, Shlain B: Acid Dreams: The CIA, LSD and the Sixties Rebellion. New York, Grove Press, 1985

Lindsay DS, Read JD: Psychotherapy and memories of childhood sexual abuse. Appl Cogn Psychol 8:281–338, 1994

Loftus EF: Eyewitness Testimony. Cambridge, MA, Harvard University Press, 1979

Loftus E: Memory. Reading, MA, Addison-Wesley, 1980

Loftus EF: The reality of repressed memory. Am Psychol 48:518–537, 1993

Loftus EF, Ketcham K: The Myth of Repressed Memory: False Memories and Allegations of Sexual Abuse. New York, St. Martin's, 1994

Lynn SJ, Kirsch II: Alleged alien abductions: false memories, hypnosis, and fantasy proneness. Psychological Inquiry 7(2):151–155, 1996

Lynn SJ, Rhue JW: Theories of Hypnosis: Current Models and Perspectives. New York, Guilford, 1991

Lynn SJ, Milano M, Weeks JR: Pseudomemory and age-regression: an exploratory study. Am J Clin Hypn 35:129–137, 1992

MacKinnon DP, O'Reilly K, Geiselman RE: Improving eyewitness recall for license plates. Applied Cognitive Psychology 4:129–140, 1990

Malpass R, Devine P: Guided imagery in eyewitness identification. J Appl Psychol 66:343–350, 1981

Mann J: Murder, Magic and Medicine. Oxford, UK, Oxford University Press, 1992

Mantwill M, Aschermann E, Koehnken G: Kognitives Interview und schemageleitete Erinnerung (The Cognitive Interview and memory retrieval). Universitat Kiel: Abschussbericht fur die Deutche Forschungsgemeinschaft Ko 882/3-1, 1992

Mantwill M, Koehnken G, Aschermann E: Effects of the Cognitive Interview on the recall of familiar and unfamiliar events. J Appl Psychol 80:68–78, 1995

Marks J: The Search for the Manchurian Candidate. New York, Times Books, 1979

McCann T, Sheehan PW: The breaching of pseudomemory under hypnotic instruction: implications for original memory retrieval. British Journal of Experimental and Clinical Hypnosis 4:101–108, 1987

McCann T, Sheehan PW: Hypnotically induced pseudomemories—sampling their conditions among hypnotizable subjects. J Pers Soc Psychol 54:339–346, 1988

McCauley MR, Fisher R: Improving children's recall of action with the Cognitive Interview. Paper presented at the meeting of the American Psychology and Law Society, San Diego, CA, March 1992

McCauley MR, Fisher R: Enhancing children's memory with the revised Cognitive Interview. J Appl Psychol 4:510–517, 1995

McConkey KM: The effects of hypnotic procedures on remembering: the experimental findings and their implications for forensic hypnosis, in Contemporary Hypnosis Research. Edited by Fromm E, Nas MR. New York, Guilford, 1992, pp. 405–426

Memon A: Telling it all: the Cognitive Interview, in Psychology and Law: Truthfulness, Accuracy, and Credibility. Edited by Memon A, Vrij A, Bull R. New York, McGraw-Hill, 1998, pp 170–187

Memon A, Cronin O, Eaves R, et al: The Cognitive Interview and child witnesses. Paper presented at the NATO Advanced Study Institute: The Child Witness in Cognitive, Social and Legal Perspectives. Lucca, Italy, May 1992

Memon A, Holley A, Milne R, et al: Towards understanding the effects on interviewer training in evaluating the Cognitive Interview. Applied Cognitive Psychology 8:641–659, 1994

Memon A, Holley A, Wark L, et al: Reducing suggestibility in witness interviews. Applied Cognitive Psychology 10:503–518, 1996

Memon A, Wark L, Bull R, et al: Isolating the effects of the cognitive interview. Br J Psychol 88:187–198, 1997a

Memon A, Wark L, Holley A, et al: Eyewitness performance in cognitive and structured interviews. Memory 5:639–656, 1997b

Moenssens AA, Starrs JE, Henderson CE, et al: Scientific Evidence in Civil and Criminal Cases, 4th Edition. Westbury, NY, Foundation Press, 1995

Munsterberg H: On the Witness Stand. New York, Doubleday, Page, 1908

Murray GJ, Cross HJ, Whipple J: Hypnotically created pseudomemories: further investigation into the "memory distortion or response bias" question. J Abnorm Psychol 101:75–77, 1992

Ofshe R, Watters E: Making Monsters: False Memories, Psychotherapy, and Sexual Hysteria. New York, Charles Scribner's Sons, 1994

Orne MT: The nature of hypnosis: artifact and essence. Journal of Abnormal and Social Psychology 46:213–225, 1959

Orne MT: The construct of hypnosis: implications of the definition for research and practice. Ann N Y Acad Sci 296:14–33, 1977

Orne MT: The use and misuse of hypnosis in court. Int J Clin Exp Hypn 27:311–340, 1979

Orne MT, Whitehouse WG, Dinges DR, et al: Memory liabilities associated with hypnosis: does low hypnotizability confer immunity? Int J Clin Exp Hypn 44:354–467, 1996a

Orne MT, Whitehouse WG, Orne EC, et al: "Memories" of anomalous and traumatic autobiographical experiences: validation and consolidation of fantasy through hypnosis. Psychological Inquiry 7(2):168–172, 1996b

People v Ackerman, 132 Ill App 2d 251, 269 NE2d 737 (1971)

People v Heirens, 4 Ill2d 131, 122 NE2d 231 (1954)

Perry C: The false memory syndrome (FMS) and "disguised" hypnosis. Hypnos 22:189–197, 1995

Perry JC, Jacobs D: Overview: clinical applications of the Amytal interview in psychiatric emergency settings. Am J Psychiatry 139:552–559, 1982

Pettinati HM (ed): Hypnosis and Memory. New York, Guilford, 1988

Pezdek K: The illusion of illusory memory. Applied Cognitive Psychology 8:339–350, 1994

Piper A Jr: "Truth serum" and "recovered memories" of sexual abuse: a review of the evidence. Journal of Psychiatry and Law 2:447–471, 1994

Poole DA, Lindsay DS: Interviewing preschoolers: effects of nonsuggestive techniques, parental coaching, and leading questions on reports of nonexperienced events. J Exp Child Psychol 60:129–154, 1995

Pope KS: What psychologists better know about recovered memories, research, lawsuits, and the pivotal experiment. Clinical Psychology: Science and Practice 2:304–315, 1995

Ramona v. Ramona: Superior Court, County of Napa, California, Case No. C61898 (September 12, 1991). Plaintiff's verified second amended complaint for slander per se, negligent infliction of emotional distress, and intentional infliction of emotional distress

Ramona v. Ramona: Superior Court, County of Napa, California, Case No. C61898 (May 12, 1993). Order of Judge W. Scott Snowden

Ramona v Superior Court, 57 Cal App 4th 107, 66 Cal Rptr 2d 766 (2nd Dist 1997)

Reiser M: Handbook of Investigative Hypnosis. Los Angeles, CA, Lehi Publishing, 1980

Rolin J: Police Drugs. New York, Philosophical Library, 1956

Saywitz KJ, Geiselman RE, Bornstein GK: Effects of cognitive interviewing and practice on children's recall performance. J Appl Psychol 77:744–756, 1992

Scheflin AW: Narrative truth, historical truth and forensic truth, in The Mental Health Practitioner and the Law: A Comprehensive Handbook. Edited by Lifson L, Simon RI. Cambridge, MA, Harvard University Press, 1998, pp 299–328

Scheflin AW: Informed consent. Lunch lecture, 42nd annual meeting of the American Society of Clinical Hypnosis, Baltimore, MD, February 26, 2000

Scheflin AW: Hypnosis and the courts: a study in judicial error. Journal of Forensic Psychology Practice 1:101–111, 2001

Scheflin AW, Frischholz EJ: Significant dates in the history of forensic hypnosis. Am J Clin Hypn 42:93–94, 1999

Scheflin AW, Opton EM Jr: The Mind Manipulators. New York, Paddington, 1978

Scheflin AW, Shapiro JL: Trance on Trial. New York, Guilford, 1989

Scrivner E, Safer M: Eyewitnesses show hypermnesia for details about a violent event. J Appl Psychol 73:371–377, 1988

Sedgwick v Kawasaki Cycleworks, Inc., 71 Ohio App 3d 117, 593 NE2d 69 (1991)

Sheehan PW, Perry CW: Methodologies of Hypnosis: A Critical Appraisal of Contemporary Paradigms of Hypnosis. Hillsdale, NJ, Lawrence Erlbaum, 1976

Spanos NP: Hypnotic behavior: a social psychological interpretation of amnesia, analgesia and trance logic. Behav Brain Sci 9:449–467, 1986

Spanos NP, McLean J: Hypnotically created pseudomemories: memory distortions or reporting biases? British Journal of Experimental Hypnosis 3:155–159, 1985–1986

Spanos NP, Barber TX: Towards a convergence in hypnosis research. Am Psychol 29:500–511, 1974

Spiegel H: The grade 5 syndrome: the highly hypnotizable person. Int J Clin Exp Hypn 22:303–319, 1974

Spiegel H, Spiegel D: Trance and Treatment: Clinical Uses of Hypnosis. Washington, DC, American Psychiatric Press, 1978/1987

State v Bianchi, No. 79-10116 (Wash Super Ct 1979)

State v Hudson, 314 Mo 599, 289 SW 920 (1926)

State v Pitts, 116 NJ 580, 562 A2d 1320 (1989)

Tellegen A: On measures and conceptions of hypnosis. Am J Clin Hypn 21:219–236, 1979

Thorner MW: The psychopharmacology of sodium amytal in catatonia. J Nerv Ment Dis 52:299–303, 1935

Townsend v Sain, 372 US 293 (1963)

Trear v Stills, 69 Cal App 4th 1341, 82 Cal Rptr 2d 281 (4th Dist 1999)

Turtle JW, Yuille JC: Lost but not forgotten details: repeated eyewitness recall leads to reminiscence but not hypermnesia. J Appl Psychol 79:260–271, 1994

United States v Solomon, 753 F2d 1522 (9th Cir 1985)

Weitzenhoffer AM: Hypnotism: An Objective Study in Suggestibility. New York, Wiley, 1953

Weitzenhoffer AM, Hilgard ER: Stanford Hypnotic Susceptibility Scale, Form C. Palo Alto, CA, Consulting Psychologists Press, 1962

Yapko MD: Suggestions of Abuse. New York, Simon & Schuster, 1994

Yuille JC, McEwan NH: Use of hypnosis as an aid to eyewitness memory. J Appl Psychol 70:389–400, 1985

14

Competence and Mental Impairment

Daniel W. Shuman, J.D.

The Nature of Assessments of Competence

In this chapter I address the substantive legal standards governing competence and its relevance to mental impairment. The standards for the admissibility of expert testimony that are the subject of the United States Supreme Court's decisions in *Daubert v. Merrell Dow Pharmaceuticals, Inc.* (1993), *General Electric Co. v. Joiner* (1997), *Kumho Tire Co. v. Carmichael* (1999), and the myriad of state court decisions that followed in their wake (discussed in Shuman, Chapter 2, in this volume) shape how, when it is relevant, proof of mental states may be made. These decisions, however, do not purport to alter the substantive legal standards that determine when and how proof of mental state is relevant. I address the substantive law that determines the relevance of competence.

How Competence Is Different

Often evidence of a party's mental state is used circumstantially in legal proceedings to infer what occurred. For example, when a life insurance company refuses to pay benefits on the death of the insured, claiming that the death resulted from suicide specifically excluded by the policy, the insured's mental state immediately preceding death is admissible to help predict (retrospectively) the insured's behavior (i.e., did the insured lose control of her vehicle, or did she purposefully steer it into the tree?). Similarly, when a criminal defendant claims self-defense, evidence of the victim's mental state may assist in judging the necessity for the defendant's use of deadly force by helping to ascertain whether the victim was the aggressor (also a retrospective prediction). In other legal contexts evidence of a party's mental state is used circumstantially to infer what will occur. For example, in a child custody dispute, evidence of a parent's mental state is admissible to predict that person's future parental behavior. Similarly, in a personal injury claim, evidence of the claimant's current mental state is admissible, among other things, to predict future mental suffering or loss.

Competence is different. When the law makes competence relevant, it demands an assessment of an actor's legal capacity to act, not to determine through circumstantial reasoning what did or will occur, but to determine directly the legal significance of an actor's behavior. Thus an inquiry into a criminal defendant's competence to stand trial does not address whether the defendant committed the act charged or will likely commit future acts of violence if not executed but his or her mental ability to participate in his or her defense so as to make meaningful the constitutional rights to counsel and confrontation. Similarly, a challenge to testamentary competence does not address whether the testator actually signed the will but whether he or she had the mental capacity to understand what he or she was doing and its legal consequences when he or she signed it. When the law makes competence relevant, it asks for a determination of the capacity to act, independent of the question of whether an act did or will occur.

When the law makes competence relevant, it also demands an assessment of the capacity to act separate from an objective assessment of the wisdom of the act. Thus an unusual disposition of property in a will is not an appropriate basis for finding the person who directed it incompetent to do so. Similarly, an inquiry into a patient's competence to consent to treatment should not turn on societal agreement with the choice made but instead with the patient's capacity to make a rational choice. Although it may be tempting to use a choice that seems objectively unreasonable as evidence of incapacity to make a rational choice, this syllogism frustrates the principle of autonomy that competence is intended to further. Principles of privacy and autonomy, arising out of both constitutional and common law, protect the right to make a wide range of personal choices independent of their concurrence with societal norms (Warren and Brandeis 1890). A competent actor is legally entitled to make unconventional choices, and an incompetent actor is not legally entitled to make even conventional choices (Saks 1991). "Law makes the power of individual choice legally contingent on competence" (Stefan 1996, at 765). Conflating the choice made with the capacity to make that choice limits the right of competent individuals to exercise their autonomy and weakens the protections the law provides for incompetent individuals.

What Competence Assesses

The competence of an actor to engage in a particular act or function is germane in numerous contexts across the legal spectrum. For example, the Constitution prohibits the trial (*Dusky v. United States* 1960) or execution of incompetent criminal defendants (*Ford v. Wainwright* 1980); legislatively created regulatory schemes require that lawyers, psychologists, and physicians possess the mental competence to practice their profession safely (Shuman 1996); and judge-made common law of informed consent doctrine permits only competent patients to give effective consent to health care (*Canterbury v. Spence* 1972; *Cobbs v. Grant* 1972) and competent testators to execute enforceable wills (*Banks v. Goodfellow* 1870). The law requires assessments of competence to address both the right to act and the responsibility for those actions.

Although competence or legal capacity to act is contextual, common issues are raised when these questions are presented. Whether assessing the adequacy of a waiver of a constitutional right (*Johnson v. Zerbst* 1938) or consent to health care (*Canterbury v. Spence* 1972), courts have required that the exercise of these rights be knowing, intelligent, and voluntary to be given legal effect. Physical performance of an act purporting to waive constitutional rights or consent to health care is not alone sufficient to give these acts legal effect; the capacity of the actor to waive or consent also is required. To assess whether behavior is knowing, intelligent, and voluntary, the law has considered as many as four different capacities: "(a) the ability to understand relevant information, (b) the ability to appreciate the nature of the situation and its likely consequences, (c) the ability to manipulate information rationally, and (d) the ability to communicate a choice" (Winick 1996, p. 4).

Although not all courts recognize or require all four capacities in all settings, these capacities represent the universe of criteria that courts apply to assess the capacity to make a rational decision. The legal relevance of these capacities is reflected in "The Law of Competence" later in this chapter. The various legal standards for competence discussed in that section indicate the law's recognition, to a greater or lesser extent, of the importance of these capacities.

Competence requires that the actor have the ability to understand relevant information. The capacity to make a rational decision requires an ability to understand information relevant to that decision. Thus in assessing competence to consent to medical care, the patient must be able to understand the risks and benefits of the proposed treatment as well as alternative treatments. A patient asked to consent to surgery who cannot understand information presented about an equally effective alternative nonsurgical treatment does not meet the threshold for competence to consent to treatment. In assessing competence to stand trial, a defendant must be able to understand information about what takes place in a criminal trial and the roles of the actors in the criminal justice system (judge, jury, prosecutor, and defense attorney). A criminal defendant who does not understand after an explanation what a judge or jury is or that he or she is at risk for incarceration does not meet the threshold for competence to stand trial.

Competence also requires that the actor have the ability to appreciate the nature of the situation and its likely consequences. The capacity to make a rational decision requires an appreciation of the context in which the decision is being made and the effect of the decision in that context. In assessing competence to execute a will, the testator must be able to understand how the will would distribute his or her property and who would normally be expected to benefit from the distribution. A testator who does not appreciate that his or her will excludes his or her children, who might normally be expected to benefit from his or her testamentary distribution, does not meet the threshold for competence to execute a will. In assessing competence to consent to medical care, the patient must have the capacity to appreciate the seriousness of the condition for which treatment is being contemplated. A patient who does not appreciate, after explanation, that his or her illness would be terminal if untreated does not meet the threshold for competence to consent to treatment. In assessing the competence of a criminal defendant to stand trial, the defendant must be able to appreciate his or her situation. A criminal defendant who does not appreciate, after explanation, that the result of the trial decision is final and will not be revisited at some later date does not meet the threshold for competence to stand trial.

Competence also requires that the actor have the ability to manipulate information rationally. The capacity to make a rational decision requires an ability to manipulate the information relevant to that decision and assess that information in the context of the decision. In assessing the competence of a criminal defendant to stand trial, the defendant must be able to understand the strength of the evidence against him or her, its effect on the likelihood of conviction, and the reasonableness of a plea bargain. A criminal defendant who does not appreciate that a videotape of his or her criminal behavior renders acquittal less likely and the correlative appeal of an offer of a minimal sentence does not meet the threshold for competence to stand trial. In assessing the competence of a patient to consent to treatment, the patient must be able to understand the relation of the risks of a treatment to its benefits. Thus a patient who does not have the ability to appreciate that the treatment that offers the greatest opportunity for a cure also has the greatest risks associated with it does not meet the threshold for competence to consent to treatment.

Competence also requires that the actor have the ability to communicate a choice. Because competence is assessed in contexts in which courts or other parties are asked to act on a decision, the ability to communicate that decision in some rational manner (i.e., orally, in writing, with sign language) is required. In assessing the competence of a criminal defendant to stand trial, the defendant must be able to communicate his or her choices. Thus a defendant who does not or cannot communicate whether he or she wishes to accept a proposed plea bargain does not meet the threshold for competence to stand trial. Similarly, a patient who does not or cannot communicate his or her treatment choice does not meet the threshold for competence to consent to treatment.

A Matter of Perspective

Many assessments of competence or capacity are current or forward looking. Thus an assessment of competence to manage one's affairs in the context of a guardianship or conservatorship proceeding asks about the proposed ward's current and future abilities. Similarly, an assessment of a convicted defendant's competence to be executed asks about current capacity, not capacity at the time of the offense or trial. The law also often makes relevant retrospective assessments of competence. For example, an assessment of testamentary capacity in a probate proceeding (i.e., after the testator has died) asks about the testator's capacity at the time the will was executed. Similarly, an attack on a conviction challenging the defense counsel's failure to raise the defendant's competence to stand trial at the time of trial asks about the defendant's competence at the trial, after the trial has been completed.

Retrospective assessments of competence present the same methodological concerns present in any retrospective assessment, and then some. When evidence of mental state is used retrospectively to infer whether an act occurred, the goal of the assessment is one-dimensional. The assessment seeks to learn what the actor was thinking at an instant in time, an issue of historical fact. Although assessing the historical accuracy of an event from mental state is precarious business, it pales in comparison to the difficulty of assessing competence retrospectively. When evidence of mental state is used retrospectively to determine competence or capacity, the goal of the assessment is multidimensional. The assessment seeks to learn not what the actor was thinking but how the actor was thinking at an instant in time, a matter of systemic functioning. Thus particularly in the retrospective context, this multidimensional goal is inherently more complex and demanding than an assessment of mental state to determine the occurrence of an act.

Role of Mental Disorder or Disability in Assessing Competence

Although the effect of a mental disorder may justify a finding of incompetence, the law neither demands proof of a mental disorder as the sole basis for a finding of incompetence nor renders incompetent for all purposes all persons with a mental disorder. Mental disorder is neither necessary nor sufficient proof of incompetence. For example, a testator is not necessarily incompetent to execute a will because he or she has a mental disorder, and the absence of a mental disorder does not necessarily mean that a testator will be found competent to execute a will (Shuman 1994). Nonetheless, the law has closely linked competence and mental disorder. Mental disorder often has been assumed, without more, to yield incompetence, and incompetence often has been assumed, without more, to be global (Perlin 1992).

Understanding of the effect of mental disorders on decision-making capacities has been significantly aided by the MacArthur Treatment Competence Study (Appelbaum and Grisso 1995; Grisso and Appelbaum 1995). Reviewing the literature on mental disorders and decision-making capacities, the study authors remind us that mental illness is not a homogeneous category (i.e., whatever effect mental disorders may have on decision-making capacities, all mental disorders cannot be expected to affect decision-making capacities similarly) and that the severity of a mental disorder may influence its effect on decision making (i.e., because a diagnosis communicates information about a category of disorder but not its severity, a diagnosis alone provides limited information about decision-making capacities).

The research literature reviewed by the MacArthur Treatment Competence Study describes little about the effect of mental disorder on the ability to communicate choices (Appelbaum and Grisso 1995). Because noncommunicative patients cannot give informed consent to participate in studies of informed consent, it is hardly surprising that little research has examined the relation of mental disorders to the ability to communicate choices. Thus although the ability to communicate a choice is essential to competence, no research base exists for predicting the effect of mental disorder on this ability.

The research literature reviewed by the MacArthur Treatment Competence Study is more informative about the effect of mental disorder on the ability to understand relevant information (Appelbaum and Grisso 1995). Several studies found significant comprehension deficits in mentally disordered patients questioned about treatment information provided to them during the study. Specifically, researchers examining thought disorders, psychosis, and schizophrenia found that these disorders predicted poor comprehension of treatment information. Nonetheless, studies comparing mentally disordered and non–mentally disordered patients' comprehension of information relevant to treatment found similar deficits.

The research literature reviewed by the MacArthur Treatment Competence Study is also informative about the effect of mental disorder on the ability to appreciate the nature of the situation and its likely consequences (Appelbaum and Grisso 1995). Most studies have addressed this issue in patients with schizophrenia and depression. Numerous studies have documented impairments in the abilities of patients with schizophrenia to appreciate their illness, although the percentage of patients with schizophrenia lacking insight has varied widely. The studies examining the effect of depression on the ability to appreciate the nature of their situation suggest the significance of the severity of the disorder: patients with mild depression appear to experience "depressive reality," whereas patients with severe depression appear to show cognitive distortions of the appreciation of their situation.

The research literature reviewed by the MacArthur Treatment Competence Study is less informative about the effect of mental disorder on the ability to manipulate information rationally (Appelbaum and Grisso 1995).

The research conducted by the MacArthur Treatment Competence Study found that the understanding, appreciation, and reasoning of patients with mental disorders were impaired as compared with medically ill and non–medically ill groups (Grisso and Appelbaum 1995). They found that these impairments were consistently more pronounced in patients with schizophrenia than in patients with depression. Nonetheless, "the majority of patients with schizophrenia did not perform more poorly than other patients and nonpatients. The poorer mean performance of the schizophrenic group for any particular measure was due to a minority within that group...with greater severity of psychiatric symptoms" (Grisso and Appelbaum 1995, p. 169). While emphasizing the role that mental disorder should play in competence assessments, this research highlights the risks of equating, without more information, mental disorder and incompetence.

The Law of Competence

Substantive Criteria for Determining Competence

Questions of competence arise, literally, in dozens of legal settings. The following discussion does not attempt to review each and every setting but instead presents the substantive criteria for determining competence and its relation to mental impairment in some of the most frequently litigated settings, particularly when the issue is often raised in a retrospective context. The substantive legal criteria emphasize, to varying degrees, the ability to understand, appreciate, and manipulate relevant information and to communicate a choice, as discussed in the previous section, as components of rational decision making (Winick 1996).

Competence to Stand Trial

To make meaningful the right to counsel and the right to confront adverse witnesses contained in the Sixth Amendment of the United States Constitution, the defendant must be mentally capable of actively participating in pretrial preparations as well as the trial itself. Thus the defendant's competence to stand trial is integral to the conduct of a fair trial. The test that the Supreme Court has articulated to assess the defendant's competence to stand trial, which binds federal and state courts, is as follows:

> It is not enough for the district judge to find that "the defendant is oriented to time and place and [has] some recollection of events," but that the "test must be whether he has sufficient present *ability to consult with his lawyer* with a reasonable degree of rational understanding—and whether he has a rational as well as a factual *understanding of the proceedings against him.*" (*Dusky v. United States* 1960, at 402; emphasis added)

Slightly embellished in a subsequent decision, the Supreme Court noted the following:

> It has long been accepted that a person whose mental condition is such that he lacks the capacity to understand the nature and object of the proceedings against him, to consult with counsel, and to assist in preparing his defense may not be subjected to a trial. (*Drope v. Missouri* 1975, at 171)

The Supreme Court's test for competence to stand trial is functional and addresses two related, conjunctive sets of considerations—communication and understanding. One set of considerations in assessing the competence of a defendant to stand trial is the ability to communicate with counsel, which addresses not only the act of communication but also the ability to work cooperatively with counsel. The other set of considerations in assessing the competence of a defendant to stand trial is the ability to understand the proceedings, which addresses not only the comprehension of the actors and their legal roles (judge, jury, prosecutor, defense attorney) but also the charges and the consequences of conviction.

Although the presence of a mental disorder is clearly relevant to and may result in an inability to satisfy the *Dusky* and *Drope* standards, the standards neither require nor explicitly mention mental disorder. Defendants with major mental disorders have been found competent to stand trial (Shuman 1994). A defendant with a mental disorder diagnosis who can communicate with counsel and understand the proceedings is competent to stand trial. The test for competence to stand trial is functional and asks about the defendant's capacity at the time of trial. Thus the effect of a mental disorder on the defendant's capacity to communicate and understand is critical rather than the diagnosis itself.

Although the standards for incompetence to stand trial and criminal responsibility are often confused, they are fundamentally different tests. The test for incompetence to stand trial differs from the test for criminal responsibility (i.e., the insanity defense) in terms of both the time frame addressed (time of trial vs. time of the offense) and the substance of the test (i.e., ability to participate meaningfully in the proceedings vs. knowledge or appreciation of the wrongfulness of the act).

Although the issue of the defendant's competence to stand trial is often raised at the time of trial, requiring an assessment of the defendant's current capacity, errors in addressing competence to stand trial are often the basis for an attack on the conviction, demanding a retrospective assessment of the defendant's competence at the time of trial. In part this is precipitated by the presumption of competence, which is not rebutted unless there is bona fide question of the defendant's competence to stand trial (*Pate v. Robinson* 1966). Competence to stand trial is not invariably (or adequately) addressed at trial.

Competence to Waive Right to Silence, Right to Counsel, and Right to Trial

The Constitution grants a suspect in a criminal investigation the right not to assist the police in their investigation by providing incriminating information about himself or herself (*Miranda v. Arizona* 1966). Once a defendant in a criminal case is charged with an offense punishable by imprisonment, the defendant enjoys a constitutional right to counsel, at government expense if the defendant is indigent (*Gideon v. Wainwright* 1963). Both the United States and the individual state constitutions provide a right to trial by jury for serious criminal charges (*Duncan v. Louisiana* 1968). The defendant may, however, waive these rights by choosing to provide incriminating information to the police (*Miranda v. Arizona* 1966), represent himself or herself (*Faretta v. California* 1975), or plead guilty (*Godinez v. Moran* 1993), if he or she is competent to do so.

Although many courts and commentators have maintained that the standard for competence to plead guilty or waive the right to counsel should be measured by a more demanding standard than that imposed for competence to stand trial, because of the gravity of those choices, the Supreme Court has rejected the need for such a distinction:

> We begin with the guilty plea. A defendant who stands trial is likely to be presented with choices that entail relinquishment of the same rights that are relinquished by a defendant who pleads guilty: He will ordinarily have to decide whether to waive his "privilege against compulsory self-incrimination"…, by taking the witness stand; if the option is available, he may have to decide whether to waive his "right to trial by jury"…; and, in consultation with counsel, he may have to decide whether to waive his "right to confront [his] accusers"…by declining to cross-examine witnesses for the prosecution. A defendant who pleads not guilty, moreover, faces still other strategic choices: In consultation with his attorney, he may be called upon to decide, among other things, whether (and how) to put on a defense and whether to raise one or more affirmative defenses. In sum, *all* criminal defendants—not merely those who plead guilty—may be required to make important decisions once criminal proceedings have been initiated. And while the decision to plead guilty is undeniably a profound one, it is no more complicated than the sum total of decisions that a defendant may be called upon to make during the course of a trial.…This being so, we can conceive of no basis for demanding a higher level of competence for those defendants who choose to plead guilty. If the *Dusky* standard is adequate for defendants who plead not guilty, it is necessarily adequate for those who plead guilty.…Nor do we think that a defendant who waives his right to the assistance of counsel must be more competent than a defendant who does not, since there is no reason to believe that the decision to waive counsel requires an appreciably higher level of mental functioning than the decision to waive other constitutional rights.
>
> …
>
> A finding that a defendant is competent to stand trial, however, is not all that is necessary before he may be permitted to plead guilty or waive his right to counsel. In addition to determining that a defendant who seeks to plead guilty or waive counsel is competent, a trial court must satisfy itself that the waiver of his constitutional rights is knowing and voluntary.…In this sense there is a "heightened" standard for pleading guilty and for waiving the right to counsel, but it is not a heightened standard of competence. (Godinez v. Moran 1993, at 398)

Thus the standard for competence to waive the privilege against self-incrimination, the right to counsel, or the right to be tried is the same as the standard for competence to stand trial, with the additional proviso that the defendant knowingly and voluntarily chooses to waive these specific rights. Although a mental illness may be relevant to the capacity to waive these rights, the Supreme Court concluded that the existence of a mental illness alone, in the absence of official coercion, does not necessarily invalidate a waiver of these rights (*Colorado v. Connelly* 1986).

These competencies may be, and often are, raised at trial, calling for an assessment of current capacity. However, allegations of errors in the failure to address or adequacy of addressing these issues at trial are often the basis for attacking a conviction, which demands a retrospective assessment of these competencies.

Competence to Be Executed

In *Ford v. Wainwright* (1986), the United States Supreme Court held that the execution of an incompetent defendant violates the Eighth Amendment's ban on cruel and unusual punishment. The Supreme Court reasoned that not only is execution of a person who is "insane" inhumane, but it does not serve the deterrent or retributive purposes of punishment; and the court concluded that "[t]he Eighth Amendment prohibits the State from inflicting the penalty of death upon a prisoner who is insane" (*Ford v. Wainwright* 1986, at 410). The Supreme Court was less clear as to the criteria that should apply to assess competence to be executed. Its limited guidance, provided later in the opinion, notes the following:

> Today we have explicitly recognized in our law a principle that has long resided there. It is no less abhorrent today than it has been for centuries to exact in penance the life of one *whose mental illness prevents him from comprehending the reasons for the penalty or its implications.* (Ford v. Wainwright 1986, at 399; emphasis added)

This language has been interpreted to bar the execution of those who are "unaware of the punishment they are about to suffer and why they are to suffer it" (*Penry v. Lynaugh* 1989, at 333). Applying this standard, which is, of course, applied contemporaneously, the courts have not found the fact that the convicted person has a mental disorder dispositive, so long as it does not prevent him or her from understanding the nature and purpose of the punishment about to be imposed (*Shaw v. Armontrout* 1989). "Insanity" is necessary but not sufficient to support a finding of incompetence to be executed. The insanity or mental illness must prevent the prisoner from understanding what he or she is about to suffer and why he or she is about to endure it to render a prisoner incompetent to be executed.

Related to the question of competence to be executed is the prisoner's competence to waive appeals of his or her death sentence. In some instances prisoners have sought to halt further legal attempts to challenge their sentence of death. The standard that the Supreme Court articulated to assess the prisoner's competence to make this ultimate decision requires that the prisoner "has [the] capacity to appreciate his position and make a rational choice with respect to continuing or abandoning further litigation or on the other hand whether he is suffering from a mental disease, disorder, or defect which may substantially affect his capacity in the premises" (*Rees v. Peyton* 1966, at 313).

Competence to Contract

Most contracts are executed and enforced without the invocation of any formal legal mechanism. Indeed, in the era of e-commerce, many contracts are entered into between people or businesses who never have met and never will meet face to face. Ordinarily only when a dispute arises does a party to a contract invoke formal legal mechanisms. Thus the competence of the parties to contract is not typically addressed at the time a contract is entered into but, if at all, at some later date.

To be competent to contract requires the capacity to understand the nature and effect of the act in which the person is engaged. Quoting from a summary of approaches taken by courts to the subject, one court noted the following:

> The test of mental capacity to contract is whether the person in question possesses *sufficient mind to understand, in a reasonable manner, the nature, extent, character, and effect of the act or transaction in which he is engaged;* the law does not gauge contractual capacity by the standard of mental capacity possessed by reasonably prudent men....On the other hand, to avoid a contract it is insufficient to show merely that the person was of unsound mind or insane when it was made, but it must also be shown that this unsoundness or insanity was of such a character that he had no reasonable perception or understanding of the nature or terms of the contract. The extent or degree of intellect generally is not in issue, but merely the mental capacity to know the nature and terms of the contract....In the final analysis, contractual capacity is a question to be resolved in the light of the facts of each case and the surrounding circumstances. (*Roberts v. Roberts* 1991, at 791; emphasis added)

Mental disorder is relevant to contractual capacity, but proof of mental disorder alone is not sufficient to void a contract. "Incidents of mental illness alone will not incapacitate a person from making a valid contract provided that person is able to understand the nature and effect of his or her acts" (*Landmark Medical Center v. Gauthier* 1994, at 1158).

Some courts have expanded this cognitive test for capacity to contract, requiring an ability to understand the transaction, to include a volitional (i.e., affective) test for incapacity that may render cognitively intact persons incompetent to contract.

> The law does, however, recognize stages of incompetence other than total lack of understanding. Thus it will invalidate a transaction when a contracting party is suffering from delusions if there is "some such connection between the insane delusions and the making of the deed as will compel the inference that the insanity induced the grantor to perform an act, the purport and effect of which he could not understand, and which he would not have performed if thoroughly sane."...Moreover, it holds that understanding of the physical nature and consequences of an act of suicide does not render the suicide voluntary within the meaning of a life insurance contract if the insured "acted under the control of an insane impulse caused by disease, and derangement of his intellect, which deprived him of the capacity of governing his own conduct in accordance with reason."...*Thus, capacity to understand is not, in fact, the sole criterion. Incompetence to contract also exists when a contract is entered into under the compulsion of a mental disease or disorder but for which the contract would not have been made.* (*Faber v. Sweet* 1963, at 767–778; emphasis added)

Testamentary Competence

A person who wants to execute a will is not required to prove his or her competence before doing so. Unless an assessment of the testator's competence is sought preventively (Shuman, Chapter 2, this volume), a challenge to testamentary capacity will entail a retrospective assessment of a person who is now unavailable for examination, which enhances the complexity of the assessment (Simon, Chapter 1, this volume) and presents a classic legal tension. The standard for testamentary capacity is an attempt to recognize the right to dispose of one's property as one chooses, which the law guards jealously, and society's interest in protecting individuals whose capacity to make those choices is fundamentally impaired, which the law also zealously protects.

Although the standard for testamentary capacity is a creature of state law, the standards from state to state are remarkably similar. The standards treat testamentary capacity as a specialized contract and apply a standard for contractual capacity, taking into account the testamentary context. The Texas standard that follows is representative of those applied across the United States:

The person at the time of the execution of the [w]ill has sufficient mental ability to understand the business in which he is engaged, the effect of his act making the [w]ill, and the general nature and extent of his property. He must also be able to know his next of kin and natural objects of his bounty. He must have memory sufficient to collect in his mind the elements of the business to be transacted and to hold them long enough to perceive at least their obvious relation to each other, and to be able to form a reasonable judgment as to them. (*Rich v. Rich* 1980, at 796)

No mere weakening of the mental powers—no mere impairment of the faculties—will invalidate a will so long as the maker has mind enough to know in a general way the natural objects of his bounty, the nature and extent of his estate, and the disposition he wishes to make of it. It is not necessary that he be competent to make contracts or transact business generally. (*In re Estate of Hollis* 1944, at 580)

Thus the diagnosis of a mental disorder, in and of itself, does not suffice to justify a finding of testamentary incapacity, and, conversely, the absence of a diagnosis of mental disorder does not ensure a finding of testamentary capacity. The test is functional and requires an assessment of the testator's cognitive capacity with regard to this act (Shuman 1994).

Another ground for challenging the validity of a will is the presence of undue influence. Although the absence of testamentary capacity invalidates a will without regard to the actions of any other person, undue influence resulting in the substitution of the wishes of another person for those of the testator may be found even if the testator possesses testamentary capacity. Indeed, if the testator lacks testamentary capacity, that, without more, should result in invalidation of the will. However, the absence of testamentary capacity and undue influence are often alleged jointly when the expected beneficiaries of the estate believe that an heir took advantage of the testator's condition for his or her own benefit.

When is influence undue? In the eyes of the law the critical distinction between influence and undue influence is the matter of coercion. Persuading the testator to draft his or her will to make a particular bequest is not legally problematic; coercing the testator to do so when he or she does not wish to do so is legally problematic. Only when the effect of the influence exerted is to destroy the testator's freedom to choose is the will the result of the person exerting the influence (*Mackie v. McKenzie* 1995). "In signing a will that is the result of undue influence, the testator is said to be in such a condition that if he could speak his wishes to the last, he would say, 'This is not my wish, but I do it'" (Madoff 1997, p. 579). Although some courts articulate specific sets of considerations that make out a case of undue influence, such situations in which there was a confidential relationship, the confidant played a role in the preparation of the will, the testator was vulnerable to undue influence, and the will made an unnatural bequest to the confidant (Madoff 1997), other courts reject the notion that it is possible to define the limitless possibilities for undue influence.

Competence to Marry

Parties to a marriage need not, as a matter of course, prove their mental competence to marry as a precondition to marriage. Indeed, the law presumes that the parties to a marriage are competent and that a marriage entered into is valid (*Geitner v. Townsend* 1984). However, incompetence to marry is often raised retrospectively in actions to annul a marriage. A marriage entered into by a person who does not meet the requirements for competence to marry is void. Typically the test applied to determine mental capacity to marry asks whether the party whose mental capacity is at issue, at the time the marriage was entered into,

> had at the time sufficient mental capacity to enable him to understand the nature of the marriage relation, the nature of the marriage contract, and to understand that upon himself he took with it all the duties, obligations and responsibilities which the law would impose upon him as a result of that contract on his part, whatever they were. (*Knight v. Radomski* 1980, at 1214–1215)

Like the test for capacity to contract, which it mirrors, competence to marry is not defeated by the presence of a mental disorder, in and of itself, and the absence of a mental disorder does not ensure that competence to marry exists.

Guardianship and Conservatorship

A finding of incompetence and the appointment of a guardian or conservator is a formal legal determination that addresses the proposed ward's current capacity. Unlike a retrospective competence assessment seeking to invalidate the purchase of an unaffordable luxury car by a patient with bipolar disorder during the manic phase of his or her illness, the appointment of a guardian or conservator is intended to act prescriptively. It is intended to provide protections for individuals unable to protect themselves by the mechanism of an adjudication of the ward's incompetence and the appointment of guardian to protect the person of the ward or a conservator to protect the property of the ward.

One common articulation of the standard for appointment of a guardian or conservator asks whether the person alleged to be incapacitated "is impaired by reason of mental illness, mental deficiency, physical illness or disability, chronic use of drugs, chronic intoxication, or other cause (except minority) to the extent of lacking sufficient understanding or capacity to make or communicate responsible decisions" (Uniform Probate Code 1992). Thus an assessment of incompetence claiming to rest on mental disorder must address first whether such a disorder exists and next its effect on the person's capacity to make or communicate responsible decisions. The two prongs of the test are conjunctive—mental illness or deficiency, without more, is insufficient to support a finding of incompetence.

Some states have feared that this test may measure normative decision-making consensus rather than decision-making ability, confusing capacity with conformity. These states have chosen an approach that addresses functional limitations as contrasted with normative measures of competent behavior. For example, in Texas, a guardian may be appointed for "an adult individual who, because of a physical or mental condition, is substantially unable to provide food, clothing, or shelter for himself or herself, to care for the individual's own physical health, or to manage the individual's own financial affairs" (Tex Prob Code Ann 1999).

Competence to Consent to and Refuse Treatment

In a succinct and often quoted statement, Justice Cardozo articulated the jurisprudence of autonomy and its incorporation into the law governing health care delivery: "Every human being of adult years and sound mind has a right to determine what shall be done with his own body; and a surgeon who performs an operation without his patient's consent commits an assault for which he is liable for damages" (*Schloendorff v. Society of New York Hospital* 1914, at 93).

This statement encapsulates two fundamental principles uniformly recognized in American courts. First, competent adults have the right to decide what health care they shall receive; concomitantly, health care rendered in the absence of a valid consent is tortious. Second, incompetent patients do not have the right to decide what health care they shall receive. Although the state may, in certain instances, have a "compelling state interest" in overriding a competent patient's decision,[1] competence is a critical

---

[1]See, for example, *Washington v. Harper* (1990) (state interest in prison safety justifies unwanted administration of psychotropic medication without a judicial determination of incompetence) and *Application of the President and Directors of Georgetown College* (1964) (court-ordered blood transfusion that patient had refused on religious grounds; based, in part, on the state's interest in patient's minor child).

component of both the right to consent to health care and the right to refuse to consent to health care.

Consent to health care, "informed consent" as articulated by most courts, must be knowing, intelligent, and voluntary (*Canterbury v. Spence* 1972; *Cobbs v. Grant* 1972). As discussed in the earlier section in this chapter "The Nature of Assessments of Competence," courts addressing capacity to consent to health care have taken into account the "(a) the ability to understand relevant information, (b) the ability to appreciate the nature of the situation and its likely consequences, (c) the ability to manipulate information rationally, and (d) the ability to communicate a choice" (Winick 1996, p. 4).

For example, in California, the

> [j]udicial determination of the specific competency to consent to drug treatment should focus primarily upon three factors: (a) whether the patient is aware of his or her situation...(b) whether the patient is able to understand the benefits and the risks of, as well as the alternatives to, the proposed intervention...and (c) whether the patient is able to understand and to knowingly and intelligently evaluate the information required to be given. (*Riese v. Saint Mary's Hosp. and Medical Ctr.* 1987, at 211)

Neither the diagnosis of a mental disorder (*Davis v. Hubbard* 1980) nor a civil commitment order (*Rennie v. Klein* 1978) by itself justifies a finding of incompetence to consent to or refuse to consent to health care. Rather, the question is whether the patient has a mental disorder that impairs his or her judgment rendering him or her "incapable of participating in decisions affecting his health" (*Goedecke v. Colorado* 1979, at 125).

Conclusion

Assessments of competence are critical to determinations of the right to perform and the consequences that flow from a wide variety of legally significant acts. Competence determinations cut across the breadth of both criminal and civil law. Yet given these varied legal settings, competence determinations have in common the necessity for a contextual analysis of the capacity to understand information relevant to the decision, to appreciate the nature of the decision, to manipulate rationally information relevant to the decision, and, ultimately, to communicate a choice.

Both the law and the research on decision-making capacity caution against simplistically equating mental disorder with incompetence. The presence of a mental disorder is undoubtedly relevant to an assessment of competence, but it is not legally or clinically sufficient to assume that the diagnosis of a mental disorder should lead to a finding of incompetence. Assessing mental impairment and competence requires a functional analysis in which the role of a mental disorder in decision-making capacity must be assessed, not assumed.

References

Appelbaum PS, Grisso T: The MacArthur Treatment Competence Study I: mental illness and competence to consent to treatment. Law Hum Behav 19:105–126, 1995

Application of the President and Directors of Georgetown College, 131 F2d 1000 (DC Cir 1964)

Banks v Goodfellow, 5 QB 549 (1870)

Canterbury v Spence, 464 F2d 772 (DC Cir 1972)

Cobbs v Grant, 502 P2d 1 (Cal 1972)

Colorado v Connelly, 479 US 157 (1986)

Daubert v Merrell Dow Pharmaceuticals, Inc., 509 US 579 (1993)

Davis v Hubbard, 506 F Supp 915 (ND Ohio 1980)

Drope v Missouri, 420 US 162, 171 (1975)

Duncan v Louisiana, 391 US 145, 156 (1968)

Dusky v United States, 362 US 402 (1960)

Faber v Sweet, 242 NYS2d 763 (NY 1963)

Faretta v California, 422 US 806 (1975)

Ford v Wainwright, 477 US 399 (1986)

Geitner v Townsend, 312 SE2d 236 (NC App 1984), review denied, 315 SE2d 702

General Electric Co. v Joiner, 522 US 136 (1997)

Gideon v Wainwright, 372 US 335 (1963)

Godinez v Moran, 509 US 389 (1993)

Goedecke v Colorado, 603 P2d 123 (Colo 1979)

Grisso T, Appelbaum PS: The MacArthur Treatment Competence Study III: abilities of patients to consent to psychiatric and medical treatments. Law Hum Behav 19:149–174, 1995

In re Estate of Hollis, 12 NW2d 576 (Iowa 1944)

In re Yetter, 62 PaD and C2d 619 (1972)

Johnson v Zerbst, 304 US 458 (1938)

Knight v Radomski, 414 A2d 1211 (Me 1980)

Kumho Tire Co. v Carmichael, 526 US 137 (1999)

Landmark Medical Center v Gauthier, 635 A2d 1145 (RI 1994)

Mackie v McKenzie, 900 SW2d 445 (Tex App 1995)

Madoff RD: Unmasking undue influence. Minnesota Law Review 81:571–628, 1997

Miranda v Arizona, 384 US 436 (1966)

Pate v Robinson, 383 US 375 (1966)

Penry v Lynaugh, 492 US 302 (1989)

Perlin ML: On "sanism." Southern Methodist University Law Review 46:373–407, 1992

Rees v Peyton, 384 US 312 (1966)

Rennie v Klein, 462 F Supp 1131 (D NJ 1978)

Rich v Rich, 615 SW2d 795 (Tex Civ App-Houston [1st Dist] 1980), no writ

Riese v Saint Mary's Hosp. and Medical Ctr., 271 Cal Rptr 199 (Cal Ct App 1987)

Roberts v Roberts, 827 SW2d 788 (Tenn App 1991)

Saks ES: Competency to refuse treatment. North Carolina Law Review 69:945–999, 1991

Schloendorff v Society of New York Hospital, 105 NE2d 92 (NY 1914)

Shaw v Armontrout, 900 F2d 123 (9th Cir 1989)

Shuman DW: Psychiatric and Psychological Evidence, 2nd Edition. Colorado Springs, CO, Shepard's/McGraw-Hill, 1994

Shuman DW: Law and Mental Health Professionals: Texas, 2nd Edition. Washington, DC, American Psychological Association, 1996

Stefan S: Silencing the different voice: competence, feminist theory and law. University of Miami Law Review 47:763–814, 1996

Tex Prob Code Ann § 601(13) (Vernon Supp 1999)

Uniform Probate Code § 5-103(7) (Supp 1992)

Warren SD, Brandeis LD: The right to privacy. Harvard Law Review 4:193–220, 1890

Washington v Harper, 494 US 210 (1990)

Winick BJ: Foreword: a summary of the MacArthur Treatment Competence Study and an introduction to the special theme. Psychology, Public Policy and Law 2:3–17, 1996

15

Remembering the Future

Policy Implications for the Forensic Assessment of Past Mental States

Daniel W. Shuman, J.D.
Robert I. Simon, M.D.

⃝f all the tasks that the legal system asks psychiatrists and psychologists to perform, retrospective assessment of mental states is likely the most problematic and, ironically, the least critically examined. How can we ever claim to have reliable knowledge of another person's past mental processes? (Sadler, Chapter 3, this volume.) Confounding the problems of performing reliable and valid contemporaneous diagnosis and assessment of mental states, retrospective assessment of mental states asks psychiatrists and psychologists to provide legal decision-makers with information about a person's mental state at a time before the mental health professional ever (and in some cases never) examined that person. The inherent limitations on obtaining contemporaneous data about past mental states render the ability to engage in this task more problematic than a contemporaneous assessment based on a concurrent examination. Although cases addressing past mental states often entail an evidentiary mosaic of lay and expert testimony (Frolik 1999), the concurrence of lay and expert testimony is not a justification for ignoring problems with the reliability of expert testimony. Neither the rules of evidence nor the decisions interpreting them distinguish the rigor with which expert testimony should be scrutinized based on the availability of nonexpert testimony or other evidence. Moreover, the absence of reported judicial decisions addressing challenges to the admissibility of expert testimony on the retrospective assessments of mental states is compelling evidence that the legal system has failed to identify the underlying issue of its reliability. Surprisingly, the inherent problems that confound the reliability of retrospective assessments of mental states have not resulted in reported challenges to the admissibility of this psychiatric and psychological evidence.

Can the immunity of expert testimony on the retrospective assessment of mental states from rigorous scrutiny of its admissibility continue (Chapter 2 in this volume)? In the wake of *Daubert v. Merrell Dow Pharmaceuticals, Inc.* (1993), and its federal and state court progeny, will the legal system eventually come to appreciate the methodological difficulties that surround the retrospective assessment of mental states and demand greater scrutiny of its admissibility? We do not know, but we choose not to remain passive observers. We recognize a moral obligation to the courts as consumers and to psychology and psychiatry as providers of assessments of past mental states to address this issue. We recognize an obligation to provide the courts with guidance in determining how to assess the reliability of retrospective assessments of mental states. And we recognize an obligation to psychiatrists and psychologists individually to suggest how to approach this task using reliable methods and procedures and institutionally to provide a basis for the development of guidelines for reliable forensic evaluations of past mental states. For psychiatrists and psychologists, it is sensible to assume that rigorous *Daubert* scrutiny will apply: 1) as a vehicle to address compliance with their ethical obligation to provide courts with information derived from only reliable methods and procedures; 2) as preparation for the rigors of cross-examination; and 3) because, as with Pascal's wager—arguing that it is best to wager on the existence of God because if one does not and is wrong, it may be too late—it is also best to weigh the application of *Daubert*, or it may be too late when the mistake is detected to correct it (Shuman and Sales 2001).

Initially we sought to respond in an article to the issues we identified about retrospective assessment of mental states. As we explored these issues, however, we came to realize the breadth of the problem and the need to call on the expertise of numerous colleagues to address the full range of issues raised. The result of that collaboration is this in-depth clinical, scientific, and legal exploration of retrospective assessment of mental states and the law. We hope that it will provide the courts, psychiatry, and psychology with an important fund of information to raise the standards for retrospective forensic assessments of past mental states.

We come away from this exploration with a serious concern for the frailties of untested clinical methodologies used in the forensic assessment of past mental states. We emphasize the importance of science both in highlighting the limits of these methodologies and in providing the foundation for the development of more reliable methodologies. Given the inherent informational limitations present in any attempt to assess past mental states, the use of reliable methods and procedures, which have not always been applied in forensic settings, is crucial. Many expected the United States Supreme Court's decision in *Daubert v. Merrell Dow Pharmaceuticals, Inc.* (1993), and its progeny to result in the trial courts demanding greater reliability in the presentation of all psychiatric and psychological evidence, but that has not come to pass (Shuman and Sales 1999). With limited exceptions, psychiatric and psychological expert testimony that had been admitted before *Daubert* has also been admitted after *Daubert*. In particular, clinical assessments of past mental states were not the subject of admissibility challenges addressing the issue of reliability before *Daubert* nor are they the subject of admissibility challenges addressing the issue of reliability after *Daubert*.

That is not to say that if *Daubert* matters less to lawyers and judges than many had thought it would, then it is unimportant for psychiatric and psychological assessment of past mental states. *Daubert's* demand that the trial court engage in a "preliminary assessment of whether the reasoning or methodology underlying the testimony is scientifically valid and of whether that reasoning or methodology properly can be applied to the facts in issue" (*Daubert v. Merrell Dow Pharmaceuticals, Inc.* 1993, at 593) is an important reminder to psychiatrists and psychologists of their clinical responsibility to do good work. Thus our efforts in this book have been, in the first instance, directed to psychiatrists and psychologists, to raise the floor for good clinical work by providing relevant and reliable information about methods and procedures for assessment of past mental states. By addressing critical sources of information and the methods for assessing them, we seek to assist in raising the quality of forensic assessments of past mental states.

Therapists, as well as forensic experts, must be able to integrate the findings of research in memory science with their clinical experience. For example, some therapists have had patients who recall traumatic childhood experiences for the first time in the absence of suggestive questioning. Such recollections are consistent with the body of research that supports the existence of repressed memories. Integration of research findings in memory science with clinical data helps the therapist walk a relatively neutral path between avoiding invalidation of patients' reports of childhood memories of abuse and the uncritical acceptance of such reports. Moreover, research-based clinical techniques and interventions help therapists avoid inappropriate defensive practices such as being afraid to ask patients about childhood abuse or refusing to treat patients who report recovered memories for fear of being sued.

In addition to the clinical responsibility of individual psychiatrists and psychologists to do good work in the forensic assessment of past mental states, much work remains to be done by the professions to raise the floor for good clinical work. First, there is the matter of the ethical rules and guidelines that address the behavior of psychiatrists and psychologists in the courtroom. Although separate ethical precepts exist for individuals who identify themselves as forensic psychiatrists or psychologists (American Academy of Psychiatry and Law 1995; Committee on Ethical Guidelines for Forensic Psychologists 1991), psychiatrists and psychologists who do not identify themselves as forensic practitioners are not ordinarily bound by them. The American Medical Association "Principles of Medical Ethics" applicable to psychiatrists does not specifically address forensic practices. The American Psychological Association "Ethical Principles of Psychologists" applicable to psychologists contains only a brief section that addresses forensic activities. Fleshing out the ethical rules that apply to all psychiatrists and psychologists who appear in the courtroom, in order to provide guidance for the professions and for the courts, is an important institutional professional responsibility. In addition to advising members of the profession about their responsibilities, ethical norms may serve "as red flags to raise potential problems of reliability in the admissibility of expert testimony" (Shuman and Greenberg 1998, p. 5).

Guidelines may provide more specific guidance for forensic assessment. Guidelines offer the profession the opportunity to review professional practice in light of the relevant research on specific tasks and to convey this information to members of the profession who might not have the opportunity to review research and current practice. An example of guidelines for a specific forensic assessment is the American Psychological Association's "Guidelines for Child Custody Evaluations in Divorce Proceedings" (American Psychological Association 1994). It addresses certain basic elements for conducting a child custody evaluation, such as obtaining informed consent from all participants, using multiple methods of data gathering, and avoiding multiple relationships that present role conflicts. Our work provides the foundation for forensic guidelines for the assessment of past mental states.

Second, there is the matter of the enforcement of the rules and guidelines. At present, professional enforcement of a profession's rules and guidelines is limited to action on formal complaints. Rarely do allegations that a psychiatrist's or psychologist's forensic activities in a particular case are unethical result in a formal complaint to a professional regulatory body. Most disputes about psychiatrists' and psychologists' forensic practices are resolved by the judge in determining admissibility of the expert's testimony or by the jury in determining the weight to be accorded the expert's testimony. The primary scrutiny of the behavior of psychiatrists and psychologists assessing past mental states occurs in the courts. The law is a blunt instrument to assess nonlegal professional competence. It is not reasonable to expect lawyers, judges, and juries to bring the same level of professional education and experience as psychiatric or psychological professional peer review of expert testimony would provide. The use of peer review of expert testimony by fellow members of the psychiatric and psychological professions to examine the behavior of their members according to the standards of their profession is, however, currently limited to voluntary submission of testimony, which is hardly likely to result in identifying questionable practices or practitioners ("American Psychiatric Association Resource Document on Peer Review of Expert Testimony," 1997). If the professions are to take self-policing of expert testimony seriously, then they must consider sampling of selected cases.

That is not to suggest that the responsibility for addressing reliable psychiatric or psychological expert testimony about past mental states should be borne by the mental health professions alone. *Daubert* recognizes the responsibility of the trial courts to serve as gatekeepers and the correlative responsibility of the trial court bar to raise these issues to the trial courts. Yet nothing in *Daubert* compels trial judges or lawyers to raise these challenges or provides them with the education or training necessary to do so. And the Supreme Court's decision in *General Electric Co. v. Joiner* (1997) instructing appellate courts to review trial court *Daubert* decisions under the "abuse of discretion" standard effectively insulates all but the most egregious trial court decisions from appellate review. Thus it is important to note that lawyers might, through this work, glean the information necessary to launch a *Daubert* challenge to the admissibility of unreliable psychiatric or psychological assessments of past mental states; however, if the challenge is unsuccessful, the same information also might provide the grist for a rigorous cross-examination. The likelihood that a rigorous cross-examination will place expert testimony in a proper light depends not only on the skills of the lawyer but also on the abilities of the jury to appreciate the issues raised on cross-examination, a matter subject to much debate.

The admissibility of reliable expert testimony about past mental states is also shaped by the substantive legal standards that call for such testimony. As discussed by Shuman (Chapter 2, this volume), substantive legal standards determine whether the parties are encouraged or permitted to offer evidence about past mental states. For example, permitting life insurance companies to limit their liability for self-inflicted injury often demands that the parties present evidence of the insured's mental state preceding the time of death (Simon 1990). One of the costs of maintaining an insanity defense is that it demands that the parties present evidence of the defendant's past mental state. Prohibiting premortem probate ensures that all challenges to a testator's competence to execute a will entail a retrospective assessment. Both the legal and the mental health professions must be alert to the way in which substantive legal standards foster unreliable psychiatric and psychological evidence of past mental states and, when possible, seek to avoid the use of legal criteria that encourage such evidence.

As we describe in this book, psychiatrists and psychologists do have the tools to conduct assessments of past mental states that are often as reliable as assessments of current mental states (e.g., Resnick, Chapter 5; Tardiff, Chapter 8; and Walker, Chapter 7, this volume). Indeed, as Rogers (Chapter 10, this volume) observes, distinguishing the reliability of evaluations based on a current-retrospective dichotomy risks "false comfort for current assessments and exaggerated concerns for retrospective assessments" because of the multiple time perspectives used in most evaluations. Relying on this same information, courts do have the tools to scrutinize the reliability of these assessments. Whether, armed with the knowledge of these tools, the quality of forensic assessments of past mental states will improve remains to be determined.

References

American Academy of Psychiatry and the Law: American Academy of Psychiatry and the Law Ethical Guidelines for the Practice of Forensic Psychiatry. Bloomfield, CT, American Academy of Psychiatry and the Law, 1995

American Psychological Association: Guidelines for child custody evaluation in divorce proceedings. Am Psychol 49:677–680, 1994

American Psychiatric Association resource document on peer review of expert testimony. J Am Acad Psychiatry Law 25:359s–373, 1997

Committee on Ethical Guidelines for Forensic Psychologists: Specialty guidelines for forensic psychologists. Law Hum Behav 15:655–665, 1991

Daubert v Merrell Dow Pharmaceuticals, Inc., 509 US 579 (1993)

Frolik LA: Science, common sense, and the determination of mental capacity. Psychology, Public Policy, and Law 5:41–58, 1999

General Electric Co. v Joiner, 522 US 136 (1997)

Shuman DW, Greenberg SA: The role of ethical norms in the admissibility of expert testimony. ABA Judges Journal 37:4–43, 1998

Shuman DW, Sales BD: The impact of *Daubert* and its progeny on the admissibility of behavioral and social science evidence. Psychology, Public Policy and Law 5:3–15, 1999

Shuman DW, Sales BD: Daubert's wager. Journal of Forensic Psychology Practice 1(3):69–77, 2001

Simon RI: You only die once—but did you intend it? psychiatric assessment of suicide intent in insurance litigation. Tort and Insurance Law Journal 25:650–662, 1990

Index

*Page numbers printed in **boldface** type refer to tables and figures.*